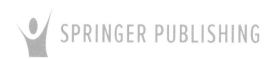

SPRINGER PUBLISHING

T0074959

GET THE MOST FROM YOUR BOOK

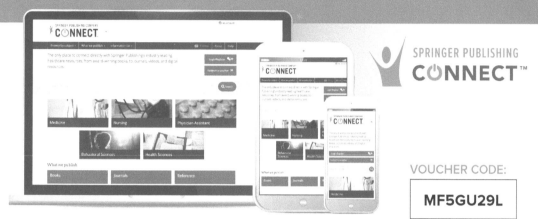

SPRINGER PUBLISHING
C●NNECT™

VOUCHER CODE:

MF5GU29L

Online Access

Your print purchase of *Healthcare Financial Management* includes **online access via Springer Publishing Connect**™ to increase accessibility, portability, and searchability.

Insert the code at https://connect.springerpub.com/content/book/978-0-8261-4475-1 today!

Having trouble? Contact our customer service department at cs@springerpub.com

Instructor Resource Access for Adopters

Let us do some of the heavy lifting to create an engaging classroom experience with a variety of instructor resources included in most textbooks SUCH AS:

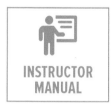

INSTRUCTOR MANUAL

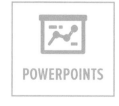

POWERPOINTS

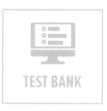

TEST BANK

Visit **https://connect.springerpub.com/** and look for the **"Show Supplementary"** button on your **book homepage** to see what is available to instructors! First time using Springer Publishing Connect?

Email **textbook@springerpub.com** to create an account and start unlocking valuable resources.

Healthcare Financial Management

Cassandra R. Henson, DrPA, MBA, is a faculty member in the Department of Health Sciences (Healthcare Management Program) at Towson University. Program courses taught include Healthcare Financial Management, Business Analytics and Statistics, Health Program Evaluation, Healthcare Law and Ethics, the U.S. Healthcare System, and Health Systems Human Resources Management. She earned a doctorate in public administration and program evaluation from the University of Baltimore, an MBA in finance from Morgan State University, and a baccalaureate degree from West Virginia University.

Prior to starting her career in academia, Dr. Henson held leadership positions in the corporate finance, local government, healthcare, and defense contracting industries. Her areas of professional specialization and expertise include financial analysis, budgeting, project management, federal and municipal contract pricing and negotiation, auditing, compliance, and strategic planning. She discovered her love for teaching while instructing clinical and other nonfinancial managers on how to properly prepare operating budgets and financial performance reports. Now she conducts and presents in-depth healthcare finance and program evaluation research, as well as teaches students the practical applications of these areas as they apply to healthcare management, public administration, and healthcare policy.

Healthcare Financial Management

Applied Concepts and Practical Analyses

Cassandra R. Henson, DrPA, MBA

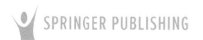 SPRINGER PUBLISHING

Springer Publishing Company, LLC
11 West 42nd Street, New York, NY 10036
www.springerpub.com
connect.springerpub.com

Acquisitions Editor: David D'Addona
Compositor: Transforma
Production Editor: Rachel Haines

ISBN: 978-0-8261-4474-4
ebook ISBN: 978-0-8261-4475-1
DOI: 10.1891/9780826144751

SUPPLEMENTS

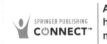

A robust set of instructor resources designed to supplement this text is located at http://connect.springerpub.com/content/book/978-0-8261-4475-1. Qualifying instructors may request access by emailing textbook@springerpub.com.

Instructor Materials:
Instructor Manual: 978-0-8261-4476-8
Chapter-Based PowerPoints: 978-0-8261-4477-5
Test Bank: 978-0-8261-4478-2
Instructor Data Sets: 978-0-8261-4481-2

Student Materials:
Answers to Practice Problems: 978-0-8261-4484-3

23 24 25 26 27 / 5 4 3 2 1

Library of Congress Cataloging-in-Publication Data

Names: Henson, Cassandra R., author.
Title: Healthcare financial management : applied concepts and practical analyses / Cassandra R. Henson, DrPA, MBA.
Description: New York, NY : Springer Publishing Company, LLC, [2024] | Includes bibliographical references and index. | Summary: "Healthcare financial management and the business processes that surround it have become a more common fixture in the academic space. Historically, the challenge has been communicating how healthcare finance impacts other functional areas within the typical healthcare organization. This text is my first contribution toward making these connections and addressing this challenge. Both instructor and student alike should be comfortable learning about and navigating the basic healthcare finance space—you have to love your numbers! Even though every student won't go on to pursue a healthcare finance career, knowing the basics of its mechanisms is a valuable and important tool to have. Hopefully, this textbook will support your teaching and learning efforts by introducing the basic elements and applying the concepts broadly"– Provided by publisher.
Identifiers: LCCN 2023007079 | ISBN 9780826144744 (paperback) | ISBN 9780826144751 (ebook)
Subjects: LCSH: Health facilities–Business management. | Health facilities–Finance. | Health facilities–United States–Business management. | Health facilities–United States–Finance.
Classification: LCC RA971.3 .H45 2024 | DDC 362.1068/1–dc23/eng/20230420
LC record available at https://lccn.loc.gov/2023007079

Contents

MODULE I: HEALTHCARE INDUSTRY FRAMEWORK

MODULE II: ACCOUNTING PRINCIPLES REVIEW

MODULE III: HEALTHCARE REVENUE CYCLE MANAGEMENT

MODULE IV: BUDGETING AND OPERATIONS

MODULE V: RESOURCE MANAGEMENT

List of Features

CHAPTER 16: COURSE PROJECT: SURGIFLEX ROBOTIC SURGERY SYSTEM

Preface

Healthcare financial management and the business processes that surround it have become a more common fixture in the academic space. Historically, the challenge has been communicating how healthcare finance impacts other functional areas within the typical healthcare organization. This text is my first contribution toward making these connections and addressing this challenge.

The underlying thought behind the book is that, no matter the department or function, you always need someone to watch the money! The discipline of healthcare finance is business-adjacent, and while all aspects of business operations are important, the patient (consumer) and the financial functions that surround them in the healthcare arena affect every part of the organization. How do you teach healthcare professionals, specifically those of nonfinance backgrounds, to recognize this? How do you keep students engaged and interested in learning more about the discipline? What do you teach them to ensure that the learned concepts are relevant, no matter the setting? Preparing the next generation of healthcare management and administration professionals is no easy feat, given the breadth of knowledge required to operate effectively and efficiently. With this in mind, I decided to approach this textbook with a simple philosophy. I used my own 20+ years of industry experience to inform my teachings in the classroom, resulting in an applied approach to healthcare finance that I carried over to this textbook. The subject needed to be approachable, accessible, and user-friendly in order to educate students and healthcare professionals from all backgrounds. This was my guiding principle for the textbook and the accompanying course project.

The five modules of the textbook are ordered in a way that meets students where they are, and then brings them along to where we need them to be. The basics of accounting and finance are discussed as the backdrop to the much broader scope of healthcare financial management. Finance is more than just the annual budget process—everything we do in healthcare has a financial impact. That is the crucial idea that needs to be conveyed; that is the idea that directly addresses the challenge of communicating how healthcare finance impacts every part of the healthcare organization. The textbook material is then applied to the course project by having students prepare various financial calculations as they would be prepared by a healthcare organization's finance department. Choosing Microsoft Excel® as the software for the project was an important and intentional consideration, because Excel serves as the support program for most accounting and finance systems. While the textbook's applied approach may present a learning curve for students unfamiliar with healthcare finance or spreadsheets, the hands-on work performed will help them develop a valuable knowledge base in different kinds of data analyses and organizational decision-making.

While every professor has their own proven teaching methods, the healthcare finance course requires more than a standard PowerPoint lecture. Healthcare finance content should be taught in a way that encourages students to engage with its complexities and not shy away from what may seem difficult or confusing. Both instructor and student alike should be comfortable learning about and navigating the basic healthcare finance space—you have to love your numbers! Even though every student won't go on to pursue a healthcare finance career, knowing the basics of its mechanisms is a valuable and important tool to have. Hopefully, this textbook will support your teaching and learning efforts by introducing the basic elements and applying the concepts broadly. Feel free to email us at chensonacademic@gmail.com with suggestions for improvement or additional content to be included in future editions of the book.

Cassandra R. Henson

Acknowledgments

I would like to gratefully acknowledge and express sincere appreciation for the expertise and meaningful feedback from Springer Publishing Company and the original manuscript reviewers. The guidance and discussions had along the way were instrumental in the drafting, revision, and subsequent completion of this project.

I'd like to thank my children, Lauryn and Leah, for understanding my seemingly endless hours of writing and reading aloud as this textbook was created. This project is dedicated to the loving memory of my parents, John and Ophelia Henson, and my aunt, Dr. Phyllis A. Wallace, who would have been proud of my accomplishments.

Available Resources

Available resources include:

INSTRUCTOR RESOURCES

 A robust set of instructor resources designed to supplement this text is located at http://connect.springerpub.com/content/book/978-0-8261-4475-1. Qualifying instructors may request access by emailing textbook@springerpub.com.

- Instructor Manual
  - Chapter-Based Solutions
  - Additional Practice Problems and Solutions
  - Sample Syllabus
- Instructor Data Sets (Microsoft Excel® Files)
  - SurgiFlex Course Project Workbook
  - Chapter Practice Problem Solutions
  - Additional Practice Problems and Solutions
    - Budgeting
    - Cost Estimation and Rate Calculation
    - Performance Measurement, Ratios, and Financial Statement Analysis
    - Time Value of Money
- Chapter-Based PowerPoint Presentations
- Test Bank

STUDENT RESOURCES

Answers to the end-of-chapter Practice Problems are available via Springer Publishing Connect™ by following the instructions on the opening page of this book and accessing Answers to Practice Problems on the Table of Contents.

Healthcare Industry Framework

CHAPTER 1

The Business of Healthcare

1. Introduce students to the foundations and core concepts of the healthcare sector.
2. Provide an overview of basic business characteristics and processes.
3. Discuss the commonalities/intersectionality between the healthcare and business sectors.
4. Understand the application of business skills in the healthcare sector as needed for problem-solving and decision-making.
5. Identify the types of business entities and their associated tax status.

FOUNDATIONS AND KEY CHARACTERISTICS OF HEALTHCARE

Healthcare and general care by a physician were initially reserved for the wealthy, especially in the formative years of the United States. Formalized healthcare for the citizenry mostly revolved around the provision of health services to military personnel, with others relying on holistic remedies provided within the community (Berridge, 2018; Sheard, 2018). From the establishment of our first medical colleges in 1765, to the creation of the United States Public Health Service Commissioned Corps in 1889, to the adoption of the U.S. Public Health Service Act of 1944, to the creation and implementation of the Patient Protection and Affordable Care Act (PPACA) in 2010, the avenues used to mandate and deliver some type of healthcare to our population have been and will continue to be ever-changing (Berger, 2019; Blank, 2012; Brandt & Gardner, 2000; Nguyen et al., 2020; Rosenberg, 2012).

Union organization and the Industrial Revolution ushered in what we would consider the earliest forms of public healthcare coverage as they sought to protect the well-being of employees in the workplace. During this period, production processes were mechanized across Europe as well as the United States, resulting in the increased need for workers in factories, mines, and mills. These dangerous and demanding environments required long workdays in hazardous conditions, with little thought given to worker safety. As factory owners and industrialists focused on increased product availability and profits, the machine-driven pace of production led to increased numbers of work-related injuries and, with it, loss of income. Employees, concerned for their safety and the well-being of their families, began to organize and demand changes be made by their employers. What came to be known as "trade unions" became the workers' first line of defense for negotiation of workplace terms and conditions. Early unions fought for coverage of lost wages due to injury, which later began to include basic medical care and, in some cases, prepaid hospital expenses. As a result of union activity, company sick benefits and medical programs began to take shape, although most employers at that time still refused to offer them.

Prior to the introduction of the Medicare Act of 1965 and managed care organizations (MCOs), approximately 80% of healthcare expenses were paid out-of-pocket by the individual seeking healthcare services (Feldstein, 2011; Hughes-Tuohy, 2019; Lyford & Lash, 2019; Speer et al., 2020), as the coverage offered by the employer was minimal. Today, no matter the health coverage method, those seeking care want it timely and at minimal cost to them. Healthcare policies and lawmakers are charged with finding the balance—satisfying individual healthcare preferences as well as the overarching needs of the public—but this all comes at a cost. Our nation's health and associated medical costs have been the focus of political and public service agendas for centuries.

To fully understand the contemporary healthcare sector and the healthcare finance discipline, we must first establish a few key definitions and foundational elements that will carry throughout our textbook discussion. There are many definitions for the healthcare sector and just as many interpretations of what the primary purpose of healthcare actually is. For the purposes of this textbook, the following definition of healthcare will be used: the practice of **healthcare** is the professional provision of medical services to address the emotional, mental, and physical well-being of a population. Healthcare covers a wide spectrum of products and services, which includes the prevention, diagnosis, treatment, and recovery of illness, disease, and injuries (Agency for Healthcare Research and Quality [AHRQ], n.d.; World Health Organization [WHO], n.d.). The look and feel of healthcare delivery varies by region in some cases as healthcare services are tailored to the population of that region, but the core purpose remains the same: preventive measures and best practices to foster overall well-being, and the treatment of illness or injury as diagnosed. A **healthcare sector** includes all of the people, organizations, and activities that contribute to promoting, restoring, or maintaining health (AHRQ, n.d.; Wendt et al., 2009; WHO, n.d.). The detailed discussion of the components of a healthcare system can be found in Chapter 3 of this textbook.

The Uniqueness of the Healthcare Sector

The healthcare sector continues to grow at a rapid pace, with an ever-changing landscape to suit a myriad of consumer needs. The quest for effective and efficient operations continuously shapes current operations, processes, and procedures. This constantly shifts the appearance of the typical healthcare organization. Of course, every industry seeks to maximize efficiencies, productivity, and profits, but there are still some fundamental differences in the operation of healthcare organizations that makes them quite unique. The first such fundamental difference is the law of supply and demand—healthcare defies it and seems to make its own rules along the way. The supply and demand theory states that a low supply of a good or service, coupled with the high demand by consumers, will actually increase the price. Conversely, high supply of a good or service paired with low demand by consumers will reduce the price (Janssen et al., 2021; Kimsey et al., 2018; Streckeisen, 2021). Supply and demand theory is applied to the original supplier of the good or service being offered, as well as competing suppliers offering a similar product or substitute. An example of this in healthcare would be name-brand medications produced and sold by a leading pharmaceutical company, with the substitutes being the generic versions of the medication being offered by a competitor. The healthcare sector has implemented several changes to improve quality and **access to care**, as well as reduce the price of care for the consumer, through measures such as increased number of providers, MCOs, accountable care organizations (ACOs), PPACA Medicaid expansions, and bundled payments. However, prices still continue to rise (Bowrey et al., 2019; Saltman, 2018; Walzer et al., 2013). A second trait that is somewhat unique to healthcare operations is the complex funding stream. Financial resource planning is not as methodical as in other industries, as consumers span numerous geographic boundaries and reimbursement includes government, private, and consumer funds, all with a different basis for payment (Janssen et al., 2021, Walzer et al., 2013). The regulations surrounding reimbursement for healthcare services also change frequently, which makes it even more difficult to plan for longer-term service delivery. A third difference between healthcare organizations and other businesses is the range of services provided. The healthcare sector does not offer one single good or service to consumers but offers a tremendous number of items to meet a myriad of needs. The provision of "healthcare" includes primary care, specialist services, dental, vision, equipment, and so forth, all with different suppliers, providers, pricing structures, and reimbursement rates. Healthcare finance professionals must therefore be agile when adjusting to this rapidly changing environment.

There is no one typical or standard type of healthcare system, but there are still some common governing aspects that remain best practice in all healthcare systems. No matter the size or scope of the organization, several items have been and will continue to be focal points of the leadership decision-making agenda. These healthcare sector goals are: (a) improving the quality of (changing) patient care, (b) maintaining sound financial operations and viability, and (c) addressing issues with access to healthcare services. Referred to as the "**Triple Aim**," these three key elements present ongoing challenges that impact every facet of the healthcare organization, including both the routine and longer-term decisions made by healthcare administrators (Bachynsky, 2019; Russo, 2016; Tasri & Tasri, 2020; Yagudina et al., 2017; Younis et al., 2009). Although these focal points work in unison to care for our population, the underlying causes and effects of each must be understood for continuous improvement and advancement of the healthcare sector.

Quality Patient Care

Delivering quality patient care is the most important aspect of what we do as healthcare professionals. Clinical or administrative, all are charged with ensuring that our population receives the care needed. The centuries-old tradition of face-to-face care is now evolving to accommodate those patients that are on-the-go, as well as those who are unable to get to standard medical facilities and offices. Of course, the clinical professionals must be the ones concerned about the actual provision of medical care given, but the nonclinical administrators must address and manage the delivery platforms, payment mechanisms, and operational feasibility of the various systems that support healthcare. Increased demand for healthcare services, long wait times, or limited availability of primary care physicians and specialists have all contributed to challenges with **quality of care** as well as the overall patient experience. There has been a great deal of improvement in providing quality of patient care, but some challenges remain. Patients' needs and preferences continue to evolve, making it challenging to improve patient and consumer satisfaction. Capacity is another challenge for healthcare organizations, as limited availability of clinicians and staff make it more difficult to meet increased needs. Resources have a direct impact on the ability to provide higher quality care, as both human resources and financial resources are needed to support improvement initiatives.

Financial Operations and Viability

The financial health of healthcare organizations is crucial to viability and stability of the sector and its supporting industries. With so many products and services being offered in healthcare, it is important to accurately capture costs incurred as well as the reimbursement that balances it. Reimbursement will be an ongoing concern as payers, rules, and regulations continue to change.

Government payers such as Medicare and Medicaid provide health insurance coverage for millions of Americans but have consistently reimbursed at a lower rate than commercial or private insurers. Implemented in 1965 during the Johnson administration, these programs were designed as amendments to the Social Security Act of 1935, extending additional health benefits for those 65 years of age and older (Medicare) and those having limited family income (Medicaid). Providers throughout the healthcare sector believe these populations to be more medically complex, thus requiring more healthcare resources which are typically not reimbursed by the government payers (Voytal & Gelburd, 2019). Commercial and private insurers, although reimbursing at a higher rate, attempt to reduce increased costs by bundling services or paying per diem (all-inclusive daily) rates. These cost-controlling measures often benefit the insurers but may result in lost revenue for the healthcare provider. Reimbursement practices and the guiding legislation are just a portion of the financial operations landscape that must be meticulously managed by healthcare organizations.

Competition from other providers is changing the overall market concentration in many areas, making viability a bit more challenging for smaller organizations, or ones that have not narrowed their focus. Medical advancements are often the result of technology-driven efficiencies designed to improve procedures or processes for providers as well as treatment and recovery time for patients. Those who cannot afford technology upgrades may lose patients to larger or newly merged entities that have more capacity and can keep up with the growing healthcare needs of the population. Increased staffing and operating costs are the standard response to meeting increased demand, but these are difficult to sustain long term. Remote areas or underserved areas often find themselves short staffed or with high turnover rates, and must rely on contracted, high-expense labor to provide care. Healthcare in the United States has proven to be expensive, and the survival of many organizations is dependent upon the consumers' ability and willingness to pay. No matter the medical issue, the financial process is initiated at the start of consultation and treatment. Most of this happens behind the scenes, as healthcare providers focus on the care of the patient.

Access to Healthcare Services

For consumers to effectively utilize healthcare services, they must be able to access the needed healthcare services. For many, it's not as simple as driving to the physician's office or taking a ride on the local public transit system. Illness, location, and clinician availability all play a role in the access to care dilemma. Decreased mobility due to health or physical condition make some unable to travel for medical care. Without medical transport or home healthcare services, those with mobility issues may go without the necessary care. For those residing in rural areas, it may take hours to get to an internal medicine physician or general practitioner, and specialist care is often unattainable. For some in urban areas, no services may be available at all if community providers lack capacity or specialization, or if providers choose practice locations based on specific socioeconomic factors. Healthcare professionals recognize this issue, but the battle to change the access to care landscape has been hard-fought. Additional providers have been added and urgent care outpatient facilities have been created to expand systems' services, ease wait times and congestion, and offer additional points of access for consumers. Increased access often results in increased costs incurred for healthcare organizations. The elements of the Triple Aim have proven to be codependent, with changes in one directly impacting the remaining two. Improvement and sustainability in the healthcare sector require continued assessment and improvement of all three elements, as all are ultimately driven by the shared mission of optimal patient care.

Technological Advancements

Technology lies at the core of healthcare operations, making it possible for many to be on the cutting edge of healthcare service delivery. The industry strives to improve treatment of existing conditions as well as prevent the onset of new ones. Advancements and innovation in equipment improve medical procedures, simplifying techniques for clinicians while reducing pain and recovery time for patients. Electronic medical records (EMRs) and electronic health records (EHRs) share patient information among providers to eliminate duplicate or unnecessary care and testing, prevent overmedication, and reduce increasingly costly internal administrative processes. With EMR and EHR information systems, providers are able to see a patient's treatments across the entire spectrum of care, with the intent of improving patient care outcomes as well as improving health system efficiencies. Telemedicine provides consultation for those seeking care for nonemergent health concerns, as well as those with limited access to care. The use of telemedicine services was proven to be particularly beneficial during the pandemic as healthcare organizations focused their efforts on those patients with more severe illnesses. Pharmaceutical treatments have expanded to not only provide traditional medications, but to incorporate wearable technology as additional treatment options. Wearable technology includes devices used for the maintenance and treatment of illnesses, as well as for general fitness tracking. Diabetes care, for example, utilizes software-enabled wearable monitors and automatic insulin pumps to help diabetics monitor glucose levels. Heartrate monitors, smart watches, and similar devices allow consumers to monitor exercise results, sleeping patterns, breathing, and so forth for personal physical fitness. Although technology has positively impacted the healthcare sector, it comes with a cost. Research and development expenses can be exorbitant, increasing the overall costs of care for both providers and consumers. The benefits of technological advancement have continued to outweigh its costs, as stakeholders from all sides of healthcare rely on these improvements for some facet of service delivery.

BUSINESS SECTOR MARKERS: WHAT ARE THEY DOING RIGHT?

The healthcare sector is indeed dynamic, with change being the only constant in this rapidly evolving and improving field. Best practices have surely been established over the years, but as change continues, so must the way by which we approach and address the current challenges in healthcare, as well as the proposed path to our future. Interprofessional collaboration has arguably worked best for the delivery of healthcare services and has been a mainstay for care delivery for generations. Should we not continue to make concerted efforts to collaborate across sector boundaries to create the most feasible and progressive healthcare operating processes? There are some who are steadfast in their opposition to using strict business practices in healthcare, but the reality of the matter is, it is already happening. The healthcare sector generates approximately $3.8 trillion in expenditure (Centers for Medicare & Medicaid Services [CMS], 2021), and that must be managed well to maintain viability and sustainability for all stakeholders involved—providers, consumers, and suppliers alike. While the discipline of medicine will always be at the forefront of healthcare provision, business practices are in fact needed for the operational soundness of the traditional back-office (nonpatient care) functions. The private/business sector has been quite successful at right-sizing its networks (adjusting the size or scope of its organizations), creating improved efficiencies, and ultimately improving performance. As healthcare expenditures continue to grow in response to changing technology and improved quality of care, our approach to the challenges in our networks must change in efforts to right-size the healthcare system as well. The overall objective of this chapter is to examine the not-so-clear sector boundaries, the commonalities between the healthcare and business sectors, and the possible operational implications of the shared best practices. These commonalities make it possible for the healthcare sector to operate and adapt as needed by society.

The field of Business has long been established as the well-oiled machine, making the most effective and efficient use of its resources. The strategies employed have been tried and revised over time, improving processes and procedures, and giving way to the established models we see today. While leadership styles and the actual governance process of business organizations are a discussion for a different course, we can in fact acknowledge the markers which help guide successful business sector organizations.

When examining the typical business structure and the related **business processes**, several distinct characteristics surface as markers or dominant traits of success that can be categorized as: (a) ongoing economic and financial activities, (b) customer/consumer-driven focus, and (c) effective and efficient resource utilization (Foster et al., 2015; McDonald et al., 2011; Northrop, 2018; Sawyer, 2018). Economic and financial activities cover a myriad of functions, all of which are crucial elements in keeping the organization running routinely, as well as securing longer-term viability. Key functions and processes in this category would include securing raw materials and the creation of finished products, distribution and sale of these finished products (goods and/ or services offered), and profit margin. The prudent analysis of risk is also included in this first category, as businesses assess risk to determine if the project or venture is worth undertaking. They have to ultimately determine if the rewards outweigh the risks of implementation. Customer/consumer-driven focus is what guides the organization—it's the reason they create the products they sell or provide the services they provide. The customer is the foundation of an organization's mission, vision, and values, with customers being both internal and external to the organization. Effective and efficient resource allocation is another characteristic of business that many other industries have adopted. The concept here is to meet the needs and established goals for consumers, as well as meeting the financial targets for the company. **Effectiveness** is a qualitative target, used as an indicator of achieving an intended outcome. Effectiveness in healthcare can be represented as the measured outcomes of a clinical intervention. For example, a cardiac treatment initiative sets a target of decreasing heart disease by 50% in a specific community or population. In a population of 100 patients with 50 patients having heart disease, a decrease to 25 patients having heart disease means the treatment initiative was effective. **Efficiency**, on the other hand, is a quantitative target, answering the question of whether or not the organization is providing the best possible product or service at the least possible cost (highest efficiency). Using the same example of the cardiac treatment initiative, efficiency would be achieving the same effectiveness using the least number of resources (financial and material). Effectiveness and efficiency targets can be established by the healthcare organization as it monitors and improves internal operations, or by the healthcare industry as it outlines standards for patient care. These characteristics, although associated with the business sector, are represented in many other sectors as a systematic approach to goal achievement. When examining the elements in this systematic approach, the business process typically resembles the path in Figure 1.1.

The business process as shown in Figure 1.1 begins with the organization's mission, vision, and values—the drivers of the organization's purpose and scope of responsibilities (Chongwatpol, 2020; Krpalek et al., 2018; Leyland et al., 2021; Lopez, 2020; Wicks & Keevil, 2014). These define the population of consumers the organization intends to serve, and exactly what products and services it intends to deliver. Goals and objectives are what the organization implements and achieves along the way, as it works toward its mission, vision, and values.

Figure 1.1

The business process

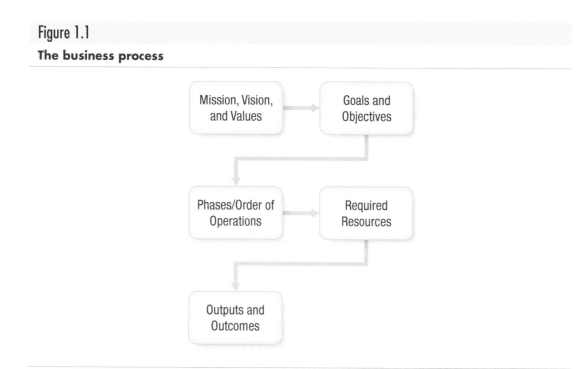

The various phases and/or order of operations is the actual creation of goods and services. This will be different for every organization and is dependent upon what the final product or service is going to be. The next part of the process is the analysis of the required resources for the entire process. Prudent business practices assess both the human resources and the material resources needed for the production of goods and services. The resources needed for production are ultimately used in the calculation of overall cost to the organization as well as the price for the consumer. Finally, the output and outcomes are the final items produced and the level of goal achievement.

INTERSECTION OF SECTORS: WHAT ARE THE COMMONALITIES?

The primary purpose of healthcare is to care for the health and well-being of a population, but the size of the sector and supporting industries forces us to implement detailed frameworks and established operating procedures. This is very familiar, as we've seen such requirements routinely implemented in the business and private sectors. All the aforementioned concerns must work in unison somehow, so as not to compromise one for the other. Operational and financial efficiencies, for example, must not be achieved by the sacrifice of quality patient care. All these functions, while healthcare focused, are implemented and maintained according to standard business processes and regulations (Black, 1995; Cebul et al., 2008; Coatney et al., 2018; Jayatilake & Ganegoda, 2021).

The healthcare sector is focused on the care and well-being of the population, addressing concerns in the preventive stages of illness, as well as the current treatment and long-term maintenance stages of care. Patient care includes more than just the physician–patient interaction, although this interaction serves as the starting point for the care process. Primary providers, ancillary services providers, specialists, suppliers, contractors, and payers are all included among the moving parts that comprise our very large system, each with its own internal operational requirements and needs. The provision of care is surely the focal point of healthcare services, but the organizational structure in many cases is solidly grounded in business ideology (Collins, 2015; Krishnamoorthi & Mathew, 2018; LeClair, 2018; Pauly, 2018). The business processes and procedures of the organization need to be defined to support and sustain the service delivery efforts. There are quite a few commonalities, as well as some very stark differences, but the establishment and reliance on routine processes and procedures is worth noting (see Table 1.1).

Table 1.1

BUSINESS SECTOR AND HEALTHCARE SECTOR COMPARISON

		Business Concepts	Healthcare Concepts
Economic and Financial		Routine financial recording and reporting	Routine financial recording and reporting
		Financial planning and forecasting	Financial planning and forecasting
		Cost control to maximize profit	Cost control to minimize overall expense
		Capital expenditures directly applicable to finished goods and services	Capital expenditures indirectly applicable to finished goods and services
Customer/Consumer Focused		Shareholder interests—profit sharing or dividends dispersed	Stakeholder interests—largely nonprofit; limited/no profit sharing or dividends for nonprofit organizations
		Meets specific product demand; mass production	Meets specific product and service demands; individual delivery
		Consumers drive what is actually demanded	Consumer and technological advancement drive what is actually demanded
		Competition includes exact product producers as well as substitutes; usually not location specific	Competition is usually dependent on location
		Individual organization approach to operations	Systematic approach to operations
Effectiveness/ Efficiency		Effectiveness is generally tied to business performance (inward focus)	Effectiveness is generally tied to consumer-specific initiatives (outward focus)
		Efficiency is maximizing the use of raw materials and resources to maximize production and revenue	Efficiency is providing the best possible services at the lowest possible cost
		Market maneuverability	Limited market maneuverability

As Table 1.1 shows, there are several commonalities among the business and healthcare sectors, with the major differences being how and to whom the final product or service is delivered. The business and healthcare sectors are both consumer-driven, but the type of consumer is what differs. Businesses, for the most part, are for-profit entities focusing on profits and returns for **shareholders**, the owners and financial investors of the company. Healthcare organizations, on the other hand, focus on both the shorter-term and longer-term healthcare improvements for its **stakeholders**, those impacted by the (nonfinancial) success of the organization. Shareholders in the business realm focus on the maximization of profits, while the stakeholders in healthcare realm focus on improvement and overall well-being of the system. Both are important, but the lens is different. The exception to this would be the for-profit healthcare entities such as pharmaceutical and healthcare technology companies. Business processes drive the underlying operations for both sectors, with detailed functions determined by the organization's mission and goals (Biermann et al., 2018; Mintz, 1995; Mintz & Palmer, 2000; Wicks & Keevil, 2014). The economic and financial indicators are relatively similar, with the major difference being the classification of capital expenditures. The business sector can map the expense directly to the production of its goods sold as a direct tie-in to volume and sales. Healthcare, on the other hand, rarely has the ability for such a connection. Capital investments in healthcare are usually advancements in technology to directly benefit the patient and improve the patient care experience. This could mean less invasive surgical procedures or rapid screening and testing and improved care for all patients not connected to any one patient's "purchase" of care.

TYPES OF BUSINESS ORGANIZATIONS AND TAX STATUS

There are several types of business organizations, which are categorized by structure, liability, and associated tax status. A **sole proprietorship** is a business entity wholly owned by one individual. These organizations can be small or large businesses, and in healthcare may include physician's offices or local neighborhood healthcare providers and pharmacies. A **partnership** is a business entity that has two or more owners and is relatively easy to form. The partnership is a common type of business arrangement in the healthcare sector, with many physicians' groups and larger practices using this business structure. The sole proprietorship and the standard partnership have unlimited liability, meaning that the business as well as the owners' assets are subject to claim for any outstanding debts or obligations. A **corporation** is a business entity that has been established to be separate from its owners. In healthcare, we see this form most often as hospitals and larger providers or manufacturers. The **limited liability partnership** (LLP) and the **limited liability company** (LLC) are business structures that combine the benefits of partnership and collaboration with the limited liability of a corporation. An example of this would be a physicians' group or community clinic having the traditional partnership structure with the liability protection of a corporation.

Any of the aforementioned business types can be for-profit or not-for-profit organizations, which will ultimately determine their tax status and reporting requirements. **For-profit** entities are investor-owned, with the focus on maximizing profits for shareholders' dividends. These companies can be publicly traded on stock markets or can be privately owned. For-profits have a corporate-level tax obligation as well as a shareholder-level tax obligation but have the ability to leverage risk and equity. **Not-for-profit** (nonprofit) entities are not investor owned but are instead owned by the community stakeholders they serve. These companies have a tax-exempt status and do not have federal tax obligations. Not-for-profits cannot sell shares or portions of the business through stock market interactions, therefore limiting their capital to donations and investments from community supporters. The Securities and Exchange Commission (SEC) regulates the financial activities and reporting for the publicly traded for-profit organizations, and the Internal Revenue Service (IRS) regulates the financial activities and reporting for the not-for-profit organizations (requiring 501c3 tax filing status). The tax code and reporting requirements are quite complex, requiring a dedicated team of accounting and finance professionals to manage this portion of the healthcare organization's business. Maintaining the designated tax status is crucial to an organization's longer-term viability, especially for those that serve the community.

APPLICATION OF BUSINESS SKILLS IN THE HEALTHCARE SECTOR AND WHAT THIS MEANS FOR HEALTHCARE FINANCE

Business acumen is necessary in most professional environments today and is considered a required knowledge base for many academic and professional training programs. This knowledge and related skillset guide the organization's internal practices as well as its external actions to ensure short-term and long-term operating effectiveness and efficiency. Although health and wellness are the overarching goals of the healthcare sector, the business end of the operations must also be managed (Brooks et al., 2015; Davey et al., 2010; Garmon, 2017; Stefl, 2008). Business competencies are required in the following areas to support the provision of healthcare: quality improvement, financial management, human resources, information management, risk management, organizational theory and governance, strategic planning, marketing, and systems theory (Brown & Rich, 2020; Burke-Smalley, 2014; Council on Linkages Between Academia and Public Health Practice, 2021; Crittenden et al., 2019; Healthcare Leadership Alliance [HLA], 2021; Ramraj & Marimuthu, 2021; Romanow et al., 2020). These routine business operations ensure that the healthcare organization is able to (a) treat and retain patients, (b) improve the patient experience and quality through technology, and (c) collect and analyze data for performance measurement and management (Bachynsky, 2019; Berwick et al., 2008; Jeyaraj, 2019; Ong & Djajadikerta, 2019; Pan & Seow, 2016; Rupert et al., 2016; Zhang et al., 2020).

As with any other type of organization, making the right business decisions is essential to keeping healthcare organizations viable (Blodgett & Melconian, 2012; Evers et al., 2007; Goldzweig et al., 2013; Hamilton et al., 2021; McCartney, 2005). Business skills such as financial statement analysis provide some of the key supporting information for the **decision-making process**. Existing information and data must be analyzed to determine the root cause of a problem, and all possible alternatives are then identified. Choosing the right alternative often means determining a solution for the present as well as outlining the necessary activities for the future state of the organization. The decisions made here include operating solutions as well as financial ones, with the best alternatives including an optimal mix of both for overall effectiveness and efficiency.

The decision-making process involves several stakeholders on multiple levels of the organization. Each step in the decision-making process as outlined in Figure 1.2 is designed to accomplish a different task toward problem mitigation and resolution. Although the tasks may be different, with each making a different contribution, they are all supported in some way by the organization's financial information (Ajani & Habek, 2021; Berger, 2019; Campanale et al., 2014; Ito & Tsutsumi, 2022; Landman et al., 2018; Munro et al., 2020; Walker & Moran, 2019; Whiteford & Striegel-Weissman, 2017). The decision-making process can be applied to an organization's operational challenges as well as patient-care flows and service bottlenecks. Success with these steps relies on the availability and interpretation of sound, reliable data, as the resulting decisions will impact the organization for both the shorter and longer terms. The data element, which provides some of the foundational information, must be well-planned and determined strategically. The thought process here must be "quality in, quality out." The information being collected from all functional and management areas must be quality information—meaningful for the assessment of the organization's performance measurement and management (Mattie et al., 2020; Menaker et al., 2020; Nix & Szostek, 2016; Peer & Rakich, 1999; Rios-Zertuche et al., 2020; Samushonga, 2021; Sariyar, 2012; Wills, 2014, Zhou et al., 2021).

Figure 1.2

The decision-making process

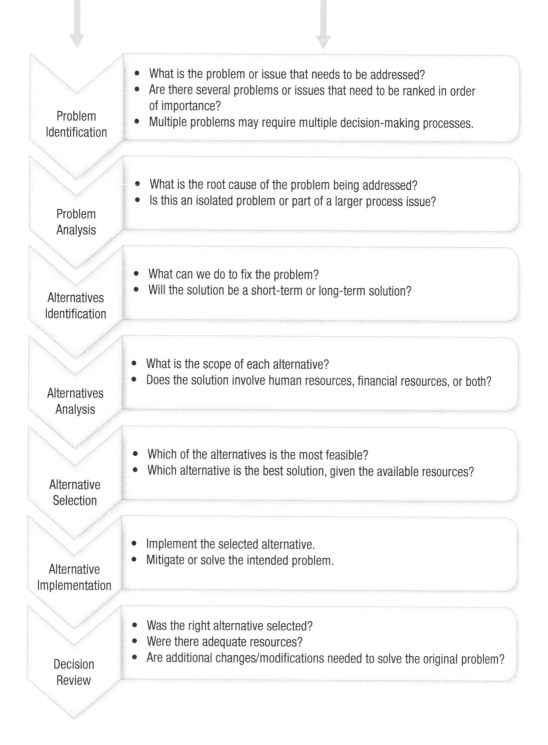

Decision-Making Steps   Questions to Ask

Problem Identification
- What is the problem or issue that needs to be addressed?
- Are there several problems or issues that need to be ranked in order of importance?
- Multiple problems may require multiple decision-making processes.

Problem Analysis
- What is the root cause of the problem being addressed?
- Is this an isolated problem or part of a larger process issue?

Alternatives Identification
- What can we do to fix the problem?
- Will the solution be a short-term or long-term solution?

Alternatives Analysis
- What is the scope of each alternative?
- Does the solution involve human resources, financial resources, or both?

Alternative Selection
- Which of the alternatives is the most feasible?
- Which alternative is the best solution, given the available resources?

Alternative Implementation
- Implement the selected alternative.
- Mitigate or solve the intended problem.

Decision Review
- Was the right alternative selected?
- Were there adequate resources?
- Are additional changes/modifications needed to solve the original problem?

The healthcare finance role is critical to the decision-making process for project-based analysis as well as larger scope organizational-level analysis. Most processes and procedures tie in some way to the organization's financial data, either retrospectively or prospectively. While managing expenses, maximizing revenues, budgeting, and reporting, healthcare finance professionals work with organizational leadership to identify and implement strategic initiatives to maintain and improve the shorter-term and longer-term operations of the health services organization. The overall impact of healthcare finance is broad and reaches beyond the routine responsibilities of the department by assisting other areas with clinical volume analysis, pricing decisions, capital purchase and project costing, and a whole other host of other crucial items.

CHAPTER SUMMARY

The business and healthcare sectors are entwined on many levels, with best practices and sound decision-making evidenced in both. The focus of the business process is the mission, vision, and values of the organization, which serve as the foundation for consumer-driven processes. The skills and knowledge needed to successfully navigate in both environments are congruent. Human resources, management and organizational theory, information technology, financial management, and so forth, are all critical to the success and achievement of the organization's goals and objectives. These commonalities (focus, skills, knowledge, etc.) create the framework which guides the provision of healthcare goods and services. There is undoubtedly collaboration between the two sectors, which is essential as we address the health needs of varying populations and keep pace with advancing technologies. While patient care is the overarching mission of the healthcare sector, we must ensure that the supporting business processes of healthcare organizations are sound, making the fulfillment of that mission possible.

KEY TERMS FOR REVIEW

access to care	for-profit	partnership
business process	healthcare	quality of care
corporation	healthcare sector	shareholders
decision-making process	limited liability company	sole proprietorship
effectiveness	limited liability partnership	stakeholders
efficiency	not-for-profit/nonprofit	Triple Aim

DISCUSSION QUESTIONS

1. What are some of the key differences between the healthcare and business sectors? How do these differences impact the operations and subsequent analysis of healthcare organizations?

2. Do you believe one sector to be more effective/efficient than the other? Why/why not? Explain.

3. What are some of the best practices that appear to be shared by both sectors? Are the best practices implemented in the same manner?

4. Discuss the importance of financial management in healthcare and the impact on the decision-making aspects of the healthcare sector.

5. Competencies and skills for both the business and healthcare sectors require knowledge of a myriad of subjects. Discuss how the knowledge of financial management supports other knowledge/subject areas.

6. The terms "effectiveness" and "efficiency" are often used interchangeably, when in fact they are two distinct concepts. Define the two terms and discuss the differences.

7. What are the various types of business organizations? Detail the differences in tax liability and the possible impacts on organizations in the healthcare sector.

CHAPTER 1 CASE: A SEAT AT THE TABLE

The Riverside Community Hospital has been a staple in the community for over 20 years, and is the only full-service healthcare facility in the area. The population served by the hospital is quite diverse and includes citizens of varying demographics and health statuses. The hospital takes great pride in meeting the healthcare needs of the community it serves and has historically been very accommodating of patient requests. Recently, the hospital has seen a decline in patient visits and has received more patient complaints than it typically does. The leadership team is unclear as to what has caused these issues, but asks you, the newest member of the leadership team, to investigate and propose viable solutions. As you begin to plan your investigation, you think of the numerous internal processes and procedures to be reviewed. You decide that the decision-making process is the best way to address concerns in multiple areas, and you realize that you cannot accomplish this task alone. The appropriate stakeholders must have a seat at the table, as the processes, procedures, and related outcomes of their respective operational areas are assessed.

1. Who are the key stakeholders within the hospital that have an interest in patient visits? How might these identified stakeholders be impacted by changes in patient visits?

2. Who are the key stakeholders within the hospital that have an interest in patient complaints? How might these identified stakeholders be impacted by patient complaints?

3. Who are the external stakeholders?

4. How would you engage the stakeholders involved in this process?

5. What would be your strategy of communicating or assigning the elements of the decision-making process?

6. Do the stakeholders identified have the ability to directly impact the issues? Here, specifically discuss what a department or unit can do to increase or decrease the number of patient visits or patient complaints (satisfaction).

7. What external factors could be the underlying cause of these issues? Do you believe that Riverside Community Hospital has the ability to influence these external factors?

REFERENCES

Agency for Healthcare Research and Quality. (n.d.). *Evidence-based practice center (EPC) reports.* https://www
.ahrq.gov/research/findings/evidence-based-reports/index.html

Ajani, T., & Habek, G. (2021). Principal component analysis for decision making in healthcare and hospital
readmissions. *Issues in Information Systems, 22*(4), 334–345. https://doi.org/10.48009/4_iis_2021_372-380

Bachynsky, N. (2019). Implications for policy: The Triple Aim, Quadruple Aim, and interprofessional collaboration.
Nursing Forum, 2020(55), 54–64. https://doi.org/10.1111/nuf.12382

Berger, Z. (2019). Metrics of patient, public, consumer, and community engagement in healthcare systems: How
should we define engagement, what are we measuring, and does it matter for patient care? *International
Journal of Health Policy and Management, 8*(1), 49–50. https://doi.org/10.15171/ijhpm.2018.94

Berridge, V. (2018). Why policy needs history (and historians). *Health Economics, Policy and Law, 2018*(13), 369–381.
https://doi.org/10.1017/S1744133117000433

Berwick, D. M., Nolan, T. W., & Whittington, J. (2008). The Triple Aim: Care, health, and cost. *Health Affairs, 27*(3),
759–769. https://doi.org/10.1377/hlthaff.27.3.759

Biermann, O., Kuchenmüller, T., Panisset, U., & Leys, M. (2018). Policy dialogues: Facilitators' perceived role and
influence. *International Journal of Health Governance, 23*(2), 120–133. https://doi.org/10.1108/IJHG-12-2017-0063

Black, D. (1995). Health care—a business or a service? *Perspectives in Biology and Medicine, 39*(1), 1–14. https://doi
.org/10.1353/pbm.1995.0021

Blank, R. (2012). Transformation of the US healthcare system: Why is change so difficult? *Current Sociology, 60*(4),
415–426. https://doi.org/10.1177/0011392112438327

Blodgett, M., & Melconian, L. (2012). Health-care nonprofits: Enhancing governance and public trust. *Business and
Society Review, 117*(2), 197–219. https://doi.org/10.1111/j.1467-8594.2012.00405.x

Bowrey, G., Smark, C., & Jones, G. (2019). The influence of economic (Ir)rationality on public sector reforms.
e-Journal of Social & Behavioural Research in Business, 10(1), 24–39.

Brandt, A., & Gardner, M. (2000). Antagonism and accommodation: Interpreting the relationship between public
health and medicine in the United States during the 20th century. *American Journal of Public Health, 90*(5),
707–715. https://doi.org/10.2105/ajph.90.5.707

Brooks, P., El-Gayar, O., & Sarnikar, S. (2015). A framework for developing a domain specific business intelligence
maturity model: Application to healthcare. *International Journal of Information Management, 2015*(35), 337–345.
https://doi.org/10.1016/j.ijinfomgt.2015.01.011

Brown, A., & Rich, M. (2020). Pedagogy and evaluation: The challenge for business and management degree
courses in the 21st century. *The Electronic Journal of Business Research Methods, 18*(2), 84–99. https://academic
-publishing.org/index.php/ejbrm/article/view/2027

Burke-Smalley, L. A. (2014). Evidence-based management education. *Journal of Management Education, 35*(5), 764–
767. https://doi.org/10.1177/1052562914529418

Campanale, C., Cinquini, L., & Tenucci. A. (2014). Time-driven activity-based costing to improve transparency
and decision making in healthcare—A case study. *Qualitative Research in Accounting & Management, 11*(2),
165–186. https://doi.org/10.1108/QRAM-04-2014-0036

Cebul, R. D., Rebitzer, J. B., Taylor, L. J., & Votruba, M. E. (2008). Organizational fragmentation and care quality in
the U.S. healthcare system. *Journal of Economic Perspectives, 22*(4), 93–113. https://doi.org/10.1257/jep.22.4.93

Centers for Medicare & Medicaid Services. (2021, December 1). *National health expenditure data.* https://www.cms
.gov/research-statistics-data-and-systems/statistics-trends-and-reports/nationalhealthexpenddata

Chongwatpol, J. (2020). Operationalizing design thinking in business intelligence and analytics projects. *Decision
Sciences Journal of Innovative Education, 18*(3), 409–434. https://doi.org/10.1111/dsji.12217

Coatney, K., Donovan, R., Whelan, D., Gill-Cox, A., & Blanton, T. (2018). The business value of information
technology. Big data analytics, and consumer health applications. *Annals of Spiru Haret University. Journalism
Studies, 19*(2), 30–52.

Collins, D. (2015). Operational best practices in business ethics: A practical and systematic benchmarking tool.
Business and Society Review, 120(2), 303–327. https://doi.org/10.1111/basr.12057

Council on Linkages Between Academia and Public Health Practice. (2021). *Core competencies for public health professionals*. The Public Health Foundation. http://www.phf.org/corecompetencies

Crittenden, W. F., Biel, I. K., & Lovelly III, W. A. (2019). Embracing digitalization: Student learning and new technologies. *Journal of Marketing Education, 41*(1), 5–14. https://doi.org/10.1177/0273475318820895

Davey, S., Brennan, M., Meenan, B., & McAdam, R. (2010). The health of innovation: Why open business models can benefit the healthcare sector. *Irish Journal of Management, 30*(1), 21–40.

Evers, S., Salvador–Carulla, L., Halsteinli, V., McDaid, D., & The Mheen Group. (2007). Implementing mental health economic evaluation evidence: Building a bridge between theory and practice. *Journal of Mental Health, 16*(2), 223–241. https://doi.org/10.1080/09638230701279881

Feldstein, P. J. (2011). *Health policy issues: An economic perspective*. Health Administrative Press.

Foster, K., Smith, G., Ariyachandra, T., & Frolick, M. N. (2015). Business intelligence competency center: Improving data and decisions. *Information Systems Management, 2015*(32), 229–233. https://doi.org/10.1080/10580530.2015.1044343

Garmon, C. (2017). The accuracy of hospital merger screening methods. *The RAND Journal of Economics, 48*(4), 1068–1102. https://doi.org/10.1111/1756-2171.12215

Goldzweig, I. A., Schlundt, D. G., Moore, W. E., Smith, P. E., Zoorob, R. J., & Levine, R. S. (2013). An academic, business, and community alliance to promote evidence-based public health policy: The case of primary seat belt legislation. *Journal of Health Care for the Poor and Underserved, 24*(3), 1364–1377. https://doi.org/10.1353/hpu.2013.0138

Hamilton, C. B., Dehnadi, M., Snow, S., Clark, N., Lui, M., McLean, J., Mamdani, H., Kooijman, A. L., Bubber, V., & Hoefer, T. (2021). Themes for evaluating the quality of initiatives to engage patients and family caregivers in decision-making in healthcare systems: A scoping review. *BMJ Open, 11*, Article e050208. https://doi.org/10.1136/bmjopen-2021-050208

Healthcare Leadership Alliance. (2021). *HLA competency directory*. http://www.healthcareleadershipalliance.org/directory.htm

Hughes-Tuohy, C. (2019). Political accommodations in multipayer health care systems: Implications for the United States. *American Journal of Public Health, 2019*(109), 1501–1505. https://doi.org/10.2105/AJPH.2019.305279

Ito, M., & Tsutsumi, M. (2022). A call to action for an inclusive model of shared decision-making in healthcare. *Nursing and Health Sciences, 24*(1), 3–6. https://doi.org/10.1111/nhs.12879

Janssen, L. M., Drost, R. M., Paulus, A. T., Garfeld, K., Hollingworth, W., Noble, S. Thorn, J. C., Pokhilenko, I., & Evers, S. M. M. A. (2021). Aspects and challenges of resource use measurement in health economics: Towards a comprehensive measurement framework. *PharmacoEconomics, 39*(9), 983–993. https://doi.org/10.1007/s40273-021-01048-z

Jayatilake, S. M., & Ganegoda, G. U. (2021). Involvement of machine learning tools in healthcare decision making. *Journal of Healthcare Engineering, 2021*, Article 6679512. https://doi.org/10.1155/2021/6679512

Jeyaraj, A. (2019). Pedagogy for business analytics courses. *Journal of Information Systems Education, 30*(2), 67–83. https://jise.org/Volume30/n2/JISEv30n2p67.html

Kimsey, L., Hoburg, A., Olaiya, S., Jones II, K. D., & Richard, P. (2018). A systems approach to person-centric health economics. *Military Medicine, 183*(11/12), 233–238. https://doi.org/10.1093/milmed/usy209

Krishnamoorthi, S., & Mathew, S. K. (2018). Business analytics and business value: A comparative case study. *Information & Management, 55*(2018), 643–666. https://doi.org/10.1016/j.im.2018.01.005

Krpalek, P., Krpalkova-Krelova, K., & Berkova, K. (2018). The importance of metacognitive strategies for building competitive business competencies. *Journal of Competitiveness, 10*(3), 69–85. https://doi.org/10.7441/joc.2018.03.05

Landman, J. H., Moore, K., Muhlestein, D. B., Smith, N. J., & Winfield, L. D. (2018). *What is driving total cost of care? An analysis of factors influencing total cost of care in U.S. healthcare markets*. Healthcare Financial Management Association. https://www.hfma.org/wp-content/uploads/2022/10/61080.pdf

LeClair, D. (2018). Integrating business analytics in the marketing curriculum: Eight recommendations. *Marketing Education Review, 28*(1), 6–13. https://doi.org/10.1080/10528008.2017.1421050

Leyland, R., Heath, M., Neve, H., & Maynard, V. (2021). Structured reflection on shared decision making. *The Clinical Teacher, 18*(1), 55–61. https://doi.org/10.1111/tct.13233

Lopez, R. (2020). Perspectives of technology competency in business instruction. *Journal of International Business Disciplines*, 15(2), 31–45.

Lyford, S., & Lash, T. (2019). America's healthcare cost crisis. *Generations*, 43(Suppl. 1), 7–12.

Mattie, A. S., Charlier, S. D., West, S., & Runyan, J. D. (2020). Educating healthcare compliance professionals: Identification of competencies. *Journal of Education for Business*, 95(6), 367–374. https://doi.org/10.1080/08 832323.2019.1664375

McCartney, J. J. (2005). Values based decision making in healthcare: Introduction. *Healthcare Ethics Committee Forum*, 17(1), 1–5. https://doi.org/10.1007/s10730-005-4946-4

McDonald, J., Powell-Davies, G., Jayasuriya, R., & Fort-Harris, M. (2011). Collaboration across private and public sector primary health care services: Benefits, costs and policy implications. *Journal of Interprofessional Care*, 2011(25), 258–264. https://doi.org/10.3109/13561820.2011.566650

Menaker, R., Ritte, R. J., & France, T. J. (2020). *Principal principles: Critical accounting and financial concepts for healthcare leaders*. Medical Group Management Association. https://www.mgma.com/resources/financial -management/principal-principles-critical-accounting-and-fina

Mintz, B. (1995). Business participation in health care policy reform: Factors contributing to collective action within the business community. *Social Problems*, 42(3), 408–428. https://doi.org/10.2307/3096855

Mintz, B., & Palmer, D. (2000). Business and health care policy reform in the 1980s: The 50 states. *Social Problems*, 47(3), 327–359. https://doi.org/10.2307/3097234

Munro, S., Kornelsen, J., Wilcox, E., Kaufman, S., Bansback, N., Corbett, K., & Janssen, P. (2020). Implementation of shared decision-making in healthcare policy and practice: A complex adaptive systems perspective. *Evidence & Policy*, 16(3), 393–411. https://doi.org/10.1332/174426419X15468571657773

Nguyen, M. T., Hua, C. L., Sun, N., & Brown, J. S. (2020). The relationship between healthcare provider density and diabetes prevalence in the United States. *Journal of Health and Human Services Administration*, 44(3), 245–259.

Nix, T., & Szostek, L. (2016). Evolution of physician-centric business models under the Patient Protection and Affordable Care Act. *International Journal of Applied Management and Technology*, 15(1), 1–20. https://doi .org/10.5590/IJAMT.2016.15.1.01

Northrop, G. (2018). Building a strong nonprofit board goes beyond best practices. *Generations*, 42(1), 56–60.

Ong, T., & Djajadikerta, H. G. (2019). Adoption of emerging technology to incorporate business research skills in teaching accounting theory. *Journal of Education for Business*, 94(7), 480–489. https://doi.org/10.1080/08832 323.2019.1574702

Pan, G., & Seow, P. (2016). Preparing accounting graduates for digital revolution: A critical review of information technology competencies and skills development. *Journal of Education for Business*, 91(3), 166–175. https:// doi.org/10.1080/08832323.2016.1145622

Pauly, M. (2018). The business of healthcare and the economics of healthcare: Shall ever the twain meet? *International Journal of the Economics of Business*, 25(1), 181–189. https://doi.org/10.1080/13571516.2017.13 95241

Peer, S., & Rakich, J. (1999). Ethical decision making in healthcare management. *Hospital Topics: Research and Perspectives on Healthcare*, 77(4), 7–13. https://doi.org/10.1080/00185869909596532

Ramraj, U., & Marimuthu, F. (2021). Preparing undergraduate learners with skills required by a transformative work environment. *International Journal of Higher Education*, 10(1), 287–294. https://doi.org/10.5430/ijhe .v10n1p287

Rios-Zertuche, D., Gonzalez-Marmo, A., Millán-Velasco, F., Schwarzbauer, K., & Tristao, I. (2020). Implementing electronic decision-support tools to strengthen healthcare network data-driven decision-making. *Archives of Public Health*, 78(33), 1–11. https://doi.org/10.1186/s13690-020-00413-2

Romanow, D., Napier, N. P., & Cline, M. K. (2020). Using active learning, group formation, and discussion to increase student learning: A business intelligence skills analysis. *Journal of Information Systems Education*, 31(3), 218–231. https://aisel.aisnet.org/jise/vol31/iss3/6/

Rosenberg, L. (2012). Are healthcare leaders ready for the real revolution? *Journal of Behavioral Health Services & Research*, 39, 215–219. https://doi.org/10.1007/s11414-012-9285-z

Rupert, D., Dillon, E. D., Teitelbaum, A. S., & Ray, S. E. (2016). Succeeding as a master's degree health communication professional: Six key skills and characteristics. *Journal of Communication in Healthcare, 9*(3), 146–150. https://doi.org/10.1080/17538068.2016.1239343

Russo, F. (2016). What is the CSR's focus in healthcare? *Journal of Business Ethics, 134*, 323–334. https://doi.org/10.1007/s10551-014-2430-2

Saltman, R. B. (2018). The impact of slow economic growth on health sector reform: A cross-national perspective. *Policy and Law, 13*(3/4), 382–405. https://doi.org/10.1017/S1744133117000445

Samushonga, H. M. (2021). Insights into research based management decision-making in healthcare: Revealing the risk of professional isolation for mobile-working community nurses. *International Journal of Healthcare Management, 14*(3), 906–913. https://doi.org/10.1080/20479700.2020.1719462

Sariyar, M. (2012). Justification of ethical considerations in health economics–Merging the theories of Niklas Luhmann and Charles Taylor. *Health Sociology Review, 21*(3), 343–354. https://doi.org/10.5172/hesr.2012.21.3.343

Sawyer, N. (2018). In the U.S. healthcare is now strictly a business term. *Western Journal of Emergency Medicine, 19*(3), 494–495. https://doi.org/10.5811/westjem.2018.1.37540

Sheard, S. (2018). History matters: The critical contribution of historical analysis to contemporary health policy and health care. *Health Care Analysis, 2018*(26), 140–154. https://doi.org/10.1007/s10728-017-0348-4

Speer, M., McCullough, K. M., Fielding, J. E., Faustino, E., & Teutsch, S. M. (2020). Excess medical care spending: The categories, magnitude, and opportunity costs of wasteful spending in the United States. *American Journal of Public Health, 110*(12), 1743–1748. https://doi.org/10.2105/AJPH.2020.305865

Stefl, M. (2008). Common competencies for all healthcare managers: The Healthcare Leadership Alliance model. *Journal of Healthcare Management, 53*(6), 360–374. PMID: 19070332.

Streckeisen, P. (2021). Medicine and economic knowledge: The relevance of career in the study of transformations in the healthcare system. *Historical Social Research, 46*(1), 112–135. https://doi.org/10.12759/hsr.46.2021.1.112-135

Tasri, Y. D., & Tasri, E. S. (2020). Improving clinical records: Their role in decision-making and healthcare management–COVID-19 perspectives. *International Journal of Healthcare Management, 13*(4), 325–336. https://doi.org/10.1080/20479700.2020.1803623

Voytal, D., & Gelburd, M. (2019). *Medicare reimbursement falls short of care delivery costs.* https://www.mgma.com/data/data-stories/2019-medicare-reimbursement-rates

Walker, K. L., & Moran, N. (2019). Consumer information for data-driven decision making: Teaching socially responsible use of data. *Journal of Marketing Education, 41*(2), 109–126. https://doi.org/10.1177/0273475318813176

Walzer, S., Nuijten, M., Wiesner, C., Kaier, K., Johansson, P. O., & Oertel, S. (2013). Microeconomic surplus in health care: Applied economic theory in health care in four European countries. *Frontiers in Pharmacology, 4*, Article 17. https://doi.org/10.3389/fphar.2013.00017

Wendt, C., Frisina, L., & Rothgang, H. (2009). Healthcare system types: A conceptual framework for comparison. *Social Policy & Administration, 43*(1), 70–90. https://doi.org/10.1111/j.1467-9515.2008.00647.x

Whiteford, H., & Striegel-Weissman, R. (2017). Key factors that influence government policies and decision making about healthcare priorities: Lessons for the field of eating disorders. *International Journal of Eating Disorders, 2017*(50), 315–319. https://doi.org/10.1002/eat.22688

Wicks, A., & Keevil, A. (2014). When worlds collide: Medicine, business, the Affordable Care Act and the future of health care in the U.S. *Journal of Law, Medicine & Ethics, 42*(4), 420–430. https://doi.org/10.1111/jlme.12165

Wills, M. J. (2014). Decisions through data: Analytics in healthcare. *Journal of Healthcare Management, 59*(4), 254–262. https://doi.org/10.1097/00115514-201407000-00005

World Health Organization. (n.d.). *Health financing.* https://www.who.int/health-topics/health-financing#tab=tab_1

Yagudina, R. I., Kulikov, A. U., Serpik, V. G., & Ugrekhelidze, D. T. (2017). Concept of combining cost-effectiveness analysis and budget impact analysis in health care decision-making. *Value in Health Regional Issues, 13*(c), 61–66. https://doi.org/10.1016/j.vhri.2017.07.006

Younis, M., Barhem, B., Hamidi, S., Inungu, J., Prater, G., & Okeefe, A. (2009). The case for regulatory reform in the business and healthcare environments. *Journal of Health and Human Services Administration*, 32(3), 324–341. https://jhhsa.spaef.org/article/1075/The-Case-for-Regulatory-Reform-in-the-Business-and-Healthcare-Environments

Zhang, L., Chen, F., & Wei, W. (2020). A foundation course in business analytics: Design and implementation at two universities. *Journal of Information Systems Education*, 31(4), 244–259. http://jise.org/Volume31/n4/JISEv31n4p244.html

Zhou, S., Zhang, R., Chen, D., & Zhu, X. (2021). A novel framework for bringing smart big data to proactive decision making in healthcare. *Health Informatics Journal*, 27(2), 1–13. https://doi.org/10.1177/14604582211024698

CHAPTER 2

The Healthcare Sector, Supporting Industries, and System Organization

OBJECTIVES

1. Identify the social determinants of health as a focus for healthcare delivery.
2. Provide an overview of the healthcare sector and supporting industries.
3. Discuss the levels of care within the healthcare delivery framework.
4. Discuss the integrated healthcare delivery system and its potential benefits.
5. Discuss the "Triple Aim" of the healthcare sector and how the various participants support it.

INTRODUCTION

The provision of healthcare goods and services is no easy feat and requires the effort of organizations in many industries. There are patients from all walks of life needing care, and in most cases there are healthcare providers and partners with the necessary skills to meet their needs. Even though we typically associate healthcare with the clinician–patient interaction, healthcare delivery involves so much more. We have clinicians, product manufacturers, healthcare insurers, and specialists all working in unison to provide the necessary care to our population, and in many cases exploring ways to expand the healthcare services currently available. The size and impact of the healthcare sector has grown exponentially over time and is showing no signs of slowing down. As medical and technological advances continue to move healthcare service delivery forward, we must pay particular attention to ensuring access for all, providing the highest quality care, and containing costs where possible. Although these goals are feasible, in a sector with so many moving parts, this can be quite daunting. There are standards of care that must be maintained for all, as well as specialized treatments and personalized services for consumers' unique health situations. The various scenarios are a lot to manage, so let us have a look at the healthcare sector and its components to see how they make it work.

THE HEALTHCARE SECTOR

The healthcare sector is comprised of the various industries and markets that supply goods and services to the healthcare network in its entirety (Angerer et al., 2021; Gottlieb et al., 2019; Henke et al., 2018; LeBlanc, 2021; Williams et al., 2022). Organizations within the sector cover the full range of healthcare needs: clinical visits and medical treatment, medical supplies and medical equipment, human resources management and contractual clinical staffing, medical research, and product development. Each supporting industry has its own production process, regulations, governing legislation, performance measurement metrics, and financial management protocols to adhere to, while considering and including the practices that govern healthcare in its entirety. In efforts to meet the healthcare needs of a population, the healthcare sector must include the delivery of products and services as well as the financial mechanisms for payment and reimbursement. In a diverse population with varied healthcare needs, the available healthcare services as well as the relative payment and reimbursement mechanisms reflect a complex range of options and an even more complex list of frameworks to manage it all. The function of the healthcare sector depends on the collaboration of sector stakeholders, dedicated to providing the products, services, treatment, support services, and financial support for the patients and other healthcare consumers. The provision of healthcare services includes multiple levels and types of care, and healthcare is one of the highest expenditures in most developed nations' economies (Braithwaite et al., 2020; Braithwaite et al., 2017; Catlin & Cowan, 2015; Di Matteo, 2003; Lippi-Bruni et al., 2021). The U.S. health expenditure in 2021 was approximately 4.2 trillion, representing 19.7% of the gross domestic product (Abásolo et al., 2017; Centers for Medicare & Medicaid Services [CMS], 2021). A professional sector of this size takes a tremendous amount of coordination and requires the concerted efforts of all participants to manage it, no matter their service or product focus (Blewett & Osterholm, 2020; Heled et al., 2019; Juhnke et al., 2016). The

Figure 2.1

The healthcare sector

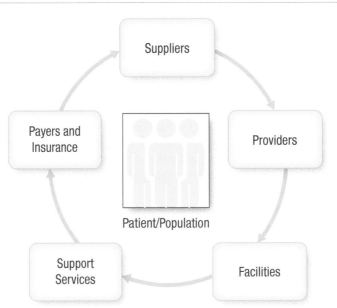

healthcare sector, as reflected in Figure 2.1, is comprised of a wide range of suppliers, providers, facilities, support services, and payers working together to provide the most effective and efficient healthcare services.

The system and its members share the common goal of addressing or supporting at least one of the patient population's **social determinants of health** (SDOH). SDOH include the nonmedical factors that impact a person's health and wellness outcomes. The main domains of SDOH are economic stability, education, healthcare, physical environment, and community (Agarwal et al., 2018; Capretta, 2016). Specifically, when it comes to healthcare, the system may provide additional options for access to quality healthcare (more providers or locations), health literacy (increased documentation or in-depth explanations), or possibly solutions to physical environment or community challenges (in-home medical equipment or mobile health screenings). In most cases, the provider is the initial point of contact for patients, with the type and acuity of illness determining the necessary medical treatment and required resources for care. The other components of the sector may be introduced at different phases of care, with each playing a distinct but very important role in the health and wellness process.

The Suppliers

The suppliers of healthcare goods cover a wide range of materials utilized in the delivery of healthcare. These items are used for both inpatient and outpatient services, spanning the entire spectrum of healthcare delivery. The flow of health information, as well as clinical interaction and treatment, are all impacted by the types of goods made available in the healthcare marketplace (Kreier, 2019; Machta et al., 2020). Medical products and medical equipment are included in this **healthcare supplier** industry, which help the clinicians and **healthcare providers** administer the proper medical care as needed. Medical product and equipment companies provide the tangible items needed for routine as well as specialized care. Bandages, syringes, gloves, and other medical office mainstays are just a few basic examples of items used during a standard office visit. These items are routinely purchased and stocked throughout the medical community, no matter the type of facility. Specialized supplies or equipment may be illness or injury specific, and the purchase and utilization of these items may vary depending on the type of provider and patient. For example, a patient with a broken bone or fracture may require crutches or specialized braces. A physical therapist may require a patient to use exercise bands or other equipment for strengthening. Surgical suppliers provide the necessary specialty items for surgical procedures, including surgical instruments (often referred to as trays) and implants, which are specific to the surgical discipline. A patient with mobility issues may require the use of a wheelchair. Inpatient facilities require a standard number of hospital beds (dependent upon licensure) as well as oxygen for patients requiring an overnight stay.

Medical device and technology companies supply instrumentation and machinery used in the diagnosis, treatment, and monitoring of patient illness and injury. These items are used by clinicians in the facilities as well as by patients during the course of their daily lives. These are more common than what many would believe and include items such as glucose monitors, pacemakers, hearing aids, and other wearable technology. Larger ticket items include implants, imaging machines, surgical robots, and information technology (IT) infrastructure, which are standard in most health systems today. All of these items provide the means for healthcare professionals to assess the patient's health condition and provide the necessary care and treatment.

Durable medical equipment (DME) is most associated with home healthcare services, as it often aids with care and treatment outside of the standard medical facility. Prosthetics, wound care products, hospital beds, walkers, and portable oxygen systems are all classified as DME and are designed for the comfort and stability of the patient. Although provided for use outside of the medical facility, these items still require an official provider's order for distribution. Some of these items will be specific or customized for a single patient (prosthetics, portable oxygen), while other items are loaned or leased based on diagnosis and need (hospital beds).

Pharmaceutical companies supply the drugs and medications that clinicians use to aid in treatment of illness and disease. These are used for standard maintenance and routine treatment of a patient's illness as well as newly diagnosed shorter-term conditions. Research and development make continuous improvement possible, as pharmaceutical companies create newer, better versions of items currently in use. Replacements of existing products improves effectiveness, efficiency, or both in terms of patient treatment and outcomes. A basic example is antibiotic treatment—the original version of the medication was designed for 7 days of treatments and outcomes. The improved version of the antibiotic replaced the original version and decreased treatment days to just 3 days. The replacement was proven to be as effective, but more efficient with the reduced treatment time.

The Providers

Providers of healthcare include a wide spectrum of professionals who provide mental, physical, and emotional care to those in need of healthcare services. Healthcare services can be rendered in an inpatient setting, an outpatient setting, or virtually via telemedicine. Providers in the inpatient setting provide services to patients during an overnight stay (hospital, rehabilitation center, long-term care [LTC] facility, etc.). The outpatient setting does not include any overnight stays, and all services are rendered during the same 24-hour period. Telemedicine allows providers to use various types of technology to deliver care from a distance. Healthcare providers come from a variety of disciplines and typically cover a specific type of healthcare need. They may work independently to care for the patient or operate as a team to provide a wider range of treatment.

Primary care physicians (PCPs) are often the first point of contact for the patient, and often see the patient before referral to a specialist or supporting healthcare service such as imaging. PCPs address the more common health issues and are often the gatekeepers of their specific specialization. Internal medicine physicians, pediatricians, licensed nurse practitioners, physician assistants, dentists, and optometrists are all examples of clinicians serving as the first point of contact during the medical visit. Depending on health insurance coverage, the PCP visit may be required before additional referrals or healthcare services are approved.

Specialists step in after the patient receives a referral from their PCP. This category of clinical professional addresses the specific health concerns identified by the PCP. Examples of those in this clinical category are cardiologists, dermatologists, gastroenterologists, orthodontists, and so forth, or any clinical professional providing specialized diagnosis and treatment. Although this care is specialized and requires specified processes, procedures, and treatments, the same suppliers are used for equipment and medication as those used by PCPs. Care by the various specialists and PCPs can in fact run simultaneously depending on the individual medical needs of the patient.

The Facilities

Our healthcare facilities are where the actual healthcare services are performed or organized (in the case of home healthcare). Patients with a variety of health needs and concerns rely on our facilities for inpatient, outpatient, and emergent healthcare services, and in some cases multiple facilities are required.

Hospital and inpatient facilities provide care in an overnight setting. An inpatient stay may be required for a specific illness, recovery following a surgical procedure, or for patient observation. Inpatient facilities usually have a full regimen of patient care services which include imaging, pharmacy, and rehabilitation, all geared to the discharge and continued recovery of the patient. Emergency departments (EDs) are usually attached to inpatient facilities and provide care in critical and crisis situations. Hospitals can be public, private, or community nonprofits or religion based, but all still have the important purpose of providing healthcare services for the communities they serve.

Ambulatory surgery centers and outpatient clinics (including urgent care centers) provide care for patients where inpatient stays are not needed. These facilities perform minor, minimally invasive surgical procedures, leaving patients to recover at home. Outpatient clinics see patients with nonemergent healthcare concerns that may be treated with standard care or standard protocol. The purpose of outpatient clinics is to help minimize the number of nonemergent patients visiting a hospital's ED by treating these patients at a separate facility. The availability of outpatient clinics in a community can improve hospital ED wait times and utilization of resources in the ED.

Private practice and medical offices are usually the place of care provided by our PCPs. This care may include physician extenders such as physician assistants or nurse practitioners, who are also licensed healthcare providers. Depending on a state's licensure and medical practice laws, nurse practitioners and physician assistants may practice independently without the supervision of a medical doctor. The private practice or medical office is the place for the basic wellness visit and consultation before seeing a specialist or seeking additional medical services.

Laboratory and diagnostic centers provide services that use technology to look inside the body. These services are usually performed at the request of the PCP or specialist, and assist with further diagnosis and treatment. Imaging can serve both screening and diagnostic purposes in attempts to detect illness or injuries early (preventive medicine) or to identify the cause or confirm a diagnosis or condition (diagnostic).

LTC and skilled nursing facilities (SNF) provide medical care for patients discharged from hospitals or other healthcare facilities who cannot care for themselves, such as older adults or those who are disabled (Grit & Zuiderent-Jerak, 2017; Schuurmans et al., 2021). Patients in these settings are considered inpatient or residential patients, relying on the LTC or SNF for the provision of all healthcare and daily living needs. Care in these facilities is an extended care scenario, not shorter-term or emergent care provided at the hospital (treated and then discharged).

Support Services

There are many support services that help keep routine healthcare operations on track. Ambulances and medical transport services provide a critical service to those in emergency situations as well as those who may be immobile. Independent claims processing and billing services help healthcare providers and facilities submit medical claims accurately and in a timely fashion, meeting the various requirements of the insurers and payers. Recruiting and staffing agencies help by supplying the system with temporary or contractual resources to help meet increased demand (Fulton, 2017; Gaynor et al., 2017). Although these services are not the primary source of care for patients, they make it possible for providers and other front-line services to operate.

The Payers and Insurers

Due to the price of healthcare services today, many rely on health insurance for funding of their healthcare. The financing of healthcare services can be accomplished in several ways and is dependent on the established national framework of the sector. The models we see in place today are predominantly: (a) the national health insurance model, (b) the national health system model, (c) the socialized health insurance model, and (d) the free-market system. In the United States, the free-market system includes a multitude of payers and insurers, many of which cover specific populations. Government payers, private insurers, and employment-related insurers are all options we see in the United States, each having different processes and reimbursement guidelines (covered in detail in Chapter 7).

HEALTHCARE TRIPLE AIM

As previously noted, the healthcare sector participants share the common focus of satisfying some facet of patient care, either directly or indirectly. Ideally, we want this care to be top-notch, and that means paying close attention to the other factors that ultimately impact patient care, even if not at the forefront of the patient visit. The Institute for Healthcare Improvement (IHI) has coined the concept of the "**Triple Aim,**" which frames healthcare organizations' efforts in providing the best healthcare possible (IHI, n.d.). The three focal points of the Triple Aim are: (a) to improve population health, (b) to improve the patient experience, and (c) to improve (reduce) the cost of healthcare. For the first aim of improving population health, the healthcare sector addresses the underlying causes of illness as well as the management of chronic conditions that impact society the most (Centers for Disease Control and Prevention [CDC], n.d.; Chen & Escarce, 2004; Galea & Vaughan, 2021; Puglisi & Shavit, 2020; Ridgley et al., 2020; Shahzad et al., 2019). Environmental factors such as neighborhood and household dynamics, employment status, and income are examples of underlying causes that impact healthcare, although not directly associated with the medical visit or clinical interaction. Population health also includes the management of chronic illnesses (such as hypertension, diabetes, and heart disease) by implementing strategies for prevention, early detection, and mitigation, as well as ongoing treatment for illnesses requiring longer-term management. There are quite a few items that impact population health that are not related to medical diagnosis, including access to healthcare services, health education and health literacy, and cultural barriers. These must also be addressed in some way, as they impact population health by influencing if and how a patient seeks healthcare services. The second aim, improve the patient experience, focuses on the quality of patient interactions with healthcare providers. This includes the medical office visit as well as the communication and information shared during the visit. The overall patient experience includes customer service and interactions with the provider, supporting services, insurance companies, and so forth, as they all contribute to the comfort and care of the patient being seen. The cost of healthcare, as addressed by the third aim, examines ways to reduce the overall cost of healthcare goods and services. There are many contributing factors to the cost of care, such as human resource expenses, material resource expenses, healthcare product research and development, and other items such as service availability and location. All three of the Triple Aim focal points influence the healthcare sector and how it approaches healthcare service delivery, with each aim having an impact on the others. The patient is the focus of the sector, with all three of the aims directly impacting the patient and the care received. Achieving the Triple Aim requires that providers, suppliers, and other stakeholders collaborate in some way to address society's population health needs, patient experience requirements, and cost of care concerns, forming the contemporary healthcare delivery system we see and utilize today.

WHAT IS A HEALTHCARE DELIVERY SYSTEM?

A **healthcare delivery system** is an organized stand-alone network of healthcare organizations providing all-inclusive care to a specific patient population. The World Health Organization (WHO) defines a health delivery system as "the organization of people, institutions, and resources that deliver health care services to meet the health needs of target populations" (Piña et al., 2015, p. 671). The interdependent network of suppliers, providers, and facilities work together to satisfy all the health needs of the population they serve. Systems can be small or large and can operate independently or collaboratively with another health system. Health systems are represented in a myriad of forms and structures, but all serve the same purpose of optimal patient care, as well as efficient and effective system operations. Figure 2.2 shows the functionality of a typical healthcare delivery system, which begins with system inputs (human and materials resources) and ends with the achievement of the desired outcomes (health outcomes or goals established through strategic planning).

The system may consist of organizations bound by ownership, contract, or referral, and may be arranged by level of care or by type of integration (horizontal or vertical). The health system, although all-inclusive, may be designed to address the needs of a specific community or group within that population (Botts et al., 2017; Cimasi, 2013; Dorrance & Phillips, 2018; Kaplan & Porter, 2011). An example of this specialist care is the "center of excellence." Some health systems have created centers of excellence to focus on the diagnosis and treatment of specific conditions, while the rest of the health system serves patients with other health needs. This includes efforts to impact determinants of health as well as more direct health-improving activities. Specialists usually step in to help with specific types of care or services, and facilities also cater to the needs of those with certain illnesses. Examples include assisted living complexes with memory care services and LTC/nursing home amenities. All healthcare needs for these populations typically take place onsite. There are scheduled physician's visits, mobile pharmacist and imaging services, and established transport for those that need to seek care at specific healthcare facilities (with larger machinery and equipment with no mobile service components). Every healthcare delivery system includes the inputs, outputs, and resources needed to provide healthcare services and ultimately achieve the organization's healthcare-related mission and objectives. Supplies and equipment, human and financial resources, and clinical care are the basic elements of care delivery and are present in some form in the healthcare delivery system. These items can be provided by the primary stakeholders within the system or contractually provided by those outside of the system.

Figure 2.2

Healthcare delivery system functionality

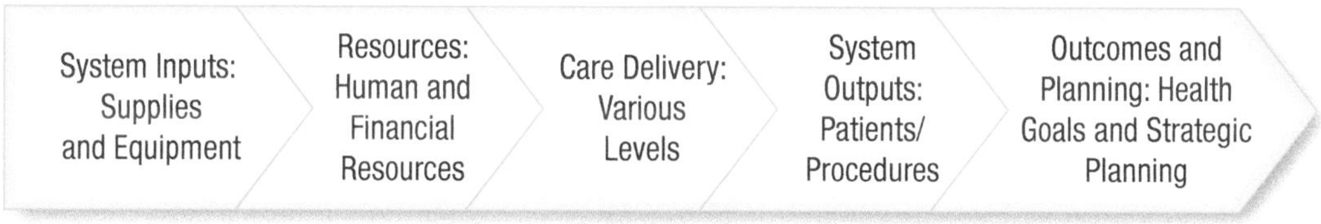

System Inputs: Supplies and Equipment → Resources: Human and Financial Resources → Care Delivery: Various Levels → System Outputs: Patients/Procedures → Outcomes and Planning: Health Goals and Strategic Planning

Levels of Care

Levels of care represent the grouping of providers and facilities organized by their typical occurrence in the healthcare process. The grouping falls into the categories of primary, secondary, or tertiary care providers. **Primary care** providers are usually the patient's first encounter or interaction for healthcare services, in an office or nonemergent setting. This initial visit allows the primary care provider to assess the patient's condition and determine if additional services may be needed. Clinicians in the primary care category are usually generalists—the gatekeepers for entry into the healthcare system. Referrals may then be given for the patient to receive specialist care and assessment, imaging, laboratory work, and so forth. **Secondary care** is provided for more serious health conditions requiring hospitalization or minor surgery. This level of care goes beyond the basic office consultation and may include ED care, outpatient surgery, or inpatient medical care. **Tertiary care** is provided by the specialists of the sector, whose focus is one specific area or type of care. Depending on the health condition, specialists may step into the primary role if specialized care is needed routinely for a period of time, even if outside of the level of care categories defined in Figure 2.3. An example of this would be an obstetrician serving as the primary care provider for an expectant mother. Under normal conditions, a general practitioner would perform the primary care role, but in the case of an expectant mother, the specialized skills of the obstetrician are needed to ensure the health of the mother and baby.

Integrated Healthcare Delivery Systems

An **integrated healthcare delivery system** is a consolidated system comprised of multiple healthcare providers and/or suppliers. The system is arranged to either meet a series of

Figure 2.3

Levels of care

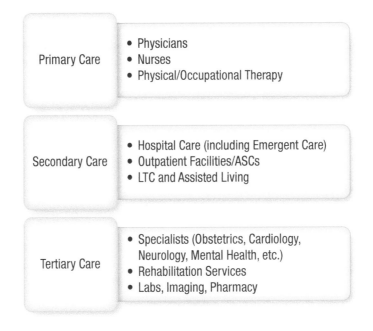

ASC, ambulatory surgery center; LTC, long-term care.

healthcare needs or to resolve access and resource issues and is organized as vertical or horizontal integration (Lintz, 2021; McCarthy & Shenghsiu-Huang, 2018; Mendoza, 2017; Owsley et al., 2020). The integrated healthcare delivery system encompasses all the various segments' roles and responsibilities to provide the best possible care for those that seek it. Care is delivered in defined settings such as homes, educational institutions, workplaces, public places, communities, hospitals, and clinics (American Medical Association [AMA], 2022; Athena Health, n.d.; Ewald & Golden, 2021). **Vertical integration** is the ownership of organizations that perform various functions at various levels within the healthcare delivery system. A very common example of this is a larger hospital buying community-based PCP practices, specialist practices, imaging facilities, and local suppliers. Essentially, the vertically integrated system has ownership of the patient's entire spectrum of care from beginning to end. The potential benefits to this approach to healthcare delivery are easy access to electronic health records, reduced contracting and outsourcing, and all-inclusive healthcare for the patient (Athena Health, n.d.; Cimasi, 2013). The vertically integrated system is self-contained and, when optimized, has the potential to improve the patient experience and reduce wait times and delays associated with processes involving internal and external entities. **Horizontal integration** is the ownership of healthcare organizations that perform the same services within the healthcare system. An example of this would be a larger nursing home chain buying smaller community-based nursing homes, or the creation of a multi-hospital system (Furukawa et al., 2020; Gaynor, 2015; Hamer & Mays, 2020). The horizontally integrated system is designed to expand current capacity and resources of the services being offered. The potential benefits to this approach to healthcare delivery are improved cost efficiency, increased productivity, and the consolidation or maximization of resources (Cutler & Scott-Morton, 2013; Hatfield et al., 2018; Lipworth et al., 2020). Depending on size and complexity, both vertical and horizontal integration, as noted in Figure 2.4, can exist within the same healthcare system. This is quite common in larger health systems striving to maximize the efficiency of clinical care (using electronic health records to coordinate all levels of care), as well

Figure 2.4

Vertical and horizontal integration

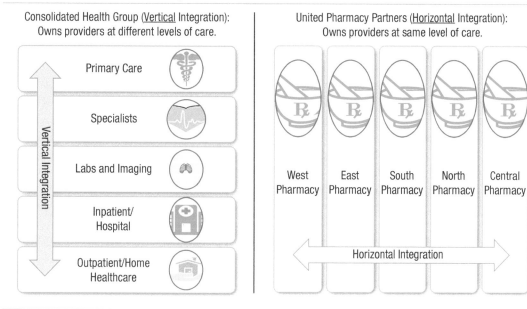

Consolidated Health Group (Vertical Integration): Owns providers at different levels of care.

United Pharmacy Partners (Horizontal Integration): Owns providers at same level of care.

as health systems with an academic component (teaching hospitals or neighborhood clinics used for medical residencies).

No matter the type of integration, healthcare delivery systems have the same goal of improving the health outcomes of the population they serve (Guo et al., 2016; Ramos et al., 2020). While providing high-quality care and an improved patient experience, organizations within the system play an important role in maintaining the system's overall effectiveness and efficiency. One such healthcare system that many refer to as the model for integration is the Kaiser Permanente System. This system reflects an all-inclusive vertically integrated health system with all of the major services provided within its network, essentially eliminating referrals to external providers (Pines et al., 2015). This eliminates lost time due to outside scheduling, eliminates duplicative services such as testing, and creates a more complete medical history and care for their patients. Healthcare visits, pharmacy services, and equipment and supplies are all provided within the network. Other integrated systems also strive to maintain a high level of efficiency, although services may not be provided by the same organization.

Assessing the performance of a health system requires the analysis of both patient-centered and nonpatient-centered practices. Ideally, all members of the system will share a common mission, goals, and objectives, with each member contributing to initiatives that help achieve the desired system outcomes. These guiding elements should be communicated throughout strategic planning and other leadership processes to ensure stakeholder buy-in and the proper trajectory of the organization. The system should be cohesive and balance the needs of the community served, improving overall health, providing quality care, and effectively utilizing resources. Sound health systems strive for increased patient satisfaction as well as support for each of its members working together to offer services at a level unattainable individually. While the operating practices within each organization may differ, the concept of Triple Aim-based performance measurements can be applied to all types of healthcare providers—individuals, group practices, and horizontally or vertically integrated systems. Routine metric measurement and performance management promote effective and efficient health system operations.

CHAPTER SUMMARY

This chapter provided an overview of the healthcare sector and the major components that comprise it. We continue to make improvements to our sector as well as how we provide healthcare services. In the short term, we must continue to provide the highest quality healthcare to consumers, meeting and even anticipating future health needs. In the long term, we must continue to explore ways to provide the necessary services as effectively and as efficiently as possible. Providers of every type play a part in care delivery, with each being unique in process, technique, market served, and costs incurred. Each supporting industry has its own regulations and best practices, all of which impact healthcare service delivery in some form. Effective healthcare leadership manages these important relationships among sector participants using integrated structures and contracting agreements to ensure quality healthcare services. Healthcare does not happen in a silo! Health services organizations rely on one another to provide services that may be outside of their current scope, available resources, or professional expertise. This collaboration is our contemporary healthcare delivery system.

KEY TERMS FOR REVIEW

healthcare delivery
   system

healthcare providers

healthcare suppliers

horizontal integration

integrated healthcare
   delivery system

primary care

primary care physicians

secondary care

social determinants of
   health

tertiary care

Triple Aim

vertical integration

DISCUSSION QUESTIONS

1. What are the various levels of care in the healthcare sector?

2. Define "healthcare delivery system."

3. Identify the major supporting industries in the healthcare sector. How do these industries work together to provide healthcare services?

4. Discuss the types of integrated healthcare systems and the focus of each.

5. What are the benefits of the integrated healthcare system?

6. Discuss the key concepts from Chapter 1 (The Business of Healthcare) and how the elements of business may impact healthcare delivery when applied to the healthcare sector's supporting industries.

7. What is the "Triple Aim"? How might the Triple Aim impact the various stakeholders within the healthcare sector and supporting industries?

CHAPTER 2 CASE: RIGHT-SIZING THE NETWORK

Your three-hospital health system has expanded rapidly over the last few years as patient healthcare needs have grown. The pandemic and associated illnesses have increased demand for even the most basic of healthcare services, exposing areas and locations with limited access to care. To help these low-access areas, you have opened three additional clinics, bringing the number of clinics in your network to five. You have also acquired three small medical groups, all of which were struggling financially due to the quarantine. One medical group offers specialty cardiac care, a second medical group offers respiratory care, and the third medical group provides traditional primary care services. The three groups add an additional 30 physicians and specialists to your network. During the course of the pandemic, federal and state healthcare agencies provided relief funding, so revenue covering specialty medical care, increased clinical staffing, and medical supplies was not an issue. The height of the pandemic has since subsided, as most medical systems have now moved to maintenance or endemic procedures. As you assess your health system's current performance, you uncover a few operating trends that may need to be addressed.

The primary payers for the recently added clinics and medical groups are Medicare and Medicaid, which offer significantly lower reimbursement than commercial or private insurers. Decreased demand has made these limited reimbursement amounts even more troubling. Financial results for the last quarter show a loss of $5 million, the first loss ever recorded for your health system. Some clinics and medical groups are still operating with full staff, even though patient visits in their area have drastically reduced. When asked to explain their location's performance, clinic and group leadership appeared to operate as if stand-alone instead of as an integral part of a larger system. All the aforementioned issues contribute to a highly inefficient and ineffective health system. In efforts to mitigate further financial losses and negative operational impacts, you have determined that now is the time to review the system's structure, and possibly right-size your network.

1. Assess the system's structure and performance in the context of the Triple Aim (high-level assessment).

2. When it comes to financial losses, what could be the drivers of the loss?

3. How might the trends noted in the case impact patients or the community being served?

4. How would you first address the leadership team to discuss the system's performance?

5. What are examples of items to assess when reviewing the performance of the clinics and medical groups?

6. How would you address the lack of cohesiveness among the clinic and medical group leadership?

7. What are some immediate changes that could be implemented to directly impact the system's financial position?

REFERENCES

Abásolo, I., Saez, M., & López-Casasnovas, G. (2017). Financial crisis and income related inequalities in the universal provision of public services: The case of healthcare in Spain. *International Journal of Equity in Health*, *16*, Article 134. https://doi.org/10.1186/s12939-017-0630-y

Agarwal, N., Chakrabarti, R., Brem, A., & Bocken, N. (2018). Market driving at bottom of the pyramid: An analysis of social enterprises from the healthcare sector. *Journal of Business Research*, *86*(2016), 234–244. https://doi.org/10.1016/j.jbusres.2017.07.001

American Medical Association. (2022). *Competition in health insurance: A comprehensive study of U.S. markets: 2022 update*. Author. https://www.ama-assn.org/system/files/competition-health-insurance-us-markets.pdf.

Angerer, S., Glatzle-Rutzler, D., & Waibel, C. (2021). Monitoring institutions in healthcare markets: Experimental evidence. *Health Economics*, *30*(5), 951–971. https://doi.org/10.1002/hec.4232

Athena Health. (n.d.). *ACO models: An overview*. http://www.athenahealth.com/knowledge-hub/aco/model

Blewett, L. A., & Osterholm, M. T. (2020). What's next for the U.S. health care system after COVID-19? *American Journal of Public Health*, *110*(9), 1365–1366. https://doi.org/10.2105/AJPH.2020.305836

Botts, S. R., Gee, M. T., Chang, C. C., Young, I., Saito, L., & Lymnan, A. E. (2017). Design and implementation of population-based specialty care programs. *American Journal of Health-System Pharmacy*, *74*(18), 1437–1445. https://doi.org/10.2146/ajhp161016

Braithwaite, J., Tran, Y., Ellis, L. A., & Westbrook, J. (2020). Inside the black box of comparative national healthcare performance in 35 OECD countries: Issues of culture, systems performance and sustainability. *Plos One*, *15*(9), Article e0239776. https://doi.org/10.1371/journal.pone.0239776

Braithwaite, J., Hibbert, P., Blakely, B., Plumb, J., Hannaford, N., Cameron Long, J., & Marks, D. (2017). Health system frameworks and performance indicators in eight countries: A comparative international analysis. *Sage Open Medicine*, 5, Article 2050312116686516. https://doi.org/10.1177/2050312116686516

Capretta, J. C. (2016). Healthcare reform. *The Linacre Quarterly*, 83(4), 375–381. https://doi.org/10.1080/00243639.2016.1247620

Catlin, A. C., & Cowan, C. A. (2015, November 19). *History of health spending in the United States, 1960–2013.* https://www.cms.gov/Research-Statistics-Data-and-Systems/Statistics-Trends-and-Reports/NationalHealthExpendData/Downloads/HistoricalNHEPaper.pdf

Centers for Disease Control and Prevention. (n.d.). *Comorbidities.* U.S. Department of Health and Human Services. https://www.cdc.gov/arthritis/data_statistics/comorbidities.htm

Centers for Medicare & Medicaid Services. (2021). *National health expenditure data: NHE summary including share of GDP. Author.* https://www.cms.gov/research-statistics-data-and-systems/statistics-trends-and-reports/nationalhealthexpenddata/nationalhealthaccountshistorical

Chen, A. Y., & Escarce, J. J. (2004). Quantifying income-related inequality in healthcare delivery in the United States. *Medical Care*, 42(1), 38–47. https://doi.org/10.1097/01.mlr.0000103526.13935.b5

Cimasi, R. J. (2013). *Accountable care organizations, value metrics and capital formation.* CRC Press/Taylor and Francis Group.

Cutler, D. M., & Scott-Morton, F. (2013). Hospitals, market share and consolidation. *Clinical Review & Education*, 310(18), 1964–1970. https://doi.org/10.1001/jama.2013.281675

Di Matteo, L. (2003). The income elasticity of health care spending: A comparison of parametric and nonparametric approaches. *The European Journal of Health Economics*, 4(1), 20–29. https://doi.org/10.1007/s10198-002-0141-6

Dorrance, K. A., & Phillips, A. A. (2018). Toward a national conversation on health: The transformative power of deregulated markets and market-driven innovation. *Military Medicine*, 183(11/12), 239–243. https://doi.org/10.1093/milmed/usy217

Ewald, B., & Golden, R. (2021). The role of care management in a changing healthcare system. *Generations Journal*, 45(1), 1–10. https://generations.asaging.org/care-management-changing-healthcare-system

Fulton, B. D. (2017). Healthcare market concentration trends in the United States: Evidence and policy responses. *Health Affairs*, 36(9), 1530–1538. https://doi.org/10.1377/hlthaff.2017.0556

Furukawa, M. F., Machta, R. M., Barrett, K. A., Jones, D. J., Shortell, S. M., Scanlon, D. P., Lewis, V. A., O'Malley, A. J., Meara, E. R., & Rich, E. C. (2020). Landscape of health systems in the United States. *Medical Care Research and Review*, 77(4), 357–366. https://doi.org/10.1177/1077558718823130

Galea, S., & Vaughan, R. (2021). Embedding prevention at the heart of the U.S. health conversation. *American Journal of Public Health*, 111(1), 17–19. https://doi.org/10.2105/AJPH.2020.306009

Gaynor, M. (2015). Efficient efficiencies analysis: False dichotomies, modeling, and applications to health care. *The Antitrust Bulletin*, 60(3), 268–273. https://doi.org/10.1177/0003603X15598592

Gaynor, M., Mostashari, F., & Ginsburg, P. (2017, April). *Making healthcare markets work: Competition policy for health care.* Brookings Institution. https://www.brookings.edu/wp-content/uploads/2017/04/gaynor-et-al-final-report-v11.pdf

Gottlieb, L., Fichtenberg, C., Alderwick, H., & Adler, N. (2019). Social determinants of health: What's a healthcare system to do? *Journal of Healthcare Management*, 64(4), 243–257. https://doi.org/10.1097/JHM-D-19-00105

Grit, K., & Zuiderent-Jerak, T. (2017). Making markets in long-term care: Or how a market can work by being invisible. *Health Care Analysis*, 2017(25), 242–259. https://doi.org/10.1007/s10728-015-0292-0

Guo, R., Berkshire, S. D., Fulton, L. V., & Hermanson, P. M. (2016). Use of evidence-based management in healthcare administration decision-making. *Leadership in Health Services*, 30(3), 330–342. https://doi.org/10.1108/LHS-07-2016-0033

Hamer, M. K., & Mays, G. P. (2020). Public health systems and social services: Breadth and depth of cross-sector collaboration. *American Journal of Public Health*, 110(52), 232–234. https://doi.org/10.2105/AJPH.2020.305694

Hatfield, L. A., Favreault, M. M., McGuire, T. G., & Chernew, M. E. (2018). Modeling health care spending growth of older adults. *Health Services Research*, 53(1), 138–155. https://doi.org/10.1111/1475-6773.12640

Heled, Y., Vertinsky, L., & Brewer, C. (2019). Why healthcare companies should become benefit corporations. *Boston College Law Review*, 60(73), 74–144. https://dashboard.lira.bc.edu/downloads/667a44fa-c263-449a-871b-55b96eab6e66

Henke, R. M., Karaca, Z., Moore, B., Cutler, E., Liu, H., Marder, W. D., & Wong, H. S. (2018). Impact of health system affiliation on hospital resource use intensity and quality of care. *Health Services Research, 53*(1), 63–86. https://doi.org/10.1111/1475-6773.12631

Institute for Healthcare Improvement. (n.d.). *IHI Triple Aim initiative.* Institute for Healthcare Improvement. http://www.ihi.org/engage/initiatives/TripleAim/Pages/default.aspx

Juhnke, C., Bethge, S., & Muhlbacher, A. (2016). A review on methods of risk adjustment and their use in integrated healthcare systems. *International Journal of Integrated Care, 16*(4), 1–18. https://doi.org/10.5334/ijic.2500

Kaplan, R. S., & Porter, M. E. (2011). How to solve the cost crisis in health care. *Harvard Business Review, 2011,* 1–18. https://hbr.org/2011/09/how-to-solve-the-cost-crisis-in-health-care

Kreier, R. (2019). Moral hazard: It's the supply side, stupid! *World Affairs, 2019,* 205–223. https://doi.org/10.1177/0043820019841436

LeBlanc, T. T. (2021). Strengthening social and economic, medical, and public health systems before disasters strike. *American Journal of Public Health, 111*(5), 842–843. https://doi.org/10.2105/AJPH.2021.306247

Lintz, J. (2021). Adoption of computerized information management systems (cims) functions: Urban versus rural primary healthcare providers. *International Journal of Healthcare Management, 14*(4), 1237–1245. https://doi.org/10.1080/20479700.2020.1756109

Lippi-Bruni, M., Ugolini, C., & Verzulli, R. (2021). Should I wait or should I go? Travelling versus waiting for better healthcare. *Regional Science and Urban Economics, 89,* Article 103697. https://doi.org/10.1016/j.regsciurbeco.2021.103697

Lipworth, W., Kerridge, I., Montgomery, K., & Komesaroff, P. A. (2020). Promoting ethics across the healthcare sector: What can codes achieve? *Internal Medicine Journal, 50*(11), 1333–1338. https://doi.org/10.1111/imj.15051

Machta, R. M., Reschovsky, J. D., Jones, D. J., Kimmey, L., Furukawa, M. F., & Rich, E. C. (2020). Health system integration with physician specialties varies across markets and system types. *Health Services Research, 55*(3), 1062–1072. https://doi.org/10.1111/1475-6773.13584

McCarthy, I., & Shenghsiu-Huang, S. (2018). Vertical alignment between hospitals and physicians as a bargaining response to commercial insurance markets. *Review of Industrial Organization, 2018*(53), 7–29. https://doi.org/10.1007/s11151-017-9609-5

Mendoza, R. L. (2017). Information asymmetries and risk management in healthcare markets: The U.S. Affordable Care Act in retrospect. *Journal of Economic Issues, 51*(2), 520–540. https://doi.org/10.1080/00213624.2017.1321451

Owsley, K. M., Hamer, M. K., & Mays, G. P. (2020). The growing divide in the composition of public health delivery systems in the US rural and urban communities, 2014–2018. *American Journal of Public Health, 110*(52), 204–210. https://doi.org/10.2105/AJPH.2020.305801

Piña, I. L., Cohen, P. D., Larson, D. B., Marion, L. N., Sills, M. R., Solberg, L. I., & Zerzan, J. (2015). A framework for describing health care delivery organizations and systems. *American Journal of Public Health, 105*(4), 670–679. https://doi.org/10.2105/AJPH.2014.301926

Pines, J., Selevan, J., McStay, F., George, M., & McClellan, M. (2015, May 4). *Kaiser Permanente—California: A model for integrated care for the ill and injured.* Center for Health Policy at Brookings. https://www.brookings.edu/wp-content/uploads/2016/07/KaiserFormatted_150504RH-with-image.pdf

Puglisi, L. B., & Shavit, S. (2020). Health disparities of people living in the community on probation: A call to action for community and public health systems. *American Journal of Public Health, 110*(9), 1262–1263. https://doi.org/10.2105/AJPH.2020.305832

Ramos, M., Bowen, S., Wright, P. C., Gomes Ferreira, M. G., & Forcellini, F. A. (2020). Experience based co-design in healthcare services: An analysis of projects, barriers and enablers. *Design for Health, 4*(3), 276–295. https://doi.org/10.1080/24735132.2020.1837508

Ridgley, M. S., Ahluwalia, S. C., Tom, A., Vaiana, M., Motala, A., Silverman, M., Kim, A., Damberg, C. L., & Shekelle, P. G. (2020). What are the determinants of health system performance? Findings from the literature and a technical expert panel. *The Joint Commission Journal on Quality and Patient Safety, 46*(2), 87–98. https://doi.org/10.1016/j.jcjq.2019.11.003

Schuurmans, J. J., van Pijkeren, N., Bal, R., & Wallenburg, I. (2021). Regionalization in elderly care: What makes up a healthcare region? *Journal of Health Organization and Management*, *35*(2), 229–243. https://doi.org/10.1108/JHOM-08-2020-0333

Shahzad, M., Upshur, R., Donnelly, P., Bharmal, A., Wei, X., Feng, P., & Brown, A. D. (2019). A population-based approach to integrated healthcare delivery: A scoping review of clinical care and public health collaboration. *BMC Public Health*, *19*, Article 708. https://doi.org/10.1186/s12889-019-7002-z

Williams, S. P., Purkayastha, S., Charurvedi, S., & Darzi, A. (2022). Organizational health and independent sector health organizations. *International Journal of Healthcare Management*, *15*(3), 196–203. https://doi.org/10.1080/20479700.2020.1870352

World Health Organization. (2022). *Thirteenth general programme of work 2019–2023*. https://www.who.int/about/what-we-do/thirteenth-general-programme-of-work-2019---2023

CHAPTER 3

Finance Department Structure, Function, and Roles

OBJECTIVES

1. Define the healthcare finance function and how it fits into the healthcare organization.
2. Identify the traditional finance department structure.
3. Discuss the various roles and responsibilities within the finance department structure.
4. Identify regulatory bodies and entities that impact the finance department and related operations.
5. Discuss how nonfinancial activities can impact the roles and responsibilities of the finance department.

INTRODUCTION

No matter the industry, there always needs to be someone watching the money! The healthcare sector is large, and watching the money here is a major responsibility. The finance department is an integral part of healthcare operations and is tied to most functions throughout the organization. Patient care, human and material resource management, reimbursement, and guest services are all tied in some way to the organization's underlying financial structure. Documentation and timing are critical to finance department responsibilities, with dedicated processes established to ensure efficiency throughout routine operations. Financial activities are divided or assigned within the department according to numerous functional units, each having specific schedules and software to assist with tasks. This chapter discusses the finance department and its key responsibilities within the typical healthcare services organization.

THE FINANCE FUNCTION

The financial function of any organization plays a significant role in the overall health and viability of that organization. Routine operations as well as future planning are focal points of the finance operation, which impacts every department and service provided in healthcare service organizations. Proper utilization of resources and sound financial planning are what organizations rely on for efficiency, with financial management central to that purpose. **Finance** as a discipline involves the control and maximization of organizational resources in efforts to achieve established goals and objectives (Menaker et al., 2020; Pina et al., 2015; Ramos-Hegwer, 2017). This involves the assessment and evaluation of financial condition, capacity, viability, stewardship, and the identification of organizational challenges as relevant to the value proposition for both internal and external stakeholders. **Financial management** is defined as the combination of accounting and finance information for decision-making purposes in achieving the organization's goals and objectives (Arduino, 2018; Bastani et al., 2016). Decision-making relative to this function includes organizing, directing, controlling, and planning for the overall optimal performance of the organization (Escobar-Perez et al., 2016; Stewart et al., 2019; Widmer, 2016). **Healthcare financial management** is the application of these financial management practices to the healthcare sector. Some of the micro-level steps may differ due to the uniqueness of healthcare, but the macro-level steps are still applicable. The concept of **value creation** becomes a primary objective of financial management, as organizations ultimately strive for both effectiveness and efficiency of operations. The process of value creation is the creation or development of a good or service that meets the needs of consumers. This could be the expansion of a healthcare network, or the implementation of electronic medical records systems and online patient access portals. Value creation in healthcare benefits both the provider and consumer of healthcare services, meaning it concerns the delivery of the best possible healthcare service and doing so as efficiently as possible (Birch et al., 2015; Lee, 2019).

THE FINANCE DEPARTMENT STRUCTURE AND RESPONSIBILITIES

The overall structure of healthcare organizations varies and is often dependent upon size, system placement, and services offered. There is always a financial component within this structure, which may also be more or less complex depending on the type of organization. Financial departments are in fact collaborative, being on both the receiving and distribution ends of the financial data process. On the receiving end of the process, finance departments rely on the other departments' data collection efforts and systems for data input (such as patient data, human resources data, supply chain data, etc.). On the distribution end of the process, finance departments disseminate information to the other areas within the system for performance management and planning purposes (actual financial results, budgeting, forecasting and projections, etc.). While the organizational structure may differ and some roles and functions may be combined or consolidated, the finance department remains an integral part of healthcare operations. Figure 3.1 shows an organizational chart for a typical hospital, as well as the executive responsible for each area. The organizational structure varies by organization, and may be different due to size, medical focus, or even location. Figure 3.2 provides a more detailed picture of the finance department structure and the functions performed.

The primary role of finance in health services organizations, as in all businesses, is to plan for, acquire, and utilize financial resources in such a way as to maximize the efficiency and value of the enterprise. In general, finance activities include planning and budgeting, financial reporting, long-term investment decisions, financing decisions, working capital management, contract management, and financial risk management. When most healthcare providers were reimbursed on the basis of costs incurred, the role of finance was minimal. At that time, the most critical finance function was cost accounting, because it was more important to account for costs than it was to control them. Today, however, healthcare providers are facing an increasingly competitive environment as well as rapidly changing reimbursement guidelines. Payers, covered services, and reimbursement can vary a great deal, with all of these variations managed by the healthcare finance department. There are a lot of moving pieces in the financial management process, and healthcare

Figure 3.1

Typical hospital organizational chart

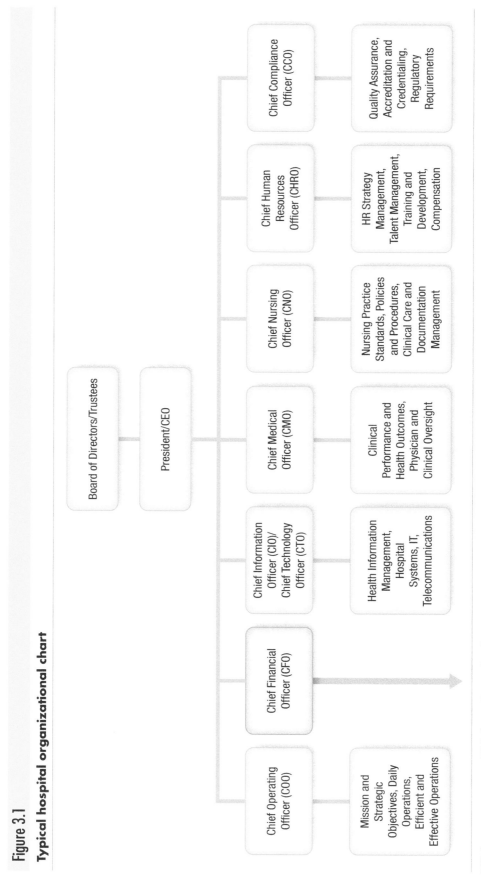

HR, human resources; IT, information technology.

Figure 3.2

Typical finance department organizational chart

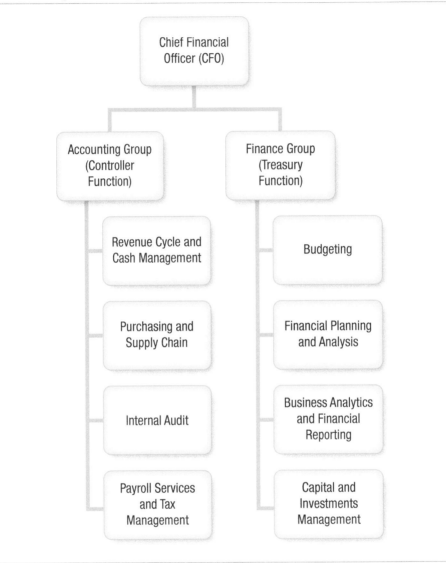

finance professionals must effectively and efficiently coordinate it all—quite the daunting task. Sound coordination requires knowledgeable leadership and a deeper understanding of the organization's structure. Many leaders within the healthcare organization have a more focused purview, with the majority of their efforts dedicated to specific operations. Finance department leadership, however, must have a broader lens with an in-depth understanding of the intersectionality of all functions—patient-centered as well as nonpatient-centered operations.

The Chief Financial Officer

The **chief financial officer** (CFO) provides oversight to financial functions, which ultimately include the operation and performance of every unit and subunit within the organization. The

CFO works in conjunction with other senior leadership to manage and improve all areas of the organization (as shown in Figure 3.1). This senior leadership team, commonly referred to as the "C-Suite," includes the chief operating officer (COO), chief information officer or chief technology officer (CIO/CTO), chief medical officer (CMO), and several other key positions often determined by the scope of the organization and its core functions. The CFO directs two senior managers who help manage finance activities: (a) the controller, who is responsible for accounting and reporting activities such as routine budgeting, preparation of financial statements, payables management, and patient accounts management; and (b) the treasurer, who is responsible for the acquisition and management of capital (funds). In large organizations, the controller and treasurer have managers who have responsibility for specific functions, such as the patient accounts manager, who reports to the controller, and the cash manager, who reports to the treasurer. In small businesses, many of the finance responsibilities are combined and assigned to one individual. In the smallest health services organizations, the entire finance function is managed by one person, often called the practice (business) manager. While the roles may be different, they are equally important in maintaining reliable, consistent, and accurate operations of the finance department functions. Longer-term financial strategy, investments, and profit maximization are also responsibilities of the CFO, which are largely dependent on the controller and treasury functions, as well as the data collected throughout these processes. Critical thinking and decision-making skills are needed for the financial planning initiatives and ongoing business development work of the CFO, but these skills are also essential for the finance professionals performing the controller and treasurer roles.

The Finance Manager: Controller Functions (The Accounting Group)

The typical finance department is divided into clear, distinct functions which address specific financial needs of the organization. One side of the department is led by the **controller** (also called the comptroller in some industries). Controller-related functions capture the financial position of the organization at a given point in time. This is the primary mechanism for accounting, data capture, and routine reporting of the actual asset and debt activity. Accounts receivable (money and assets coming into the organization) and accounts payable (money and debt for the organization) are key responsibilities on the controller side of the department. All of these functions are discussed in detail in later chapters of this textbook (Module II), with an overview of each provided in the sections that follow.

The **revenue cycle and cash management** functions fall within the controller responsibilities, and include all billing and collections activities as well as short-term cash transactions. Efficient revenue cycle management is important for the success of any organization but is critical to the viability of most healthcare organizations. The revenue cycle can be complex depending on the health services offered, as well as the designated payer for those services. Generated revenue is what keeps an organization afloat, with the patient–medical professional interaction serving as the primary driver for the generated revenue. Efficient revenue cycle management maximizes the amount of revenue an organization generates by closely monitoring claims acceptance and reimbursement, as well as errors, denials, and resubmissions. The cash management process records and manages cash inflows and cash outflows, paying particular attention to overall liquidity of assets. Cash-related accounts are short-term accounts and are highly liquid, serving as the accounts for routine daily operations. Examples of cash accounts are accounts payable (for expenses), accounts receivable (for income), petty cash, and (noncapital) supplies and inventory.

Purchasing and supply chain functions secure the products and goods needed to provide services within the healthcare organization. In many instances, this includes contract management and price negotiations, as these are key elements in securing the items needed for the provision of healthcare. The importance of this function has evolved from simply maintaining the basic warehouse or stockroom, to building a network that includes raw material supply, processing or product creation, and transportation to the final point of sale. Purchasing and supply chain activities constitute a large portion of a healthcare organization's expenditure, second only to salaries and wages, and must therefore be accomplished as efficiently as possible. Ideally, services and supplies are secured for the entire system to get volume discounts, where applicable, to minimize waste and excessive ordering.

Internal audit provides the checks and balances within an organization, ensuring effectiveness and efficiency, as well as compliance to regulatory guidelines and reporting requirements. With so many individual processes happening simultaneously, it's definitely possible to lose sight of how things work together. Internal auditors provide the routine spot-checks to ensure that things are being done according to documented policies and procedures, and are as effective as possible. Internal controls, as implemented and assessed by internal audit, are reviewed in different types of audits. Compliance audits review adherence to industry compliance regulations. Information systems audits ensure that healthcare data capture is both accurate and private. Operations audits assess the organization's routine processes and procedures. Financial audits analyze financial recording and reporting (Bell-Buchbinder, 2004; McGhee et al., 2003; Menaker et al., 2020). Internal audit findings are usually the catalysts for process redesigns, as areas for improvement are identified.

Payroll services and tax management include compensation of employees and contractors, as well as annual filing of the organization's income taxes. Recording of hours worked, gross pay calculations, benefits and tax withholding, and leave time accrual are all included in these services (Grogan et al., 2021; Herbst et al., 2020; Shortell et al., 2021). Payroll may seem like a basic function, but for larger organizations with thousands of employees, this can be a time-consuming responsibility. Most organizations utilize a timekeeping and payroll system that communicates directly with the cost accounting and other financial systems. Hospitals with emergency departments and some larger health systems have 24-hour operations, which translates to a wide variety of employees, positions, and pay rates. Accurate and timely processing of payroll is crucial to keeping the organization running—employees must be paid for the hours or work performed.

The Finance Manager: Treasury Functions (The Finance Group)

Treasury functions utilize some of the same accounting data as created by the controller group, but use the data for very different purposes. The treasury function activities, led by the **treasurer**, include financial decision-making and the projection of anticipated financial performance for maximizing organizational effectiveness and efficiency as well as moving the organization forward. Initiatives include both internal and external stakeholders, examining and impacting operations at all levels of the organization. These functions are introduced here, and further detailed throughout the Module IV chapters of this textbook.

Budgeting is the way by which an organization estimates its revenues and expenses for the upcoming fiscal year or other specified time period. This process includes a healthcare organization's projected patient volume and revenue as well as the revenue and expense for all other service lines. Every department within the organization and system prepares an operating budget, in most cases based on prior actual performance. Seasonality and other factors are also considered, to make budgets and estimates as accurate and as realistic as possible. The budgeting cycle occurs annually, and requires input and participation from every department within the healthcare organization, even those with no direct patient contact. The goal of the budgeting process is to anticipate expenses for a given period, and to generate enough revenue to cover those expenses with at least marginal profit. The process requires a more in-depth look at operations and the drivers of the financial position, providing insight on activities with the most influence on performance and outcomes. This makes it possible for leadership to prioritize initiatives and organizational goals in preparation for financial planning and determining the future of the organization. Budgeting assists with the allocation of resources and the longer-term performance measurement and management of the organization.

Financial planning and analysis (FP&A) uses the budgeted information to assess the healthcare organization's financial health and develop strategies for sustained growth and viability. Those in the FP&A role analyze how the organization actually performs, using various methods to forecast the future state. Both qualitative and quantitative methods are used in the analyses, with the findings and final reports used by leadership for informed decision-making. Ideally, this process is structured to identify possible improvements to organizational effectiveness and efficiency, and is integrated into the existing budgeting and accounting systems. This integration makes it easier to collect the necessary data from multiple areas throughout the organization and compare the data over time.

Business analytics and financial reporting are closely tied to the core FP&A function and are often performed by the same group of professionals. In business analytics, the organization's past performance is investigated to identify strengths, challenges, and opportunities for improvement. When it comes to identifying new services, products, partnerships, and so forth, the business analytics group can assess current resources to determine the feasibility and time frame of the possible implementation or expansion. The **capital investments and management** function determines the likelihood of success for new investments and large projects. "Capital" refers to the value of a project or initiative, and is typically defined by the dollar value of the investment, both initial and longer-term. Capital projects and purchases are organized and presented in a separate budget with funding allocated from a separate pool of money. Examples include large construction projects for new facilities or expansions, new diagnostic and treatment technologies, and major financial investments that span an extended period of time.

Risk management is often a finance department function that involves the accounting group as well as the finance group to identify and mitigate threats to the organization's operations. These nonpatient care risks (patient safety and care risks are usually handled by a clinical team) include (a) ethics and fraud, waste, and abuse of funds; (b) systems breaches impacting medical record privacy and confidentiality; (c) health information technology, data collection, and security; and (d) instances of noncompliance. These concerns are ongoing and can be larger initiatives, depending on the organization or network size as well as the patient or service volume. Risks may derive from an internal or external source, with the source playing a major role on the areas of the organization impacted by the risk. Internal risks can impact the entire organization, and once identified can be resolved, eliminated, and prevented from reoccurring. External risks, on the other hand, are often outside of the organization's control, so mitigation rather than elimination may be the only course of action. The risk management team works closely with internal audit to proactively identify potential risks (internal and external), determine the appropriate path forward, and improve processes and/or systems to handle similar situations in the future.

Common Skills for the Healthcare Finance Professional

As noted in the previous sections, the accounting and finance professionals within the finance department are extremely important to the overall operations of the healthcare organization. To perform the critical tasks required of the healthcare finance professional, role-specific education or certification, accounting knowledge (including financial statement preparation), and financial reporting are needed, as well as analytical and problem-solving skills. The healthcare finance professional is not only responsible for the collection and entry of data, but also for the analysis, interpretation, and communication of the results to leadership throughout the organization—an all-inclusive approach as shown in Figure 3.3. Since many leaders outside of the finance department are not directly involved in the process, the finance department representative must have the ability to convey the relevant information in a way that is understood by those receiving it. Routine data collection from the various internal systems—compilation, analysis, reporting, budgeting, and projections—are just some of the responsibilities of the finance department professionals that assist leadership with shorter-term and longer-term management decisions for the overall effectiveness and efficiency of the healthcare organization.

Figure 3.3
The healthcare finance function

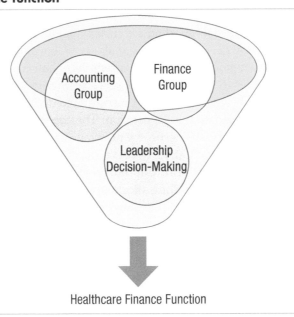

Healthcare Finance Function

Many academic programs have incorporated these essential skills into their curriculum to ensure that future healthcare professionals have at least a basic understanding of financial activities. Though most will not be directly responsible for finance department operations, the basics of payroll, budgeting, volume and visit capture, and patient billing are needed for the management of their respective functional areas. Healthcare management and healthcare administration majors require a more immersive exposure to healthcare finance, as these disciplines prepare graduates for nonclinical roles within the healthcare sector. The business of healthcare has a broad scope, so our healthcare finance professionals must have the skill and ability to apply the core concepts of the discipline to all facets of the healthcare organization.

Medical Practice Management: A Consolidated Model

The finance department and roles discussed so far resemble the standard structure used by hospitals and larger healthcare organizations. There are, however, some organizations that utilize a different, more consolidated staffing model. Smaller medical practices and physicians groups may not be large enough to employ the standard finance department structure, and instead rely upon a practice manager. The practice manager handles the daily operations and all of the supporting functions for the business, serving as the primary point of contact for all clinicians of the practice. This consolidated role performs the key finance functions such as billing, budgeting, and payroll processing, as well as human resources, patient services, nonclinical staff supervision, and administrative responsibilities. The same core elements of healthcare finance are still performed, but the personnel and systems that house the necessary information may be quite different. Larger organizations typically have more complex software systems which are often specialized according to function (e.g., medical records, billing, and inventory are separate systems). Smaller medical and physicians' practices would typically have an integrated system with data and information for the various functions existing in the same system (represented as different modules). The overarching goals remain the same for all types of healthcare organizations, as they prioritize the patient experience. They must still perform the required business functions to make the healthcare services possible.

PROFESSIONAL LICENSING AND REGULATORY ORGANIZATIONS

As with other professions, healthcare and the healthcare finance function rely on the guidance of numerous professional and regulatory organizations, all of which help to maintain quality performance as well as accurate and transparent reporting. Regulatory organizations ensure industry standards are followed, relying on categorization and recording requirements established to maintain data and financial reporting quality. The American Accounting Association (AAA), the American Institute of Certified Public Accountants (AICPA), the Healthcare Financial Management Association (HFMA), and the American Health Information Management Association (AHIMA) are a few professional organizations that promote continuing education and professional development among accounting and finance professionals. These organizations are dedicated to helping professionals apply traditional theoretical concepts of the discipline to real-world situations and scenarios. Other organizations, such as the American College of Healthcare Executives (ACHE) and the Association of University Programs in Health Administration (AUPHA) are comprised of high-level leaders from healthcare organizations and health administration academic programs.

Together, these organizations work to inform university academic content and training for preparing the next generation of healthcare professionals, ensuring the highest quality and standards for the healthcare sector. The Healthcare Leadership Alliance (HLA) includes some of these organizations (and a few others) that share this common mission of advancing the healthcare management discipline. The HLA is comprised of the following organizations:

- American College of Healthcare Executives (ACHE)
- American Organization of Nurse Executives (AONE)
- Healthcare Financial Management Association (HFMA)
- Health Information and Management Systems Society (HIMSS)
- Medical Group Management Association (MGMA)

While the aforementioned organizations provide organization-level guidance, they also provide discipline-specific certifications, licensure, and career guidance.

CHAPTER SUMMARY

The accounting group and the finance group work together to maintain the financial operations of the healthcare organization. Although the functions of each are distinct, they are closely tied, and in many cases interdependent, when it comes to maintaining the financial viability of the organization. One side of the department cannot feasibly exist without the other, as both are needed to maintain the organization and the goal of patient care. Patient-centered care is the focus of the health services organization, as it should be. However, the continuum of care is made possible over the longer term by prudent financial management and sound leadership and decision-making, which are all significantly impacted by the work of the finance department. The key finance functions will be further detailed throughout Modules II and III of this textbook to discuss the details of the relevant roles and the overall contribution to sustaining the healthcare sector.

KEY TERMS FOR REVIEW

budgeting

business analytics and financial reporting

capital investments and management

chief financial officer

controller

financial management

financial planning and analysis

healthcare financial management

internal audit

payroll services and tax management

purchasing and supply chain

revenue cycle and cash management

risk management

treasurer

value creation

DISCUSSION QUESTIONS

1. Discuss the similarities and differences between the accounting and finance functions within a healthcare organization's finance department.

2. Identify the key data elements/concepts that connect the controller and treasury functions. How might the overlaps benefit the healthcare organization?

3. How does the financial function within a healthcare organization inform the decision-making of leadership?

4. Discuss the controller functions and how they work together to perform the accounting-focused responsibilities.

5. Discuss the treasury functions and how they work together to perform the finance-focused responsibilities.

6. Discuss the finance function for medical practices and physicians' practices. How does it differ from other healthcare organizations?

7. Reflect on the role of healthcare finance and its key responsibilities. How might inefficiencies or errors in the finance function impact the larger healthcare sector?

CHAPTER 3 CASE: OUT OF SORTS

An independent physician's practice has been acquired by a larger health system and must now begin the process of consolidating its core business processes. Historically, the routine business operations for the practice were handled by the practice manager, who has been with the practice for the past 5 years. The health system has adequate resources to handle the business aspects of the practice, leaving the practice manager with the administrative tasks. The CFO has asked the practice manager for a list of typical financial activities, organized by the functional unit that will be responsible for those activities. This request is a bit confusing for the practice manager because in small physicians' practices, the manager handles everything, with very little delineation among responsibilities. As an experienced finance manager who's been with the health system for quite some time, you've offered to help the practice manager sort through the organization's financial responsibilities.

1. Review the list of activities in Table 3.1 to determine:
   a. Is the activity administrative or financial in nature?
   b. If the activity is financial, would it be assigned to the controller group or the treasurer group?
   c. Which functional unit within the assigned group (controller or treasurer) is responsible for routinely performing the activity?

2. For activities that are administrative in nature, provide guidance on how these activities may impact finance department operations.

Table 3.1

FINANCE DEPARTMENT ACTIVITIES: ADMINISTRATIVE OR FINANCIAL?

	Practice Activity	Administrative (A) or Financial (F)	Controller Group (C) or Treasurer Group (T)	Functional Unit	Admin Impacts/ Guidance Comments
1	Annual budgeting				
2	Imaging equipment purchase				
3	Insurance company billing				
4	Insurance payment receipts				
5	Office space rent payment				
6	Patient copay receipts				
7	Patient scheduling and registration				
8	Physician's notes/ medical record documentation				

(continued)

Table 3.1

FINANCE DEPARTMENT ACTIVITIES: ADMINISTRATIVE OR FINANCIAL? (*continued*)

	Practice Activity	Administrative (A) or Financial (F)	Controller Group (C) or Treasurer Group (T)	Functional Unit	Admin Impacts/ Guidance Comments
9	Rate (amount charged) adjustments				
10	Staff payroll processing and payments				
11	Staff scheduling				
12	Supply invoice payment				

HEALTHCARE FINANCE COURSE PROJECT: PREPARATION

The healthcare finance course project is designed to help students think critically about the healthcare finance function and how other areas within the organization are impacted by finance data and associated responsibilities. This chapter is an important first step in framing the course project, by giving context to the finance role and how it supports the delivery of healthcare services. Successful course project implementation and completion will require students to assume the vantage point of a healthcare finance professional, with key responsibilities for data consolidation, data visualization, and financial reporting using Microsoft Excel®. As an introduction to the course project, please review "Course Project: An Introduction," presented in Chapter 16 (the last chapter of the textbook), which gives an overview of the project, as well as the objectives and desired outcomes. Subsequent chapters will include information on the application of chapter concepts into the various parts of the course project.

REFERENCES

Arduino, K. (2018). *The increasing importance of strategic capital planning.* https://www.hfma.org/topics/hfm/2018/february/59164.html

Bastani, P., Abolhallaje, M., & Sadeghi, A. (2016). Experts' analysis of the improvement spaces of the first phase of reform in health system financial management: A qualitative study. *Journal of Qazvin University of Medical Sciences, 20*(1), 47–55. http://journal.qums.ac.ir/article-1-1985-en.html

Bell-Buchbinder, S. (2004). Serendipity, propinquity and the science of healthcare financial management. *Research in Healthcare Financial Management, 9*(1), 1–2.

Birch, S., Tomlin-Murphy, G., MacKenzie, A., & Cumming, J. (2015). In place of fear: Aligning health care planning with system objectives to achieve financial sustainability. *Journal of Health Services Research and Policy, 20*(2), 109–114. https://doi.org/10.1177/1355819614562053

Escobar-Perez, B., Escobar-Rodriguez, T., & Bartual-Sopena, L. (2016). Integration of healthcare and financial information: Evaluation in a public hospital using a comprehensive approach. *Health Informatics Journal, 22*(4), 878–896. https://doi.org/10.1177/1460458215595259

Grogan, C. M., Lin, Y.-A., & Gusmano, M. K. (2021). Health equity and the allocation of COVID-19 provider relief funds. *American Journal of Public Health, 111*(4), 628–631. https://doi.org/10.2105/AJPH.2020.306127

Herbst, J. L., O'Brien, S. J., & Chumas, E. G. (2020). Hospital taxes, Medicaid supplemental payments, and state budgets. *Journal of Legal Medicine, 40*(2), 135–170. https://doi.org/10.1080/01947648.2020.1822243

Lee, D. (2019). Effects of key value co-creation elements in the healthcare system: Focusing on technology applications. *Service Business, 13*(2), 389–417. https://doi.org/10.1007/s11628-018-00388-9

McGhee, C. R., Glasser, J. H., Chan, W., & Pomeroy, N. (2003). Forecasting health care expenditures and utilization based on a Markov process and a deterministic cost function in managed care settings. *Institute of Mathematical Statistics, 42*(2003), 229–238. https://doi.org/10.1214/lnms/1215092404

Menaker, R., Witte, R. J., & France, T. J. (2020). *Principal principles: Critical accounting and financial concepts for healthcare leaders.* https://www.mgma.com/resources/financial-management/principal-principles-critical-accounting-and-fina

Pina, I. L., Cohen, P. D., Larson, D. B., Marion, L. N., Sills, M. R., Solberg, L. I., & Zerzan, J. (2015). A framework for describing health care delivery organizations and systems. *American Journal of Public Health, 105*(4), 670–679. https://doi.org/10.2105/AJPH.2014.301926

Ramos Hegwer, L. (2017). The future of healthcare finance: Focusing your strategies amid uncertainty. *Healthcare Executive, 32*(3), 11–16.

Shortell, S. M., Rundell, T. G., & Blodgett, J. C. (2021). Assessing the relationship of the human resource, finance, and information technology functions on reported performance in hospitals using the lean management system. *Healthcare Management and Revenue, 46*(2), 145–152. https://doi.org/10.1097/HMR.0000000000000253

Stewart, C. C., Yu, L., Wilson, R. S., Bennett, D. A., & Boyle, P. A. (2019). Healthcare and financial decision making and incident adverse cognitive outcomes among older adults. *Journal of the American Geriatrics Society, 67*(8), 1590–1595. https://doi.org/10.1111/jgs.15880

Widmer, A. (2016). Of means and ends: The financialization and regulation of health care. *The Linacre Quarterly, 83*(4), 382–386. https://doi.org/10.1080/00243639.2016.1248168

Accounting Principles Review

CHAPTER 4

Financial and Managerial Accounting

1. Explain the various compliance regulations and accounting standards.
2. Provide working definitions of financial accounting and managerial accounting.
3. Explain the differences between and utility of both accrual-based accounting and cash-based accounting.
4. Define revenues and expenses, and describe how these impact the healthcare organization's financial position.
5. Discuss the difference between inward-facing management metrics and outward-facing measurement metrics.

INTRODUCTION

Accounting and financial management are important to every organization for short-term and long-term viability as well as soundness of practice. This information is used in a variety of ways, and the focus, or purpose of use, will often dictate which type of accounting will be the most appropriate. Data from routine operations, which in healthcare means patient care and the supporting elements of patient care (pharmaceuticals, supplies, equipment, etc.), drives the accounting and financial management processes. The various types of accounting and reporting methods are used collaboratively to record, report, manage, and predict current and future activities—activities which support the organization's mission, vision, and values. Financial accounting and managerial accounting are the two dominant types of accounting used in the healthcare sector (with other methods applied to organizations that manufacture tangible goods), with each playing an important role in the healthcare finance function. Although the type of services provided and captured in the financial statements may vary by organization, the key elements of the healthcare finance function exist in all healthcare organizations. This chapter discusses the regulations that govern the financial functions, the differences between financial and managerial accounting, and the types of results produced by each.

COMPLIANCE AND ACCOUNTING STANDARDS

Before discussing the types of accounting, we must first understand the rules. Financial and managerial accounting, to be accurate and well-governed, must adhere to the established guidelines set forth by the industry's regulatory bodies. There are in fact multiple layers to this governing structure, with a broad hierarchy to oversee the various sector-specific accounting needs. The Financial Accounting Foundation (FAF) governs the Financial Accounting Standards Board (FASB), which creates and enforces the accounting practices we use today. These generally accepted accounting principles (commonly referred to as GAAP) determine the accounting best practices used in both financial accounting and managerial accounting. The foundational data itself does not change, but the way that the information is used does. Table 4.1 shows the list of items included in GAAP, all of which are incorporated in some way into an organization's accounting system.

Table 4.1	
GAAP PRINCIPLES LIST	
GAAP Principle	**Definition**
Principle of regularity	Regularly follow all accounting rules and regulations
Principle of consistency	Accounting standards must be consistently applied to the accounting process
Principle of sincerity	Truthfulness and sincerity in financial reporting
Principle of permanence of method	Use the same accounting methods across all reporting periods
Principle of noncompensation	Assets and liabilities should be reported separately
Principle of prudence	Financial performance should not be overstated
Principle of continuity	Stability of the organization; continuity of operations without assumptions
Principle of periodicity	Report at regular intervals to allow for comparison and analysis
Principle of materiality	Full disclosure; anything that affects the company's financial standing must be reported
Principle of utmost good faith	Honest recording and reporting of financial data

GAAP, generally accepted accounting principles.

Although most accounting software packages will have many of these requirements included as standard, much of the reporting and disclosure is still left to the accounting and finance professionals. Transparency, accountability, and ethical reporting are critical to the accounting and finance roles, and these core elements are embedded within the principles required for training and certification. While GAAP serves as the accounting foundation within the United States, the principles are applied in different (but similar) ways depending on the industry and the users. FASB regulates the application of GAAP for public, nongovernmental organizations (NGOs). The Governmental Accounting Standards Board (GASB) regulates the application of the principles to state and local government entities. The International Accounting Standards Board (IASB) incorporates a lot of the core GAAP concepts but applies international accounting rules and regulations as accepted by the countries and jurisdictions that subscribe to IASB practices.

These compliance and governing bodies contain many of the same regulations and work together in instances of multinational operations. In today's global economy, many organizations and governments conduct business in several locations using multiple currencies. Accounting and financial reporting must satisfy their home-country requirements as well as those of the country in which they're doing business. The standards boards are, however, working together to ensure some continuity in financial reporting, due to what we see today as a global economy with corporations operating in any number of countries.

These foundational principles provide the framework for an organization's financial recording and reporting practices, which ultimately assist with the attainment of its goals and objectives. While both the financial and managerial accounting functions utilize this data, they are used in very different ways to accomplish very different tasks. Ideally, all efforts should work toward the organization's benefit, but the implementation of the core principles and processes will surely vary and serve different purposes. The GAAP principles provide the regulations for financial accounting, which supplies foundational data for managerial accounting–making it GAAP compliant by default. Internal reports and analyses produced for decision-making purposes are not regulated by external organizations, although various operating areas may have regulations from professional accrediting organizations.

FINANCIAL ACCOUNTING

Financial accounting is the reporting of an organization's financial position at a given point in time and is what we generally think of when we hear the term "accounting" referenced. This information is primarily used for regulatory purposes outside of the organization, such as auditing and financial reporting. The financial accounting process annotates and summarizes an organization's financial standing for a given reporting period. Monthly, quarterly, and annual reporting intervals are the norm, but accounting departments have the ability to "pull" this information at a moment's notice for any calendar period of interest. The "financial close" period is the time frame allotted for this process, which finalizes all transactions (incoming, ongoing, and related adjustments) for the reporting period (this process, and the steps involved, are detailed in this chapter and Chapter 5). The final financial reporting package is made available for auditors, investors, creditors, and other stakeholders. The financial data alone is not substantial enough for decision-making but must be analyzed in conjunction with additional financial and operational indicators for decision-making and strategic planning. This is where the managerial accounting process steps in.

Accrual Accounting Versus Cash Accounting

When it comes to financial accounting, there are two primary bases by which key accounting tasks are accomplished: accrual accounting and cash accounting. **Accrual accounting** records the financial transaction at the time it occurs. This means that we recognize the debit (expense/payment made) and the credit (revenue/payment received) in the actual accounting period that it takes place. Accruals are "reversed" at the beginning of the next accounting period, as the previously accrued amount has been actualized. **Cash accounting**, on the other hand, records the financial transaction when the item is paid or reflected on the banking/account statements. An everyday example of these concepts could be their application to our personal finances. If we were to purchase a household good and pay for it using a check, we would theoretically write this as a debit in our checking account journal and subtract the amount from our current balance. This simulates the accrual accounting process and provides us with a real-time idea of our checking account available balance. If we wait to deduct the amount from our current balance until the check clears the bank, we will be overstating our available balance by that amount, and be in jeopardy of overspending or overdrawing the account. The real-time status provided by the accrual accounting process is the method most utilized throughout the healthcare finance field. Depending on the size of the organization, the transaction recording in the general ledger and accrual processes can be quite involved; therefore, most organizations will utilize a dedicated software package, even if only a basic one. These standardized systems will have the ability to record all transactions and summarize the information on the financial statements for reporting purposes.

BOX 4.1

Accrual Versus Cash Accounting

Mrs. Smith purchases three prescriptions from her local pharmacy and decides to pay by check. Her bank balance is $500, so the $100 total for the prescriptions can be covered. She wants to get her health errands out of the way early, so she can go shopping later on that day (she doesn't realize that the check for the prescriptions won't be cleared/processed by the bank for 1–2 weeks).

Accural Accounting:		Cash Accounting:	
Bank Balance:	$ 500	Bank Balance:	$ 500
Prescriptions:	$ (100)	Prescriptions:	$ -
Net Balance:	$ 400	Net Balance:	$ 500

In the example in Box 4.1, you can see the difference between the accrual method of accounting and the cash method of accounting. With the accrual method, Mrs. Smith would have a real-time account balance after deducting the pharmacy expense at the time it occurs. With the cash accounting method, Mrs. Smith's account includes the $100 that she has technically already spent by not recognizing the pharmacy expense until the check clears the bank. Although both methods are acceptable, the cash accounting balance would show $500 available when Mrs. Smith really only has $400 available, possibly causing an overdrawn account or other banking penalties. In healthcare, transactions are accrued by recording them when they occur, not when the payment is posted by the bank. This real-time view of the organization's account balances shows the accounting and finance professionals exactly how much revenue has been generated as well as how much expense has been incurred. This data provides the support for departmental and organizational budgets, supply and technology purchases, volume projections, and other management accounting responsibilities.

Revenues and Expenses

Determining a healthcare organization's financial position (or that of any type of organization, for that matter) involves the analysis of its routine financial activities and its profitability. The accounting and finance functions are designed to perform the needed analyses using the data collected by the various systems, showing the resources coming into the organization as well as how those resources are utilized. **Revenue** is the income generated by the provision of healthcare goods and services. This includes patient services revenue, sale of medical supplies and products, and other (nonpatient) operating revenue such as gift shop sales or parking fees. **Expense** is the cost the organization incurs for the production of the goods and services provided. Expenses include salaries and wages, raw materials and supplies, marketing and advertising, and utilities. **Profit** is the remaining income after all expense obligations have been satisfied (as calculated in Box 4.2). Profitability analysis is used to assess financial standing, but it may also identify issues with internal processes or practices that ultimately impact efficiency. Decreased or insufficient revenues could mean billing and reimbursement process delays, or possibly an outdated fee schedule. Increased expenses could be the result of ineffective staffing, internal staff shortages (relying on agency staffing), increased vendor and supply pricing, or inefficient internal work processes.

BOX 4.2

Profit Calculation

$$\text{Revenues} - \text{Expenses} = \text{Profit}$$

Financial Statements and Reporting

Accounting information is summarized into a series of routine monthly **financial statements** for the purposes of external reporting and compliance. The standard **financial reporting package** will typically include the following: (a) statement of financial position or balance sheet, (b) statement of operations or income statement (also called the profit and loss statement), (c) statement of cashflows, and (d) statement of shareholder's equity (or change in equity statement). These reports are included in the period-end financial reporting package, and present consolidated data on the organization's operating, financial, and investing activities to stakeholders in the context of the organization's mission and strategic goals. Additional notes and verbiage accompany the standard financial statements to explain the various accounting methods used and other events that may have impacted the financial results. The financial reporting package also includes detailed supporting data on labor-related expenses, volume and patient visits, capacity, and inpatient occupancy. Various finance and healthcare sector compliance regulations play a major role in how the information is reported and what should be included to ensure accuracy, transparency, and appropriate internal controls. The accounting information and financial reports, although prepared for external purposes, provide the foundational data for internal use by the organization's leadership. This begins the managerial accounting process.

MANAGERIAL ACCOUNTING

Managerial accounting is the analysis and utilization of accounting data for decision-making purposes. The decision-making process is closely tied into the organization's goals, with the managerial accounting information primarily used for purposes internal to the organization. Managerial accounting (often called cost accounting) uses the available financial information for informed organizational decision-making. Financial information alone is rarely sufficient for larger, more complex analysis; however, when paired with management accounting methods, it provides sound foundations for decision-making in the areas of budgeting, strategic planning and forecasting, activity-based costing and project analysis, effectiveness, and efficiency management. The managerial accounting process and related techniques help the leadership to assess the current state of the organization's operations and prepare for the future. It interprets the accounting data and explains it in the context of routine activities for the purposes of directing and controlling the organization's trajectory. The types of managerial accounting techniques will vary and align with the industry, service, or goods provided, but most methods are applicable to the healthcare sector in some way. The focus of managerial accounting can be represented by the three Ps: Products, Projects, and Projections. These three categories of activity (shown with examples in Figure 4.1) cover all aspects of the healthcare organization by considering the historical performance, current operations, and future planning. In the text that follows, we'll broadly discuss these categories within the context of managerial accounting applications. Detailed analyses and calculations will be presented in subsequent chapters of the text.

Figure 4.1

Managerial accounting's three Ps

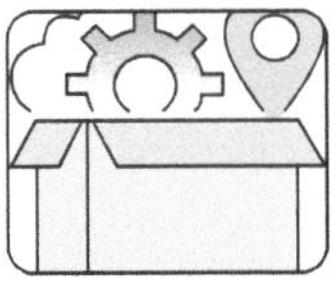

Products
- Healthcare Services Offered
- Pharmaceuticals
- Routine Supplies and DME

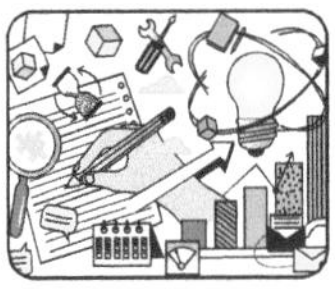

Projects
- Capital Projects or Expansions
- New Medical Equipment
- Investments or Financial Ventures

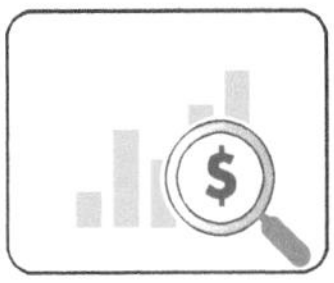

Projections
- Volume and Utilization Trend Analysis
- Resource Requirements (Human and Material)
- Budgeting and Financial Forecasts

DME, durable medical equipment.

Managerial Accounting for Products

A **product** is defined as an item created for sale or consumption. In healthcare, the professional service provided by a clinician or specialist and the materials used for that service are considered products. Managerial accounting for products involves the cost analysis of all phases of production: sourcing, production, and sales. In the context of healthcare, this means the analysis of both human and material resources necessary for the delivery of healthcare services. Clinical providers, specialists, healthcare supplies, pharmaceuticals, and durable medical equipment are all considered in the analyses, with data for these items reflected in the operations budget and the sales forecasts. The data collected helps with the decision-making process by providing clear information on what products are consumed the most in comparison to those with little or no consumption. A healthcare provider or supplier could use this data to determine what items to continue offering routinely, what items to offer sporadically, or what items should be phased out.

Product consumption and utilization data is used not only for ensuring that consumer and community needs are met, but for financial operations as well. Utilization and market analysis is used for pricing decisions, which help an organization determine how much to charge consumers for their products. The economics of supply and demand come into play, with pricing strategies having a direct impact on revenue and longer-term financial planning. At the operations level, contract negotiations can also be impacted by pricing, particularly those contracts associated with supply chain and contracted staffing. Initial costs of materials and contracted staffing prices (which tend to be above and beyond standard in-house labor costs) have a direct correlation to pricing for consumers. Healthcare providers throughout the industry are often faced with make-versus-buy decisions. This not only involves the decision on making an actual product or purchasing it, but also a decision on using in-house/permanent personnel or agency/contracted personnel. Price is not the only determining factor, as capacity and efficiency have proven to be equally as important. To illustrate product analysis, let's consider the scenario in Box 4.3, which shows the comparison of three different products.

BOX 4.3

Basic Product Analysis

The finance director and the director of supply chain management are analyzing data for the expansion of the respiratory services department. Prior to 2019, pulmonologists saw very few patients with sleep apnea and only had one vendor for continuous positive airway pressure (CPAP) machines and associated supplies. Since then, volume has drastically increased and the single-vendor product and pricing no longer work for the facility. They have decided to offer an in-house product solution but still need to choose the best product. All product options have the same level of quality, so the determining factor will be the cost of production per unit and patient demand. Special order units may also be an option.

	Mini/Travel (Product 1)	Full-Size (Product 2)	w/ Humidifier (Product 3)
Raw Materials	$ 545	$ 699	$ 725
Assembly Labor	$ 100	$ 125	$ 125
Quality Check Labor	$ 75	$ 50	$ 100
Final Packaging	$ 25	$ 25	$ 25
Cost Per Unit	$ 745	$ 899	$ 975

The calculations in Box 4.3 show Product 1 as the lowest-priced option when comparing the three different types of CPAP units, so based on price alone the choice would be to offer the Mini/Travel unit as the standard option for patients. If anticipated annual patient demand is determined to be 30 requests for the Mini/Travel CPAP units, 250 requests for the Full-Size CPAP units, and 20 requests for the CPAP Humidifier units (300 total requests), the standard option choice would indeed change. In a scenario where demand is the driver for the selection, the Full-Size CPAP would be the standard unit for patients because 83.33% of the patients (250 out of the 300 total requests) prefer this model. The remaining 16.67% of requests (10% for Mini/ Travel units and 6.67% for Humidifier units) could be special ordered.

Managerial Accounting for Projects

Healthcare **projects** can include a number of initiatives to expand service lines, improve organizational efficiency, or restructure current operations. Project costing and cost–benefit analysis techniques are both used to determine if the project is financially and operationally feasible, as well as the probability of reaching the intended outcomes. An example of a service-line expansion is the addition of an in-house function that was previously outsourced. Imaging and laboratory-work services are often outsourced, and the purchase of imaging equipment or laboratory-processing equipment would be a way for an organization to offer these services for their patients. Changes and additions to the organization or health system structure is another example of a major project which could expand existing service lines or expand the system/ network to offer additional services or offices/locations.

The accounting data is part of a larger **project analysis**, which examines all of the factors impacting the project's implementation and expected outcomes. All key stakeholders are included in the analysis, as their inputs and needs must be considered. This collective information can be used to determine if a project should be initially implemented or, if already implemented, if a project should be continued. The project analysis process and its stages are reflected in Figure 4.2.

Figure 4.2

The project analysis process

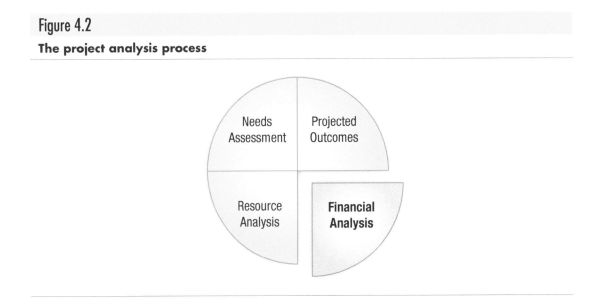

The **needs assessment** stage in project analysis examines the need or demand for a specific product or service. In healthcare, this could mean determining the need for a new clinical specialist or the need for a new pharmaceutical product or medicine. If the community served by a hospital has a large number of people with a medical condition requiring specific treatment, the hospital would then determine how to best provide the treatment. In the **resource analysis** stage, the healthcare organization reviews its current resources available for the potential implementation of the project. Every project will have items required for production, so the organization must have these resources on hand or at least have reasonable access to them. Resources review includes staffing and materials accessible within the organization or within its network of stakeholders. The **financial analysis** stage of the project analysis shows the project details in operating and financial terms. Staffing and wage information are combined to provide labor cost estimates, while supplies and purchase price information are combined to provide materials cost estimates. All other costs associated with the operationalization of the project, such as indirect costs and overhead, are calculated to give the leadership team the information needed for final decision-making. The **projected outcomes** phase uses the information gathered in the previous three phases to determine the viability of the project. The needs assessment will provide community needs for the short and long term, giving an idea of the demand for the product or service. The resource analysis will inform leadership on the availability as well as the sustainability of resources, providing important information on the overall supply chain. The financial analysis helps to determine if the project is financially feasible and what the price should be for breakeven or profit scenarios. Questions answered in the outcomes phase include: Are we meeting the needs of the community? Do we have consistent access to the resources needed to produce this healthcare service? Are we able to sustain this project financially? This information is used collectively to determine if this project will be a solid part of the organization's offerings.

The project analysis for each project informs managerial accounting for projections. Once implemented, the project's actual performance is analyzed to determine if initial project estimates were correct. If things are going according to plan, no changes may be needed, but if the project is not performing as expected, changes may be implemented to alter the trajectory of performance. There are software programs designed for detailed project analysis, used by organizations whose revenue is tied directly to project performance and data (contractors, consultants, etc.). The project analysis process is important for all phases of the project, as decision makers rely on this information to plan future operations.

Managerial Accounting for Projections

Projections include the data analysis and decision-making processes that will guide the organization forward. In unison, these activities provide a comprehensive look at all facets of operations. The analysis of the organization's historical performance helps determine what worked well and what may need to be changed or updated. Volume and utilization data provide insight on well-performing services and products as well as those items no longer deemed valuable or needed by consumers. Projections include materials resources as well as the human resources that are required to operate the organization and provide healthcare services to the patients. The project analyses from existing products and projects provide performance trends that lay the foundation for projections for pricing, revenue, and patient needs. Seasonality and other trends evident in the historical data help with the prediction and preparation for performance under similar circumstances. Trends could provide support for maintaining current processes or support for changes and improvements.

Projections can be quarterly or annual, but ideally should remain adjustable to account for any major changes in operations. In some cases, especially when data for the full reporting period has not yet been realized (still in process), the historical data must be annualized to provide a sound basis for projections. To annualize a figure, the average for the reported periods is calculated, then multiplied by the remaining periods before calculating the total. To illustrate data **annualization** calculations, we can use the data provided in Box 4.4.

BOX 4.4

Data Annualization

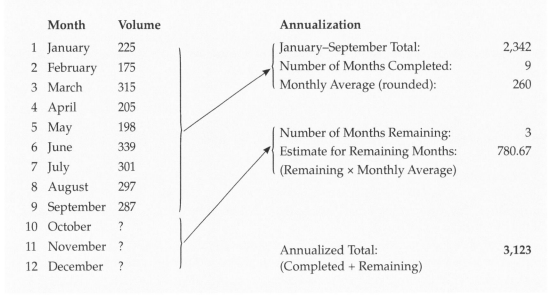

	Month	Volume		Annualization	
1	January	225		January–September Total:	2,342
2	February	175		Number of Months Completed:	9
3	March	315		Monthly Average (rounded):	260
4	April	205			
5	May	198		Number of Months Remaining:	3
6	June	339		Estimate for Remaining Months:	780.67
7	July	301		(Remaining × Monthly Average)	
8	August	297			
9	September	287			
10	October	?			
11	November	?		Annualized Total:	**3,123**
12	December	?		(Completed + Remaining)	

The example in Box 4.4 shows the annualization of volume using 9 months of actual recorded data, which serves as the basis for predicting the final 3 months. This process can be used for volume, supplies, salaries, or any other expense. If the actual data were to be simply divided by 12 months, the average would be understated, causing errors in all related projections. The annualized total then provides the foundational data needed for projections. When we think about projections, we also consider other important internal processes such as budgeting, financial planning, strategic planning, and other contracting initiatives, which leadership uses to guide and adjust business operations. Paying close attention to projections, and the actual performance they are based upon, allows the healthcare organization to possibly maximize revenues, minimize (or manage) expenses, and remain agile and responsive to changes within the healthcare sector. Although projections are more closely tied to managerial accounting and related decision-making, financial accounting data still provides the foundations of the projections as it consolidates the historical financial performance of the organization. Table 4.2 compares the key concepts of financial accounting and managerial accounting, showing similarities as well as differences in data.

OTHER TYPES OF ACCOUNTING

Although financial accounting and managerial accounting are the two most common types used in healthcare operations today, there are several other specialized types of accounting that may impact how we do business within the sector. **Fund accounting** is a specialization that focuses on the financial operations of nonprofit organizations. This is important in healthcare because many hospitals and charities providing and funding care are nonprofit, and therefore must

Table 4.2		
FINANCIAL AND MANAGERIAL ACCOUNTING COMPARISON		
Historical/Performance Data	**Financial Accounting**	**Managerial Accounting**
Users/Target audience	External stakeholders (auditors, regulatory bodies, creditors, donors, investors)	Internal stakeholders (management and leadership, patient advocates, employees)
Purpose of data	Regulatory reporting and compliance, credit considerations, investment decisions	Performance measurement and management, budgeting, forecasting, strategic planning, project planning and analysis
Presentation of data	Financial statements, audit reports	Internal reports, actual-budget reports, production reports, cost reports, patient occupancy reports
Regulation of data	GAAP, IRS, FTC	GAAP (as FAF)

FAF, Financial Accounting Foundation; FTC, Federal Trade Commission; GAAP, generally accepted accounting principles; IRS, Internal Revenue Service.

follow the appropriate guidelines. **Tax accounting** is another accounting specialization that may be used in healthcare organizations to manage the complex tax scenarios that arise. In larger healthcare delivery systems, there may be several types of stakeholders with different structures and tax classifications. This may require a tax accounting professional to manage tax calculations and reporting when there are different types of organizations contributing to the system's overall financial picture. **Internal auditing** can also be included in the list of accounting types because it (like other types) has specific focal points. Internal auditors examine the organization's internal processes, procedures, and systems to identify areas of improvement. These are identified by uncovering any evidence of misuse or misallocation of resources, as well as missed opportunities caused by inefficiencies. Review of processes and procedures is crucial to maintaining an efficient healthcare delivery system. Internal audit may be a function within an organization's infrastructure, or it may be performed by an external internal audit consulting firm. **Forensic accounting** is closely tied to the internal audit function, as it examines accounting and financial records for erroneous, missing, or fraudulent data, ultimately helping with the improvement of internal controls. Along with regulatory bodies, insurance companies and payers also use forensic accounting services.

CHAPTER SUMMARY

Financial accounting and managerial accounting, although based on the same foundational information, serve two very different purposes. Both are equally important in the financial operation of healthcare organizations, requiring skill and industry knowledge to make it all come together. Effective and efficient management of current operations is necessary, as well as future planning and projections of financial activity. Accounting data is often used in performance measurement and management, assisting with decision-making that maximizes the organization's effectiveness and efficiency initiatives. Healthcare finance focuses on the decision-making and projections aspects of the business, performing the routine functions of budgeting, forecasting, and financial and strategic planning. There are many underlying activities and reports that accompany the healthcare finance functions that provide great insight to what actually drives the organization and how. Finance and leadership work together to utilize this information to improve the patient experience and the organization.

KEY TERMS FOR REVIEW

accrual accounting	financial statements	profit
annualization	forensic accounting	project
cash accounting	fund accounting	project analysis
expense	internal auditing	projected outcomes
financial accounting	managerial accounting	projections
financial analysis	needs assessment	revenue
financial reporting package	product	tax accounting

DISCUSSION QUESTIONS

1. What are the primary uses for financial accounting?

2. What are the primary uses for managerial accounting?

3. Is one type of accounting more useful than the other? Explain your answer.

4. In today's healthcare environment, organizations must be very strategic in their efforts to maximize services while minimizing expenses. Discuss how both financial accounting and managerial accounting can be used to realize strategic goals and objectives.

5. Define the acronym GAAP. How is it applied to the field of accounting?

6. Discuss the differences between accrual accounting and cash accounting, as well as which method has proven to be more beneficial to healthcare organizations.

7. Identify the "three Ps" of management accounting and how they may be applied to a healthcare organization.

8. What is annualization? How does it support the various accounting and finance functions?

9. How might the other forms of accounting (not financial or managerial) be used or represented in the healthcare sector? Would they be used individually or in conjunction with financial and managerial accounting methods?

PRACTICE PROBLEMS

Answers to this chapter's Practice Problems are available via Springer Publishing Connect™ by following the instructions on the opening page of this book and accessing Answers to Practice Problems on the Table of Contents.

1. HealthMed Claims Processing is the company contracted to process medical claims for your physicians' medical group. Although most of the industry uses the accrual method of accounting, HealthMed offers its clients the option of choosing the accrual method or cash method. Your group's current bank balance (end of July) is $500,000 and you have billed an additional $10,000 in revenue for the month. You have also paid several medical supply invoices (paid by check, clearing in approximately 15 days), totaling $3,500.

   a. Using the accrual basis of accounting, what is the group's bank balance for the month of July?
   b. Using the cash basis of accounting, what is the group's bank balance for the month of July?
   c. If the bank account yields 5% interest, what are the new bank balances for both the accrual and cash bases for the month of July?
   d. After all calculations (revenues, supplies, and interest), which accounting method shows the greatest balance for the month?

2. There are three orthopedic implant vendors competing for the community hospital's knee implant business (see Table 4.3). Anticipated surgical volume for each of the next 3 years is 250, 285, and 325, respectively. All vendors offer the same, high-quality product so the final decision will come down to price. Each vendor has administrative fees (as a percentage of cost) and offers volume discounts for knee implant orders. Using the data that follows, determine the: (a) base price per year and contract total for each vendor, (b) adjusted/discounted price per year and contract total for each vendor, and (c) the most feasible vendor choice (explain your choice).

Table 4.3

VENDOR ANALYSIS DATA

	Vendor #1	Vendor #2	Vendor #3
Implant Unit Cost	$5,610	$5,565	$5,705
Admin Fee	2.5%	2.5%	2.5%
Volume discounts	3.0%, 201–250	10%, >250	5.0%, 201–300
	4.5%, 251–300		7.0%, >300
	5.0%, 301–350		

3. You are the manager of operative services. You have spent the following amounts so far this year, and it is the end of August. What do you think your annual expenses will be in each category?

Telephone	$2,366
Housekeeping	$18,522
Medical waste	$4,523
Sterile processing	$25,320
Agency staffing	$120,000

4. Pantheon Health System has implemented a solution to address the problem of access to care for patients in rural environments. They have implemented mobile units for healthcare services, which can be utilized by patients anywhere in its health system, including its subsidiaries. After a year of actual performance, the mobile healthcare service must now be analyzed for profitability as leadership determines which of the organization's projects will be continued in the coming years.

Using the revenue and expense data in Table 4.4:

a. Calculate total revenue and total expenses using the accrual-basis of accounting.
b. Calculate total revenue and total expenses using the cash-basis of accounting.

Table 4.4

REVENUE AND EXPENSE DATA

Transaction	Amount
Billed revenue	$4,241,580
Clinical staff salaries (earned)	$655,000
Clinical staff salaries (paid)	$525,000
Collected revenue (cash)	$1,485,650
Medical supplies	$975,025
Purchased medical equipment (cash)	$1,159,350

5. Calculate profit using the revenue and expense data in Table 4.5:

Table 4.5

REVENUE AND EXPENSE DATA

Transaction	Amount
Patient services revenue	$325,000
Supply costs	$110,000
Salaries and wages	$50,000
Professional subscriptions	$1,000
Rent	$15,000
Utilities	$5,000
Parking revenue	$1,250
Cafeteria sales	$3,500

6. The chief operating officer (COO) of a large health system is considering a horizontal merger with the purchase of two existing community health clinics. There are three clinics currently seeking consolidation, and the COO has to determine which two clinics would be the best fit for their business venture.

- Northwest Clinic pays $69,000 annually for office space rental. All healthcare services are provided in an outpatient setting, so there are no hospital or room charges to consider. Ancillary services such as imaging, phlebotomy, and physical therapy are contracted at a rate of $75 per patient, $50 per patient, and $125 per patient, respectively. Direct clinical staffing (physician, nurse) is $235 per patient. All patients receive all three of the ancillary services.
- Eastside Clinic pays $75,000 annually for office space rental. All healthcare services are provided in an outpatient setting, so there are no hospital or room charges to consider. Ancillary services such as imaging, phlebotomy, and physical therapy are contracted at a rate of $70 per patient, $50 per patient, and $150 per patient, respectively. Direct clinical staffing (physician, nurse) is $210 per patient. All patients receive imaging and phlebotomy services, but only 50% of patients receive physical therapy.
- Downtown Clinic pays $85,000 annually for office space rental. All healthcare services are provided in an outpatient setting, so there are no hospital or room charges to consider. Ancillary

services such as imaging and phlebotomy are contracted at a rate of $125 per patient and $75 per patient, respectively. Direct clinical staffing (physician, nurse) is $265 per patient. Approximately 75% of patients receive imaging services and all patients receive phlebotomy services. The Downtown Clinic does not provide/offer physical therapy services.

a. If annual patient visits for each location are estimated to be 1,800 patients and current reimbursement is $875 per patient, which of the three clinics has the highest profit?

b. If insurance reimbursement rates are renegotiated and revenue per patient increases to $950 per patient, how much additional profit will each clinic earn?

CHAPTER 4 CASE: THE PRICE IS RIGHT! OR IS IT?

A healthcare financial advisory firm has hired you as a financial consultant and you've just been assigned to your first client, a large healthcare system. The system includes several hospitals, outpatient facilities, and suppliers, as well as multiple subsidiaries. The financial picture for the system has grown to be quite complex, and the leadership team now seeks a professional analysis of its operations. Specifically, they want you to analyze key components such as labor/salary and wage information, expenses, patient volume, and revenues to determine if they are charging enough to meet their financial goals. The leadership team has supplied the most recent 9 months of data, which will provide you with a clear picture of how things are going so far this fiscal year.

Staffing

The healthcare system is a full-service entity, offering services for both the adult and pediatric populations, with the ability to provide the required services, supplies, and materials within its network. Some clinicians are contracted (specifically, psychology services and radiology services), but most are full-time employees of the organization, with their base salary and fringe benefits covered by the system. The full-time staff cover multiple specializations (all have inpatient and outpatient capacity) and have varying salaries; however, the associated benefits package is applied at a standard rate of 33% of base salary. Base salaries for each specialization are shown in Table 4.6, with the respective number of full-time equivalents (FTEs).

Table 4.6

FULL-TIME EQUIVALENT AND SALARY DATA

Specialization	# of FTEs	Total Base Salaries (9 mos.)
Internal medicine	55	$9,721,800
Emergency medicine	25	$6,481,875
OB/GYN	15	$3,440,250
Cardiology	7	$2,443,875
Nursing	125	$8,586,563
Urology	5	$1,454,438
Orthopedic	10	$3,877,500
Anesthesiology	12	$3,717,900
Pulmonology	7	$1,523,813
Neurology	12	$3,253,500
Pediatrics	17	$3,114,315

FTEs, full-time equivalents.

Expenses

The nonsalary data expenses incurred by the healthcare system are the same as those incurred by any other similarly sized organizations and include items for the inpatient facilities/hospitals, outpatient clinics, and items utilized for homecare services. Nonsalary expenses for consideration are reflected in Table 4.7.

Table 4.7

NONSALARY EXPENSE DATA

Expense Type	Total Expense (9 mos.)
Medical supplies	$10,294,159
Surgical supplies	$5,661,975
Office rent	$93,750
Utilities	$50,887
Housekeeping supplies	$30,000
Equipment maintenance	$262,500
Contracted services	$131,250
Transportation—patient	$18,750
Transportation—employee shuttle	$11,250

Patient Volume

The healthcare system's patient volume for the last 9 months is shown in Table 4.8 and includes all inpatient and outpatient visits. The data is aggregated by visit type, instead of clinical

Table 4.8

PATIENT VOLUME DATA

	Jul-22	Aug-22	Sep-22	Oct-22	Nov-22	Dec-22	Jan-23	Feb-23	Mar-23
Medical inpatient days	19,586	18,607	17,676	16,793	18,472	20,319	22,351	20,786	19,331
Surgical inpatient days	881	893	859	995	918	885	893	838	967
Outpatient visits	3,589	3,410	3,239	3,077	3,385	3,723	4,096	3,809	3,542
Total discharges	4,498	4,273	4,059	3,856	4,242	4,666	5,133	4,774	4,440
Outpatient ancillary	2,984	2,835	2,693	2,558	2,814	3,096	3,405	3,167	2,945
Total patient activity	31,538	30,017	28,527	27,280	29,831	32,689	35,878	33,374	31,225
Total licensed beds	750	750	750	750	750	750	750	750	750
Occupancy rate	88.03%	83.87%	82.38%	76.51%	86.18%	91.20%	99.97%	102.97%	87.30%
Average length of stay (days)	4.55	4.56	4.57	4.61	4.57	4.54	4.53	4.53	4.57

specialization or facility location. The data table shows the distribution of visits monthly as well as the corresponding occupancy rate and average length of stay (for inpatient capacity).

Total discharges in this data represent the number of discharges for both medical and surgical inpatient activity. Outpatient ancillary patient volume represents outpatient visits from services outside of the hospital setting, such as physical and occupational therapy, speech and language therapy, substance abuse treatment, homecare and wound care services, and behavioral health and imaging services.

Current Fee Schedule

The current fee schedule for services offered by the healthcare system are shown in Table 4.9.

Table 4.9

FEE SCHEDULE DATA

Service Type	Per Service
Standard outpatient visit	$500
Ancillary outpatient visit	$250
Inpatient stay	$3,500
amount or fees applied to each discharge	

Using the data provided for this case, determine if the current fee schedule provides adequate revenue for the healthcare system. As you do this, be sure to answer the following:

1. Calculate the remaining monthly and annualized salary for each clinical specialization, and the grand total for all clinician salaries and wages.

2. Calculate the annualized totals for each of the nonsalary expenses.

3. Calculate the annualized patient volume data for each item shown in Table 4.8.

4. Calculate revenue using the annualized data for the items shown in the fee schedule.

5. Does the healthcare system generate enough revenue to cover its salary and nonsalary expenses? If there is an excess, what is the remaining profit?

6. Are there trends evident in the patient volume data?

7. How would you interpret the occupancy rate and how might the occupancy rate impact the healthcare system's revenue?

MICROSOFT EXCEL: LET'S PRACTICE

This first chapter in Module II of the textbook begins the ongoing healthcare financial analysis purview of this text and our work for this course. All of the Practice Problems and the case study can be done using Microsoft Excel® to hone students' skills with the software. Why is Microsoft Excel used throughout the lessons of this textbook? There are many accounting and finance software packages used by healthcare organizations today, with some being customized or specifically designed for the organization and some being standard or basic packages off-the-shelf. Microsoft Excel is used as the common thread between them all, due to its ease of configuration and analysis. Most software packages today are designed to import data from spreadsheets or "roll data up" into the system, as well as export system data or "download" data into an Excel spreadsheet. This allows accounting and finance professionals to share information with those who do not have routine access to the system. An example of this would be budget season, when nonfinancial managers are responsible for reviewing their department's actual performance to use as a basis or benchmark for estimates and projections. The managers often receive an Excel spreadsheet containing their department's historical data. The revised spreadsheet containing their estimates and projections is then returned to the finance department, then rolled up into the system for inclusion in the organization's consolidated budget.

To begin our Excel practice, we'll use the data provided for the Chapter 4 case, The Price Is Right! Or Is It? The data tables used for case analysis include a myriad of data entry and formatting changes, all of which will help students become familiar with the Excel software. After reviewing the Microsoft Excel® Reference Guide (provided in the Appendices):

1. Open the Microsoft Excel program and create/save a workbook titled "Chapter 4 Case Study Data Analysis."

2. Create and label three worksheets within the workbook, one for each data table (staffing/salary and wage, expenses, patient volume).

3. Recreate the Full-Time Equivalent and Salary Data (Table 4.6), Nonsalary Expense Data (Table 4.7), and Patient Volume Data (Table 4.8) tables as shown for the case study. Be sure to duplicate the shading and formatting as shown in the tables and place each table in its own spreadsheet within your workbook.

4. Once the tables have been duplicated, expand the tables using the required basic functions to calculate the annualized figures and analyses required for the case. Be sure to add both monthly totals and annual totals using basic Excel functions.

HEALTHCARE FINANCE COURSE PROJECT: SETUP

After reviewing the Microsoft Excel basics and the background information for the course project, it's time to set up the project workbook. Be sure to set your computer to Auto-Save or save your file regularly to avoid losing data!

Step 1: Create and save a workbook, using your last name and the name of your healthcare organization to be used for the duration of the project (Example: Smith—Smith General Hospital).

Step 2: Create and label a worksheet within your workbook for each item listed in the "Course Project: Excel Workbook Setup" section of Chapter 16.

Step 3: For each worksheet created within your workbook, add a title block/title section as required for financial reporting, using the example shown in the "Course Project: Excel Workbook Setup" section of Chapter 16 (can be left-justified or centered; can be changed later).

CHAPTER 5

General Ledger Categorization and Recording Transactions

1. Understand the accounting equation and its categories.
2. Understand the accounting cycle in the context of healthcare organizations and related activities.
3. Properly categorize debits and credits as required for basic accounting bookkeeping.
4. Categorize assets, liabilities, and equity appropriately according to basic accounting rules.
5. Prepare supporting documents (ledgers, worksheets, etc.) for the accounting close process.

INTRODUCTION

Chapter 4 (the beginning of Module II) introduced the types of accounting and the compliance regulations that govern accounting and finance activities. One of the ways an organization maintains its compliance is by keeping very detailed, accurate financial records. This ensures that everything is being done according to industry regulation, while capturing the important elements of the business. Formal recordkeeping allows the organization to analyze financial performance over time and adjust where necessary to meet its goals and objectives for strategic planning. Many daily decisions are based on financial information, even if we don't realize the connection to the larger-scale accounting information. Office supply purchases, payment for deliveries, or copayments received for an office visit are all examples of daily activities that tie back into the accounting data in some way. Financial information is not only important for internal leadership and decision makers, but for the organization's external stakeholders as well. Aside from the required financial reporting and disclosures, sound financial performance is one of the ways an organization shows market value, which is used for industry/competitive positioning and creditor assessment. In a sector as large as healthcare, this information provides the basis for potential investments in nonprofits, credit lines for supply chain contracts, or partnership in an integrated healthcare delivery system. All transactions must be captured and categorized in the healthcare organization's financial statements that begin with the accounting equation.

THE ACCOUNTING EQUATION

Accounting summarizes the financial position of the organization, which can be represented by the accounting equation. The **accounting equation** summarizes all facets of the company's financial activity and states them in terms of three broad categories, as shown in Table 5.1.

Table 5.1
THE ACCOUNTING EQUATION
Assets = Liability + Equity

Assets are items of economic value that are owned by the organization. These may include cash, equipment, property, supplies and inventory, trademarks, or patents that the organization has paid for and is in possession of that are expected to be of use or benefit in the future. Healthcare assets include medical supplies, purchased equipment or machinery, and facilities used to conduct patient visits or secure additional assets. Organizations such as pharmaceutical companies or research and development companies may hold trademarks or patents on medications or medical devices, which give them great value for market and competitor positioning. **Liabilities** are debts owed by the organization to creditors. These may include loans, notes payable, or any other accounts payable item. For healthcare organizations, this could be balances owed to suppliers, mortgage payments for purchased land or medical facilities, or possibly wages owed to employees. Liabilities represent outflows of cash payments in the shorter or longer term. **Equity** represents the net worth of the organization, or the remaining assets after all liabilities are paid. Table 5.2 lists examples of the accounts that may be included in each category of the accounting equation. The accounts may vary by organization, dependent upon their financial standing or their product or industry within the healthcare sector. These are just examples, realizing that some organizations may have many more categories and supporting accounts.

Ideally, a company will have more assets than liabilities for sound financial positioning. Positive equity usually indicates that the organization manages its accounts correctly, with stable operations and effective decision-making. Many healthcare organizations are not-for-profit or nonprofit organizations not publicly traded in the financial markets, and will therefore have no shareholders with stock or ownership in the organization. Instead, they will have stakeholders who have an interest in the overall success of the organization. Stakeholders are the community members, including citizens and patients, who collaborate for the organization's short-term and longer-term stability and success. In for-profit organizations, the equity section may include shareholder dividends and payouts, or purchase and sales of stock. Further discussion of assets and liabilities is included in Chapter 6 within the context of the financial statements and related analyses. Let's have a look at how the accounting system and the recorded activity keeps things balanced.

TRANSACTION BASICS: DEBITS AND CREDITS

Accounting transactions capture incoming as well as outgoing financial activity, with all information recorded as entries into the accounting system. Routine operating activities such as salaries, purchases, rentals, marketing, product sales, patient visits, insurance reimbursement, and

Table 5.2

ACCOUNTING EQUATION CATEGORIES AND ACCOUNTS

Account Name	Account Description
Asset Accounts	
Cash	Bank balances; money coming into and out of the organization
AR	Payments received
FF&Es	FF&Es owned and/or used by employees/providers; leased assets
Buildings/Land	Patient care buildings; warehouses/storage
Prepaids	Items paid in advance
Notes receivables/Accrued receivables	Promises to pay (patients/customers); contracts
Liability Accounts	
Accounts payable	Credit purchases to be paid
Loans/Lease payments	Outstanding debts/borrowed money
Notes payable/Accrued expenses	Promises to pay (healthcare organization)
Salaries	Employee wages and benefits
Utilities (and other monthly items)	Electricity, gas, and so forth
Unearned revenue	Payments received before goods/services are delivered
Equity (Owner's Equity)	
Capital	Shareholder's/Owner's contributions
Withdrawals	Withdrawals/Payments to owners

AR, accounts receivable; FF&Es, furniture, fixtures, and equipment.

so forth, are documented meticulously in the accounting system. All entries must be posted to the correct account (asset, liability, or equity, as noted in the accounting equation) and the accounts must remain balanced. To ensure balance, accounting systems are designed for double entry, with every transaction impacting at least two accounts. The two entries, one showing an increase to an account and the second showing a decrease to an account, are **debits** and **credits.** We often see this represented visually as the basic "**T-account**," with debits on the left side and credits on the right side. The debits and credits for every financial transaction must balance, or cancel each other out, with the resulting increase or decrease dependent on the type of account. Determining if a debit entry or a credit entry is needed to increase the account value depends on the normal balance of that account. The normal balances outline the behavior of the accounts, and become the entry required to increase it. A snapshot of account balances and associated behaviors are reflected in Table 5.3 to provide guidance on when to increase or decrease each type of account.

With so many transactions happening simultaneously, the normal balance helps establish a standard for each account type. The standard categorization of accounts is put in place when the accounting system is designed, with the ability to create additional accounts as needed. The accounting standards outline the following rules for assigning debits and credits to various accounts:

1. Debit the amounts coming in and credit the amounts going out.
2. Debit expense accounts and credit income accounts.
3. Debit the receiving account and credit the giving account.

Table 5.3

DEBIT AND CREDIT BALANCES GUIDE (INCREASES AND DECREASES)

	Normal Balances Guide		
Account Type	Normal Balance	To Increase, Record As	To Decrease, Record As
Assets	Debit	Debit	Credit
Liabilities	Credit	Credit	Debit
Equity	Credit	Credit	Debit
Revenues	Credit	Credit	Debit
Expenses	Debit	Debit	Credit

These rules are applied across account types as well as within account types, as items or values are transferred from one account to another. These may seem counterintuitive, but they work together to maintain balance of the accounting equation. Remember that the categories in the accounting equation have subaccounts to record activity for specific functions within the organization and could therefore be shown as multiple debits and credits for a single transaction. The system structure is static, with the core account classifications remaining the same every accounting period. Asset and expense accounts are increased by a debit entry and decreased by a credit entry. Liability, equity, and revenue accounts are increased by a credit entry and decreased by a debit entry. The key is to accurately determine where the funds are coming from and where the funds are going. If items are posted to the incorrect account, corrections can be made during the accounting cycle. However, as with any other change or update to the system, they have to be properly documented. For clarity, let's review the following examples for varying account types and entries.

BOX 5.1

Rule #1 (Debit Incoming, Credit Outgoing)

Community Hospital is expanding and needs additional equipment for its imaging department. To avoid long-term payments, the hospital seeks donations from its current partners and stakeholders. MediCore, a long-standing contributor, has donated $50,000 in cash for the equipment purchase.

Account Name	Debit	Credit
Cash	$50,000	
MediCore		$50,000
OR		
Account Name	Debit	Credit
Cash	$25,000	
Equipment	$25,000	
MediCore		$50,000

In the example of Rule #1 (shown in Box 5.1), the (incoming) donation will be applied to Community Hospital's asset account as a debit, coming from the MediCore account (outgoing) applied as a credit. In the first part of the example, the entire donation is applied to the cash account (an asset account), where it will stay until the purchase is made or until additional donations are received. In the second part of the example, the donation is split between two asset accounts, representing an equipment purchase posted to the equipment account and the remaining donation amount in the cash account. For a double-entry accounting system, there must be a minimum of two entries for each financial transaction (one debit entry and one credit entry), but it can include multiple entries to accurately reflect the breakdown and entry of the full transaction amount. Both T-accounts in the Box 5.1 donation example are permitted, as long as the debits and credits for the adjusted accounts are balanced, canceling out to zero. Accrual amounts are also included in the debit and credit entries, capturing activities at the time they are incurred but not finalized. Goods sold or services provided would be accrued if payments have not yet been received. Another example is the purchase of medical equipment by a provider, but with a check or payment that has not yet been processed by the supplier. All activities that have been initiated during the current accounting period but will not be finalized until the next accounting period must be included as accrual entries during the current accounting cycle and financial close period.

BOX 5.2

Rule #2 (Debit Expense, Credit Income)

Account Name	Debit	Credit
Salary expense	$100,000	
Patient services revenue		$100,000

OR

Account Name	Debit	Credit
Salary expense	$75,000	
Contracted labor	$25,000	
Patient services revenue		$100,000

In the scenario for Rule #2 (shown in Box 5.2), $100,000 in patient services revenue was received as payment for services rendered. The salary expense can be entered as one consolidated figure as shown in the first part of the example or entered to reflect internal/employee salary expense and contracted/agency expense as shown in the second part of the example. Patient services revenue would also have subaccounts and could show the $100,000 split by payer. Medicare, Medicaid, and commercial insurance plans are often represented individually to track the payer mix, which details the coverage and reimbursement percentages for each payer. Keep in mind that this salary example is indicative of personnel who are directly linked to revenue generation, not indirect or administrative personnel.

In the example for Rule #3 (shown in Box 5.3), cash is used as payment for outstanding loan balances or notes payable. Here, the liability accounts are receiving the payments and the asset account is giving the payment. Auto loans and bank loans are just two types of liability accounts; others include salaries, supply purchases, raw materials, subcontracting, or other accounts payable items that are considered short-term or current obligations.

BOX 5.3

Rule #3 (Debit Receiving, Credit Giving)

Account Name	Debit	Credit
Notes payable	$100,000	
Cash payments		$100,000

OR

Account Name	Debit	Credit
Auto loan	$50,000	
Bank loan	$50,000	
Cash payments		$100,000

THE GENERAL LEDGER AND THE ACCOUNTING CYCLE

Every part of an organization's routine operations is captured in some way in the accounting data. Collecting and organizing this data requires a defined process with built-in checks and balances, as well as a meticulous time schedule. The **accounting cycle,** as outlined in Figure 5.1, is the process that guides this data collection and organization effort. This basic framework is present in some form in most organizations. The accounting cycle is completed every **accounting period**, which in most cases is monthly, with consolidated activity processed quarterly and annually.

Figure 5.1

The accounting cycle

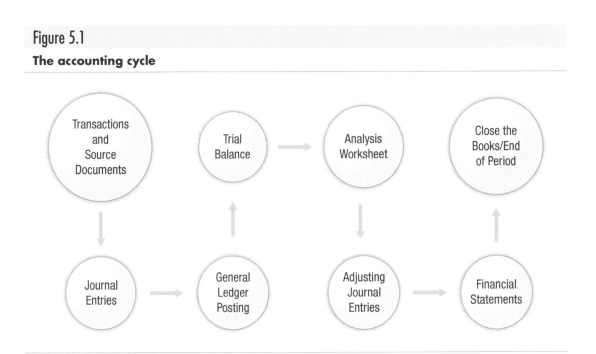

The entire process begins with the initial activities that drive the organization, the transaction. A **transaction** is the interaction between providers and consumers—the sale and/or purchase of a good or service. In healthcare, the transaction is the provision of care, the purchase of a medication, or the leasing of medical care devices. The office visit, healthcare procedure, purchase of equipment, and so forth, launches the accounting and finance activity for the organization. There is a detailed process for getting the organization's transactions to the final published financial statements, which all begins with the chart of accounts and the general journal. The **chart of accounts** is a numbering system that organizes the accounts and types of transactions specific to the organization. The accounts are listed as they would be shown in the financial statements, with each account providing structure for the related subaccounts. This system of organization helps the accounting professionals manage all of the routine accounting activity, which is the foundation for so many other systems and reporting functions. The **general journal** is a listing of all transactions as evidenced by the **source documents**. Source documents in accounting are the actual evidence of the transaction—receipts, invoices, purchase orders, checks received, cash payments, and so forth. The **journal entries** are listed chronologically and are applied to at least two accounts, one as a debit and one as a credit. The purpose of this double-entry accounting system is to ensure that the debits and credits have the same total, balancing the accounting equation. The accounting journal will often have supporting journals, which are specific to the types of transactions captured. For example, larger organizations may have payroll, accounts receivable (AR), or cash supporting subjournals to organize transactions before transfer to the main accounting journal. These are often reconciled first to reduce the number of errors in the main accounting journal. Upon review and reconciliation of all journal entries, the information is organized by account in the **general ledger** (GL).

The GL is the summary of all account activity, which includes all journal entries as well as the account balances. Accounts included in the GL include asset and liability accounts, income and expense accounts, and capital and investment accounts. The GL is organized by account type and contains the detailed information relevant to the account: account number, account name, account balances, and other information from the chart of accounts. After everything has been transferred to the GL, a **trial balance** is run to review the account balances to assess the debit and credit totals. If entered correctly, all accounts will have a zero balance, as the corresponding debits and credits cancel each other out. Any accounts that do not have a zero balance will have to be adjusted to ensure balance. The trial balance does not contain detailed transaction or account information like the GL, only the account balances.

The remaining steps in the accounting cycle focus on the analysis and correction of postings, ensuring balance within accounts. The **analysis worksheet** is a spreadsheet created to reconcile the account debits and credits. The reconciliation process reviews all of the debits and credits posted and compares them with the source documents to ensure accuracy. This process can be done by account, service line, or project, which may have additional guidelines for utilization, timing, and allowability (specifically for grants and contracts). Any discrepancies found in the GL are corrected by reversing the incorrect journal entry, then making **adjusting journal entries** and rerunning or recalculating the GL. Adjusting journal entries correct the financial records by inserting any revenues or expenses previously unrecognized (or applied) such as accruals, deferred items, or prepaid items. These are transactions that were begun when the current accounting period was being closed but will not be finalized until the next accounting period. After all adjusting entries have been identified and corrections have been posted to the GL, another trial balance is run to check the account balances and to ensure that the adjustments were entered properly, with all accounts being reconciled. The **financial statements** are then created to reflect all of the activity for the reporting period (the financial statements and the line items and accounts included in each are discussed in Chapter 6). The financial statements summarize all business activity for the reporting period, and often show these results in comparison to the previous period. The key financial statements are the income statement (often called the statement of operations), balance sheet, statement of cash flows, and change in equity statement. Each statement conveys different information with data often presented in its consolidated form, to show all affiliated entities (parent and subsidiaries) as one unified organization.

At the end of the reporting period, the accounts are taken to zero to "close the books" in preparation for the next accounting cycle, typically in 5 days (or more, depending on complexity and accounting staffing levels). The categories of accounts remain the same, with all activity in the new accounting period being entered into the system under the appropriate accounts using accrual accounting methodology. These activities are processed on the financial accounting side of the department, with the resulting financial statements beginning the analyses performed by the finance side of the department. The fiscal year is the 12-month period of performance included in the organization's accounting, tax, budgeting, and financial recording process, and may not be the same as the calendar year. Most companies have a July to June fiscal year (nonprofits), with the federal fiscal year being October to September.

GRANT ACCOUNTING

Depending on the structure and services offered, some healthcare organizations rely on traditional funding as well as grant funding. **Grants** are gifts to an organization and can take the form of money or other valuable items that support the overall mission or possibly a specific purpose. Many healthcare organizations are nonprofit or research-driven, receiving a large portion of their operational funding from grants. Grant accounting follows the standard accounting process but may include additional steps during the accounting cycle that require special attention for documentation and reporting. To capture the additional requirements, the grant will have different GL account numbers separate from the standing accounts. For example, if a hospital receives a grant for community heart health education, all revenues and expenses associated with the grant will be recorded separately. If the grant or program has a dedicated team of clinicians and health educators, the salary and wage expenses will be applied to the grant accounts instead of the hospital's regular salary and wage expense accounts. The grant may also have requirements for the timing and utilization of the funding, which must also be documented properly. Items within the stated requirements are considered allowable, while those outside of these requirements are deemed unallowable and cannot be posted to the grant accounts. If the grant specifically states that the funds can only be used for the community heart health education project, then no other programs or initiatives can use this **restricted funding**. If the grant states that the funds may be applied to any program at the discretion of the hospital leadership, these **unrestricted funds** can be allocated as needed. Restricted funds may become unrestricted funds if the grant requirements are only in effect for a specified time. Any items not covered by the grant must be covered by the organization's other funding. Recording items in this way allows the accountants to capture the information in the usual accounting process for organization-level analysis as well as for grant-level analysis and subsequent reporting.

DEPRECIATION

Another part of the organization's financial health is the routine monitoring of assets and other items of value as captured in the financial statements. The accounting and finance professionals keep a watchful eye on the resources that make revenue generation possible, recording the changes in value over the life span of the asset. **Depreciation** is the decrease in an asset's value over time, allowing the organization to incur the lost value gradually instead of all at once. Larger assets such as costly medical equipment or high-tech machinery would hold value longer due to maintenance but may still depreciate rapidly because of technological advancements and improved, newer models. Traditional depreciation methods include the declining balance method, unit of production method, and sum of year's digits method, but the most common method for calculating depreciation in the healthcare sector is the straight-line method. The straight-line depreciation method can be calculated using the formula presented in Table 5.4.

Table 5.4
STRAIGHT-LINE DEPRECIATION CALCULATION
(Asset Purchase Price – Salvage Value) / Life Span

There are several factors that influence the variables in this equation, ultimately impacting the depreciation amount. Asset purchase price is the initial amount paid for the asset, excluding supplies and maintenance contracts (which are captured separately). Salvage value is the amount you would receive if selling the equipment at the end of its life span. The life span of the asset is its useful life, or how long the equipment can generate revenue. All of these vary and are based on utilization, maintenance, and advancements in technology. The higher the utilization, the greater the "wear and tear" on the equipment. The longer the life span, the greater the initial purchase price, as well as the salvage value.

CHAPTER SUMMARY

The accounting cycle captures and summarizes the historical data for the organization, examining its past performance. It provides the foundation for the budgeting cycle and financial planning cycle, assisting with the short-term and long-term goals, as well as the strategies implemented to achieve them. Although accounting and finance professionals approach the analysis of this historical data very differently, the soundness and completeness of this information is equally important to both. All areas within the organization contribute to the accounting and finance data, even if they are unaware of how exactly they do so. The timing of the accounting cycle is extremely important for reporting and decision-making purposes, as well as efforts to improve effectiveness and efficiency.

KEY TERMS FOR REVIEW

accounting cycle	analysis worksheet	debit
accounting equation	assets	depreciation
accounting period	chart of accounts	equity
adjusting journal entries	credit	financial statements

general journal	liabilities	transaction
general ledger	restricted funding	trial balance
grants	source documents	unrestricted funds
journal entries	T-account	

DISCUSSION QUESTIONS

1. What is the accounting equation? Define the types of items that are included in the accounting equation elements.

2. Define debits and credits. Discuss their importance to the accounting and finance functions.

3. Outline the accounting cycle. Explain how the various stages of the accounting cycle are interdependent, as well as their impact on the accounting period.

4. Give examples of activities that would be considered transactions. What types of source documents would be generated by the transactions identified?

5. What is the relationship between the chart of accounts and the GL?

6. What stages in the accounting cycle are used to reconcile the account balances or make corrections?

7. List the key financial statements. How might the financial statements be impacted by erroneous accounting data?

PRACTICE PROBLEMS

Answers to this chapter's Practice Problems are available via Springer Publishing Connect™ by following the instructions on the opening page of this book and accessing Answers to Practice Problems on the Table of Contents.

1. Community Hospital owes MediCore $5,000 for imaging equipment and associated supplies (film, contrast materials, etc.). The shipment has been received, but Community Hospital hasn't sent the payment yet. Is the amount owed an asset or a liability?

2. The left-side of a T-account is the:
   a. Liabilities
   b. Credit side
   c. Debit side
   d. Equity side

3. At the end of the third quarter of the fiscal year, Community Hospital recorded debit entries of $12,000 and recorded credit entries of $9,500. All of the journal entries were posted to AR. The final AR balance will be:
   a. $21,500 total balance
   b. $2,500 equity balance
   c. $2,500 debit balance
   d. $9,500 credit balance

4. For each accounting equation scenario listed as a to e in Table 5.5, calculate the missing value and discuss what each equation may mean for an organization's financial position.

Table 5.5

THE ACCOUNTING EQUATION—MISSING VALUES

	Assets	Liabilities	Equity
a.	$75,000	?	$50,000
b.	?	$10,000	$35,000
c.	$100,000	$30,000	?
d.	$50,000	?	$50,000
e.	$25,000	$25,000	?

5. Which of the following items is NOT an asset?

   a. Prepaid expenses
   b. Accrued receivables
   c. Furniture and equipment
   d. Unearned revenue

6. Create T-accounts for the following transactions:

   a. Salaries paid in the amount of $75,000
   b. Surgical supplies bought with the company credit card, in the amount of $1,500
   c. Patient copayments received in the amount of $7,000
   d. Donations received from investors, in the amount of $25,000
   e. An approved staffing agency contract, for the amount of $65,000

7. Create the general journal for the transactions given in Problem 6. Be sure to follow the transaction rules as outlined in the chapter and use the standard general journal table format provided in Table 5.6.

Table 5.6

GENERAL JOURNAL ENTRIES

General Journal

Date	Account Title	Debit	Credit

8. Pantheon Health System has the following account information (see Table 5.7) to be contained in its GL.

Table 5.7

PANTHEON GENERAL LEDGER DATA

Accounts payable	$30,000	Patient service revenue	$50,000
Accounts receivable	$25,000	Prepaids	$45,000
Agency/Contract staffing	$40,000	Salaries and wages	$50,000
Cash receipts (copays)	$2,000	Utilities	$3,000
Office supplies	$750		

a. Prepare a trial balance to determine if the accounts/financial records are in balance.
b. Create any adjusting journal entries needed to balance the financial records by applying the amount of the imbalance equally to accounts payable and agency staffing.

CHAPTER 5 CASE: WHOSE LINE IS IT ANYWAY?

Central University Health System (CUHS), the largest health system in your state, is comprised of several hospitals, clinics, and specialty centers of excellence. The mission of the system is centered on the improved overall health of the state's citizens, as well as creating an expansive integrated healthcare system focused on efficient healthcare delivery and health education initiatives. University-based health systems receive traditional funding, but largely rely on grants received for academic research. Grant accounting and recordkeeping often involve strict funds allocation and utilization, which are both time-bound and purpose-bound. As an accountant with CUHS, you've just begun the monthly accounting cycle and close process, and you just received an email from the health education and promotion (HEP) department's new manager. The manager identified several transactions for the department but is unsure of which items are to be charged to the regular department's accounts and which are to be charged to the community education program (CEP) grant accounts. You ask for a copy of the grant documents so you can be sure of the requirements and limitations pertinent to the allocation of grant funds.

To get this all sorted out, you must review each transaction for the department, as well as the other line items you're responsible for, and post them to the general journal (for review and subsequent posting to the GL). The CUHS chart of accounts is organized by account category and is represented by the numbering convention provided in Table 5.8.

Table 5.8

CUHS CHART OF ACCOUNTS

Account Category	Account Number	Account Name
Asset	10010	Cash
Asset	10020	Accounts receivable
Asset	10030	Checking account
Asset	10031	Savings account
Asset	10040	Medical equipment
Asset	10041	Office equipment
Asset	10050	Inventory (on-site)
Liability	20010	Payroll (accrued)
Liability	20020	Accounts payable
Liability	20030	Loans
Liability	20031	Notes payable
Liability	20032	Credit balances
Liability	20040	Bank fees
Liability	20050	Deferred revenue
Equity	30010	Capital
Equity	30020	Dividends to owners
Equity	30030	Withdrawals by owners
Revenue	40010	Patient services revenue
Revenue	40020	Product sales
Revenue	40030	Cafeteria sales
Revenue	40040	Gift shop sales
Revenue	40050	Parking revenue
Revenue	40060	Contributions and donations
Revenue	40070	Grants
Expense	50010	Salary and wages
Expense	50020	Office space rental
Expense	50021	Utilities
Expense	50030	Agency labor
Expense	50040	Medical supplies
Expense	50041	Office supplies
Expense	50050	Transportation/Fleet

CUHS, Central University Health System.

The transactions from the HEP department that need to be properly posted are listed in Table 5.9. Use the traditional general journal format for the postings, since no account balances are given in this scenario. Any items not clearly marked for the grant should be applied to the CUHS main accounts. All work should be done using Microsoft Excel®.

Table 5.9

GENERAL JOURNAL TRANSACTION LIST

04/01/22	The following items were received from DHS for CEP start-up: $100,000 for three mobile clinics (vans), $40,000 for medical screening equipment, and $10,000 for computers and office supplies.
04/01/22	Payments received from private insurers (combined payers), $1,000,000.
04/05/22	Purchased CEP computers and office supplies, $7,000.
04/07/22	Purchased CUHS computers and office supplies, $5,000.
04/15/22	Received DHS funding for part-time CEP staff, $250,000.
04/15/22	Biweekly salary and wages, $750,000.
04/17/22	Rent community center space for CEP information sessions.
04/22/22	Paid RN To Go for agency nursing, $5,000.
04/22/22	Signed mobile clinic lease agreements and paid for the first 6 months, $60,000.
04/30/22	Biweekly salary and wages, $750,000.
05/01/22	Recorded cash from patient copays, $2,500.
05/01/22	Payments received from private insurers (combined payers), $500,000.
05/01/22	CEP staff start, $25,000.
05/10/22	Purchased CEP medical screening equipment, $37,500.
05/15/22	Paid gas, electric, and water bills, $2,500.
05/15/22	Signed 6-month agreement with oxygen tank supplier, $3,000.
05/15/22	Biweekly salary and wages, $750,000.
05/15/22	Biweekly salary and wages CEP, $25,000.
05/31/22	Recorded cafeteria sales, $5,000.
05/31/22	Recorded parking garage receipts, $7,000.

CEP, community education program; CUHS, Central University Health System; DHS, District Health Society.

HEALTHCARE FINANCE COURSE PROJECT: BEGIN PHASE I

The course project walks students through the calculations for various phases of a new healthcare service implementation. SurgiFlex is the new robotic surgical service being introduced at a local hospital, with the financial calculations completed in three distinct phases:

- Phase I: SurgiFlex Calculations

- Phase II: Organization-Level Calculations

- Phase III: Financial Statement Creation and Analysis

The first phase of the course project introduces the students to zero-based budgeting and the foundational elements of healthcare financial management. Healthcare finance begins with the "patient encounter," introduced in Phase I as SurgiFlex utilization data (surgical cases). The surgical case volume drives the surgical team labor expense (workload calculation using hourly rate and worked hours), related revenue (multiple payers), supply expense, and breakeven analysis. Review the "Course Project: Phase I: SurgiFlex Robotic Surgery System Calculations" section of Chapter 16, which contains all of the relevant information and data for completion of the course project. Phase I begins with Worksheet #1 (SurgiFlex Surgical Data) and ends with Worksheet #6 (Supply Vendor Analysis Calculations). Worksheet #1 is the starting point for the course project's calculations, and must be created to reflect the data provided in Exhibit 16A.1.

CHAPTER 6

Financial Statements Analysis, Benchmarking, and Decision-Making

1. Discuss the components of the financial statements and distinguish between the reporting purposes of each.

2. Categorize various types of financial activity into the appropriate financial statement.

3. Examine how an organization's financial performance impacts both short-term and long-term decision-making and strategic planning.

4. Understand the performance measurement process and how the results may frame process improvement.

5. Explain the differences between performance measurement and performance management.

INTRODUCTION

All elements of business operations are captured in some form during routine data collection and reporting. There are several systems in place to accomplish this, and the types of data collected for each department will vary. Previous chapters detail the accounting cycle and related analyses, which consolidate the organization's activities for a given period of time. Together, the statements provide a clear picture of financial health, operational stability, industry performance, potential profitability, and longer-term viability and success (Healthcare Financial Management Association [HFMA], 2021; Menaker et al., 2020). While the organization's mission and purpose are the initial reasons for support, the financial health of the organization is the second most common measure considered by stakeholders for determining support and potential financial investment. The various statements reflect different information and are therefore useful to stakeholders (and shareholders, in for-profit organizations) for different purposes. Internally, financial statement data act as indicators of organizational performance and the direct result of leadership's decision-making. Externally, financial statement data helps investors or potential investors decide if their relationship with the organization should continue. The statement of operations (also called the income statement or statement of profits and losses), balance sheet (also called the statement of financial position), statement of cash flows, and statement of changes in assets (also called the statement of shareholder's equity) are the statements used by most healthcare organizations, which may vary depending on service lines and nature of ownership. Activities captured in the financial statements and supporting reports are categorized depending on how they impact the organization and the achievement of its mission. The statements include data on the inflow and utilization of valued items and revenue-generating resources, as well as the outflow and investment of cash and other major capital. One thing to note is that every department or division within the organization contributes in some way to the items represented in the financial statements, even if they are not directly connected to patient care services or product sales. The examples provided in the following sections show consolidated statements, which include the activity for the parent organization as well as the subsidiaries and affiliates. Even if each organization within the system provides a different service or product, they ultimately work together to meet the needs of the population served and the overarching mission of the entire system. In this chapter, we will examine the general format of the major financial statements, the elements that comprise them, and what they reveal about the organization's financial health and business operations.

INCOME STATEMENT

The **income statement** tells the story of the production of healthcare goods and services, as well as the sale or consumption of the items produced. It reports the organization's activities as specifically related to three categories: revenues, expenses, and profit (excess revenue over expenses), and is often referred to as the statement of operations or the statement of profits and losses (see Figure 6.1 for an example). These categories summarize the organization's financial health and give stakeholders an idea of the organization's ability to generate revenue and minimize or control operating expenses, all while maintaining the effectiveness and efficiency of routine patient care operations. In the income statement, all incoming and outgoing financial transactions are captured, driven by patient activity or healthcare supply needs provided by the company.

Revenue is the income generated from the sale of healthcare goods and services. In healthcare organizations, revenue is typically generated by patient activity and other items related to providing patient care. Hospitals, outpatient health centers, emergency departments, and so forth, generate revenue by seeing the patient and providing necessary healthcare services. Most organizations will have separate accounting line items or categories for inpatient and outpatient activity, because they may require different types of healthcare services. Inpatient revenue captures financial activity of patients staying overnight at the healthcare facility, such as inpatient stays at hospitals, long-term care facilities, skilled nursing facilities, and the like. Outpatient revenue captures financial activities of patients receiving care without being admitted to the hospital. This includes urgent care centers, ambulatory or outpatient surgery centers, rehabilitation services (physical, occupational, and speech therapies), and routine healthcare visits and consultations. Patient revenue, whether inpatient or outpatient, includes monies received from patients, third-party payers, and insurance companies—all funds received to cover patient care. Some healthcare organizations will also have an "other operating revenue" category that captures revenue or sales that are not patient-care driven. Items included in other operating revenue would include gift shop sales, cafeteria sales, visitor parking fees, and so forth. These items are a result of an organization's routine business operations and do not depend on a patient's inpatient or outpatient status.

Expense is the cost of creating the goods and services that are needed to generate revenue, as well as any other outflows of money. When calculating expense, we must consider everything that

Figure 6.1

Income statement (statement of operations)

Pantheon Health System, Subsidiaries, and Affiliates
Consolidated Statements of Operations
Fiscal Years Ended June 30, 2022 and 2021

(In Thousands)

	2022	2021
Revenues:		
Inpatient revenue	$ 2,563,873	$ 2,294,666
Outpatient revenue	$ 1,709,249	$ 1,529,778
Other operating revenue	$ 299,119	$ 267,712
Total revenues	$ 4,572,241	$ 4,092,156
Expenses:		
Wages and fringe benefits	$ 1,508,840	$ 1,403,221
Purchased/contracted services	$ 1,131,630	$ 1,052,416
Supplies and other expenses	$ 497,917	$ 463,063
Interest expense	$ 32,048	$ 29,805
Depreciation and amortization	$ 213,656	$ 198,700
Total expenses	$ 3,384,091	$ 3,147,205
Operating income (loss)	$ 1,188,150	$ 944,951
Nonoperating revenues and expenses:		
Contributions (unrestricted)	$ 3,757	$ 4,020
Marketing expense (brochures and publications)	$ (67)	$ (65)
Investment income	$ 53,047	$ 50,395
Total nonoperating expenses	$ 56,737	$ 54,350
Excess of revenues over (under) expenses	$ 1,131,413	$ 890,601

goes into creating our goods and services, which includes both human and material resources. Salary and wage expense (including fringe benefit coverage) is the amount an organization pays its employees, no matter the department or location. Included in this category are employees who provide direct patient care as well as those in the operations areas who are indirect (human resources department, finance department, customer service, housekeeping, etc.). Contracted labor and purchased services are also considered an expense, and are captured separately from the standard salary and wage category. Contracted labor describes clinical or administrative professionals who are hired contractually for a specified time or purpose. Organizations hire contractual employees when they have increased demand that the scheduled staff cannot cover, or for a specified time frame for operations or events that may not be ongoing. An example on the clinical or patient-care side would be the contracting of additional nurses to provide care for a sudden influx of patients resulting from a natural disaster or public health crisis. On the administrative side, if an employee is out of the office for short-term or long-term medical leave, contractual or temporary staffing could be used to maintain process workflow and department productivity. Supplies and other purchased materials are considered expense, but this does not include larger purchases or items that would be included in the capital budgeting process. Routine office supplies as well as medical supplies would be included in this category (although medical supplies may be categorized by service type at the department or unit level). Interest expense, depreciation, and amortization are also expenses representing outflows of money from the organization. Interest expense is the cost incurred for borrowing money. Lenders (banks, investors, etc.) impose interest (a fee usually represented by a percentage) to be paid back on top of the amount originally borrowed (principal). Interest-based loans include an interest amount to be paid that does not get applied to the principal balance owed. Depreciation is the decrease in asset value, realized over the life span of an asset (Financial Accounting Standards Board [FASB], 2022). An imaging machine, for example, may be purchased for $50,000, but due to heavy utilization or rapid development of upgrades or alternatives, it may decrease in value over its estimated life span. Amortization is the monthly payment of loans or other debts, represented by equal payments over the borrowing period. Amortized loan repayment differs from interest-based loans because a portion of the monthly amount paid is applied to the principal amount borrowed. This decreases, over time, the amount of interest paid over the life of the loan.

Operating income or profit margin is the amount remaining after all operating expenses are covered. Ideally, this would be a positive number (or surplus), indicating that the organization has generated enough revenue to cover all of its expenses. If the operating income is a negative number (or deficit), the organization has incurred more expenses than the amount absorbed by revenue. Since the financial statements are created for each accounting period, usually monthly, a deficit could actually happen if revenues are not received in a timely fashion, or as scheduled. **Nonoperating revenue and expense categories** capture activities that may not occur routinely, or activities that may be unpredictable. Items included in this section of the balance sheet would be contributions, fundraising activities, marketing materials (print or other advertising media), and investment income, which is completely dependent on market performance.

BALANCE SHEET

The **balance sheet** summarizes the healthcare organization's assets and liabilities, showing stakeholders what is owned and what is owed. Items listed in the balance sheet can be purchased using equity (monies already available) or using borrowed funds (debt financing).

An example of a balance sheet is shown in Figure 6.2. Although this is a simple balance sheet, assets and liabilities may in fact have several types, depending on the nature of the organization. **Assets** are items that the organization owns, particularly of worth or economic value. Items included in this category can include cash and cash equivalents, equipment or machinery, inventory, furniture, and buildings. The organizations may also have intangible assets such as patents or trademarks. These items may not have an actual physical presence, but may impact revenue generation in the future through incoming cash flow or value. Assets are categorized in several ways, dependent upon liquidity and purpose. Current assets are items that will be consumed or sold within the current fiscal year, or items that can be liquidated quickly for current or short-term organizational needs. Items included in current assets are cash holdings, prepaid expenses, owned inventory (not leased or consigned), and accounts receivable balances. All of these items can be converted to cash quickly to assist with routine operations and pressing expenses. Noncurrent assets are items that hold value but are used for the longer term.

Figure 6.2

Balance sheet

Pantheon Health System, Subsidiaries, and Affiliates
Consolidated Balance Sheets
Fiscal Years Ended June 30, 2022 and 2021
(In Thousands)

	2022	2021
Assets		
Current assets		
Cash and cash equivalents	$ 756,542	$ 703,267
Accounts receivable (patients)	$ 100,000	$ 100,000
Inventory and supplies	$ 235,000	$ 210,000
Prepaid expenses	$ 75,000	$ 68,000
Short-term investments	$ 145,369	$ 186,322
Total current assets	$ 1,311,911	$ 1,267,589
Investments (long-term)	$ 4,837,510	$ 4,729,581
Property and equipment	$ 2,377,859	$ 2,238,951
Limited-use assets	$ 3,689,512	$ 3,357,628
Fundraising/charity	$ 590,000	$ 341,500
Total assets	$ 12,806,792	$ 11,935,249
Liabilities		
Current liabilities		
Accounts payable	$ 237,381	$ 215,950
Accrued expenses	$ 485,660	$ 480,000
Lease liabilities	$ 325,000	$ 300,000
Lines of credit	$ 125,000	$ 150,000
Total current liabilities	$ 1,173,041	$ 1,145,950
Insurance and pension liability	$ 275,000	$ 250,000
Long-term debt	$ 540,000	$ 585,490
Salvage receipts	$ 1,500,000	$ 1,500,000
Total liabilities	$ 3,488,041	$ 3,481,440
Net assets	$ 9,318,751	$ 8,453,809

Trademarks and patents, property (land, buildings, production facilities, or plant operations), and long-term investments are examples of noncurrent investments.

Liabilities are debts that the organization owes, either for the short term or long term. These financial obligations are outgoing cash flows and have a negative impact on the organization's overall financial position. As with assets, liabilities can be current or noncurrent depending on their due date or anticipated payoff. Current liabilities are items with payment due within the current fiscal year, such as short-term debt, accounts payable, lines of credit, or short-term loans and accrued expenses. Noncurrent liabilities are items with payment due beyond the current fiscal year, and include long-term debt, mortgages, capital leases (often for expensive equipment), and deferred taxes. Remaining assets, after the satisfaction of all liabilities, are net assets or remaining equity. Later chapters will discuss financing options, as decision-making often includes the comparison of equity financing and debt financing.

STATEMENT OF CHANGES IN NET ASSETS (OR OWNER'S EQUITY)

The tax status of an organization often impacts how data is reflected in the financial statements, with different information required in for-profit and not-for-profit reporting (FASB, 2022; HFMA, 2021; Menaker et al., 2020). In a traditional **statement of owner's equity**, information on the organization's value or net worth would be presented in the context of the shareholder's or owner's investments, stock issued (purchased by others or sold to new investors), and withdrawals (including dividends or payouts). For many healthcare organizations with a tax-exempt or not-for-profit tax status, this statement contains changes in assets as governed by donor restrictions (or lack thereof) instead of owner's equity. Most health services organizations (particularly hospitals) are not-for-profit and therefore do not have shareholders. Instead, it relies on patient revenues and donors to fund operations. Figure 6.3 shows the statement reflecting the **change in net assets** as it would be presented by a typical not-for-profit health system.

Figure 6.3

Changes in net assets

Pantheon Health System, Subsidiaries, and Affiliates
Consolidated Changes in Net Assets
Fiscal Years Ended June 30, 2022 and 2021
(In Thousands)

	2022		2021
Excess revenue over (under) expenses	$ 1,131,413	$	890,601
Change in net assets without donor restrictions			
Released for fixed assets purchases	$ 19,385	$	20,445
Pension and retirement liabilities	$ 339,500	$	310,115
Total change in net assets without donor restrictions	$ 1,490,298	$	1,221,161
Change in net assets with donor restrictions			
Contributions	$ 35,900	$	38,750
Investment income	$ 15,589	$	17,500
Released restricted assets	$ 10,000	$	12,500
Total change in net assets with donor restrictions	$ 61,489	$	68,750
Increase (decrease) in net assets	$ 1,551,787	$	1,289,911
Net assets			
Beginning of year	$ 2,389,271	$	1,099,360
End of year	$ 3,941,058	$	2,389,271

The changes in net assets statement details the increase or decrease in the value of assets over a specified period. Items included in this statement are not reflected in the statement of operations and are not included in revenue generated by routine operations or patient activity. Assets included in this financial statement are items given to the organization as contributions or other donor-related funding. Categories for these special items are **restricted assets** (includes temporarily restricted) and **unrestricted assets**, as designated by the donor. Purpose-restricted assets are to be used for a specific purpose within the organization's operations. An example would be funds specifically donated for cancer research, or cancer treatment and related activities. In such an instance, the restricted funding cannot be used for any other purpose, no matter where a shortfall or need may be occurring. Temporarily restricted assets, or time-restricted assets, are used for a specified purpose or program for a limited amount of time. After that time, they may be used for other needs as determined by the organization. Unrestricted assets are donations that can be distributed or utilized in any way the organization deems necessary. It is extremely important for the funds in each category to be captured appropriately for regulatory reporting as well as internal auditing and stakeholder account reviews.

STATEMENT OF CASH FLOWS

The **statement of cash flows** (as shown in Figure 6.4) contains consolidated information on the organization's incoming cash transactions as well as the outgoing cash transactions. This

Figure 6.4

Statement of cash flows

Pantheon Health System, Subsidiaries, and Affiliates
Consolidated Statements of Cash Flows
Fiscal Years Ended June 30, 2022 and 2021
(In Thousands)

		2022		2021
Operating activities				
Changes in net assets	$	1,551,788	$	1,289,912
Depreciation and amortization	$	100,000	$	80,000
Investment gains/losses	$	(10,000)	$	(10,000)
Restricted contributions received	$	(50,000)	$	(50,000)
Fundraising/charity	$	405,000	$	305,000
Net operating cash	$	1,996,788	$	1,614,912
Investing activities				
Property and equipment purchases	$	(125,000)	$	(90,000)
Third-party investments	$	(60,000)	$	(30,000)
Other investment activities		(40,000)		(20,000)
Net investing cash	$	(225,000)	$	(140,000)
Financing activities				
Lines of credit repayment		(175,000)		(100,000)
Finance lease payments		(1,589,970)		(1,350,645)
Other financing activities		46,457		30,000
Net financing cash		(1,718,513)		(1,420,645)
Net increase (decrease) in cash/equivalents	$	53,275	$	54,267
Cash and cash equivalents				
Beginning of year	$	703,267	$	649,000
End of year	$	756,542	$	703,267

financial statement summarizes activities in three major categories: operating activities, investing activities, and financing activities. **Operating activities** include revenue and expense items that occur during routine business practices such as asset management and contributions. Incoming cash from product sales, inventory returns and rebates, or other cash-based accounts receivable items are also included in operating activities. Cash outflows in this section of the cash flow statement would include income tax payments, payments for space rental, or cash-based interest payments for loans or notes payable. **Investing activities** include large equipment purchases (quite common in healthcare), partnership ventures, and stock market and securities investments. Increased assets from mergers and acquisitions, building and land purchases, and increases in short-term assets would also be included in the investment activities category. **Financing activities** include payments on existing debt (loans and lines of credit) as well as newly financed purchases or projects. Shareholder dividends, public bonds, and associated interest are also considered financing activities. The final section of the statement of cash flows shows the ending balance for cash and cash equivalents. This ties the cash flow statement into the balance sheet, with cash and cash equivalents being included in the assets section of the statement.

Together, the four financial statements provide a great deal of information about a healthcare organization and the nature of its operations. The financial statements are created quarterly and annually, with the final reports audited by external auditors and government agencies (like the Securities and Exchange Commission) before being made publicly available. An organization's growth potential, profitability and industry comparison can all be assessed by analyzing the data reported in the financial statements. Revenues, expenses, assets, liabilities, and cash are all key elements of organizational and financial management, providing leadership with a summary of historical data upon which to base projections.

FINANCIAL STATEMENTS ANALYSIS: WHAT DO THE NUMBERS TELL US?

After the data has been summarized and the financial statements have been created, interpretation of the results begins. Analyzing the financial statements can involve several ratios and calculations, using the data from multiple reports to determine the organization's financial position in the context of profitability, asset and debt management, and liquidity (including cash management). **Ratio analysis**, which is designed to assess the organization's overall financial position, also provides insight to operating efficiency and competitiveness. The categories for the various ratio types as well as their definitions are listed in Table 6.1. Some of the most common ratios used for financial statement analysis are:

- Operating margin: Operating Income ÷ Operating Revenues (measures profitability)

- Profit margin: Net Income ÷ Revenue (measures profitability)

- Total margin: Net Income ÷ Total Revenues (measures profitability)

- Return on assets: Net Income ÷ Total Assets (measures profitability)

- Total asset turnover: Total Revenues ÷ Total Assets (measures asset management)

- Current ratio: Current Assets ÷ Current Liabilities (measures liquidity)

- Debt ratio: Total Liabilities ÷ Total Assets (measures liquidity)

- Days cash on hand: Cash (including Cash Equivalents) + Short-Term Investments ÷ [(Operating Expenses − Depreciation) / 365] (measures liquidity)

Table 6.1

TYPES OF RATIO ANALYSIS

Ratio Category	Analysis Purpose/Questions Answered
Asset management	Does the organization have revenue-sustainable assets? Is the organization generating enough revenue using the assets on hand? Includes the analysis of inventory, fixed assets, total assets, product sales/patient services revenue, account receivable.
Debt management	Is the amount of debt the organization has reasonable? Is the organization generating enough revenue to satisfy its debt or other financial obligations?
Liquidity	Does the organization have adequate assets for quick cash conversion? Can the organization satisfy its short-term obligations?
Profitability	Does the organization's revenue exceed its expense? Is the profit margin adequate to meet the organization's investment and long-term goals? Has the level of profitability been consistent over time?

All of the measures used in the previously noted ratios come from at least one of the routinely prepared financial statements. Results from the ratios calculations can be used comparatively to determine how well an organization is performing in comparison to others in the industry, or how the organization has performed over multiple time periods. It highlights financial strengths and areas of improvement, pointing to specific line items in the financial statements. For example, when examining the current ratio, a low ratio indicates a high level of risk and the possibility of an organization's inability to cover its debts and liabilities. To further analyze and mitigate the issue, an organization could evaluate current assets and current liabilities specifically (since these are the only two measures included in the calculation) and make the necessary changes to the operational areas that impact these items. Using the balance sheet presented for Pantheon Health System:

$$\text{Current Ratio} = \text{Current Assets} \div \text{Current Liabilities}$$
$$= \$1{,}311{,}911 \div \$1{,}173{,}041$$
$$= 1.1184$$

For the current ratio, the desired result is greater than 1.0, which means that a company has enough assets to cover all of its financial obligations. This result indicates that Pantheon Health System holds enough assets to cover its liabilities. The ideal result for the various ratios is highly dependent on the type of healthcare organization, as well as the goods and services they produce. As a rule, for an organization to be financially sound, income and assets should always be greater than expenses and liabilities (Menaker et al., 2020).

The financial statements and associated ratios tell a story about the organization's common practices, its financial standing, and its ability to achieve its mission. The actual numbers are only indicators and must be interpreted within context in order to have real meaning and facilitate actionable change. **Income ratios** (often referred to as revenue ratios) analyze the money coming into the organization generated by assets and investments. Healthcare organizations recognize revenue from providing patient services, as well as other operating revenue such as visitor parking and gift shop sales, grants, and contributions. **Liquidity ratios** gauge the organization's ability to use short-term assets to cover its short-term liabilities. These ratios analyze cash-on-hand to ensure the organization has enough cash reserves to satisfy obligations quickly. Items included here are employee payroll and vendor supply payments, the critical items needed for patient care. **Debt ratios** analyze the amount of debt the organization owes. This impacts not only the short-term assets and ability to pay, but the longer-term obligations and the need for increased revenues. **Profitability ratios** measure not only the revenues retained after debts are paid, but the underlying policies that support revenue generation. An example here is product or service pricing for healthcare services rendered. An organization must periodically review its fee schedule to determine if its current rates are comparable to those charged by competitors as well as industry averages. The fee schedule must also be reviewed periodically to ensure that enough revenue is generated to cover liabilities, which may also include an analysis of patient case mix and payer mix. All of the financial statements, as well as the ratios that are based on their data, assist with management decisions designed to improve the overall effectiveness and efficiency of the organization, as well as improve projections, forecasting, and strategic planning.

PERFORMANCE MEASUREMENT AND BENCHMARKING

Healthcare organizations have a solid understanding of what they produce and of the population or consumers that rely on their goods and services. All of the inputs and inclusions to the financial statements have been established, but leadership must also analyze the overall performance of their organization in the context of its established goals, objectives, and mission. The published data only represents a part of the bigger picture, which must also include the organization's performance in comparison to others in the healthcare sector. "Performance" can be defined as the effective execution of goals or objectives, which can be quite a subjective definition. Performance is measured both internally and externally, and typically includes both financial and nonfinancial measures. The various performance measures, referred to as **key performance indicators** (KPIs), reflect actual performance of the patient care and financial and operational functions in comparison to internally established targets, as well as in comparison to competitor and industry standards. KPIs may be specific to the organization, or they may be the most common items measured in the industry or sector. The purpose of developing KPIs is to monitor the same indicators over time and identify any trends, seasonality, or anomalies in the organization's performance. It allows leadership to pinpoint specific activities or areas that impact an outcome, and make targeted, meaningful changes to processes and procedures. Performance definitely has a direct relationship to the organization's financial information, with implemented process changes impacting both. Let's first take a look at the performance measurement process, then examine some of the most common KPIs in healthcare.

The Performance Measurement Process

The performance measurement process is designed to analyze current operations and identify potential areas for improvement (U.S. Department of Health and Human Services, 2021). Because all areas of the healthcare organization contribute to the achievement of its goals, the chosen measurement metrics at the organization level encompass data and inputs from a variety of departments and functional areas. Choosing the KPIs in this manner ensures that all stakeholders are considered when determining effectiveness, making the outcomes of the performance measurement process meaningful. Like financial operations and related analyses, the performance measurement process is ongoing, and examines data over time to capture trends, seasonality, or other phenomena that may impact future performance and planning. The process is comprised of several phases, each with a specific purpose as reflected in Figure 6.5.

　　The first phase of the performance measurement process is identifying the "purpose"—discussing why the data capture for a department or process is important. Ideally, the

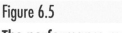

Figure 6.5

The performance measurement process

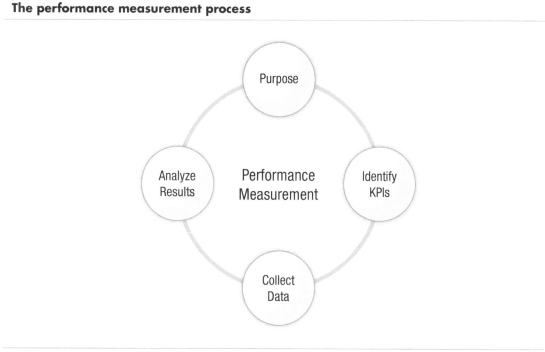

KPIs, key performance indicators.

purpose for every department should be tied to the overall goals, objectives, and mission of the healthcare organization, even though how they support these may differ. "Buy-in," and getting the stakeholders on board, is critical to the success of the process as well as the outcomes. Ideally, stakeholders will understand that the collection of the department's data can provide support for budgetary requests or for additional direct care resources. The second phase of the performance measurement process is the identification of KPIs. KPIs are the items within a department or standard operating procedure that best indicate completion and effectiveness in relation to its purpose. While all items may be important to patient care or other service delivery, all may not be measurable over time, or may not be within the stakeholders' realm of control. Items selected for the performance measurement process should be core items, not one-time or seasonal items that won't be present over time. Examples of core items used for KPIs are patient record updates, decreased medication errors, or reduced readmission rates. All of these items are central to an organization's purpose of patient care and can be measured over time.

The "collection of data" is the third phase of the performance measurement process, and is often the most complex. This phase gathers and compiles all of the data for the KPIs identified by stakeholders. Ideally, the data will cover several historical periods to ultimately provide a clear picture of previous performance, including all of the inputs used for patient care or the production of other goods and services. Current data is also included in this phase to assess how the organization or process has changed over time.

"Results analysis" is the fourth phase of the process, where stakeholders review the collected data and interpret the story that it tells. During this phase, the data should reveal what has worked and what may need to be updated or changed for the continued accomplishment of the organization's goals.

The identification of KPIs varies even within an organization, as leadership and other stakeholders determine the most important metrics for measurement and improvement. Most organizations use a combination of both qualitative and quantitative indicators to provide a more complete picture of the state of operations. Examples of KPI categories used in performance measurement include quality of service and patient experience, productivity and/or volume, process efficiency and/or production time, effectiveness and health outcomes, profitability and financial standing, and value proposition.

Common Performance Measurement Methods

There are many methods and models used for performance measurement in the healthcare sector, but there are some common methods and techniques that work well with multifaceted health services organizations (see Table 6.2). One of the most common tools used today is the **balanced scorecard** (BSC), originally introduced by Kaplan and Norton (1996). This framework focuses on four primary domains called "perspectives," each capable of containing any number of KPIs as deemed necessary by the organization. The flexibility of the BSC is what makes it applicable and effective for healthcare organizations of different types. **Total quality management**, or TQM, another common framework used in the healthcare sector, focuses on internal organizational changes as a catalyst for improved outcomes. The underlying philosophy of TQM posits overall improvement by managing internal inputs. The **pay for performance** model (often represented as P4P) is similar to the TQM premise as it focuses on quality of care and improvement. P4P incentivizes care excellence by using financial rewards, with the end goal of improved efficiency and patient outcomes. Globally, the World Health Organization (WHO) references tools such as the Health Service Database (https://www.who.int/data/collections) and the Harmonized Health Facility Assessment (https://www.who.int/data/data-collection-tools/harmonized -health-facility-assessment/introduction) to analyze availability and quality of healthcare services among partnering nations. Some performance measurement frameworks are tailored to reflect a specific facet of healthcare service delivery, such as primary care or supply chain management.

Benchmarking

When it comes to organizational performance measurement, like most other organizations, health services organizations examine internal processes as well as external standards to gauge how well they are doing. The reasoning behind this could be internal process improvement or improvements to industry standing and market share. **Benchmarking** is the process used by organizations as they compare themselves to process best practices and competitors to strive for optimal performance. The benchmarking process assists with the decision-making process throughout the entire organization, not just the financial performance. Both quantitative and qualitative measures are used in the benchmarking process as the organization seeks to improve its performance in areas of efficiency, effectiveness, and productivity. The approach to benchmarking is dependent on the purpose or desired outcomes and may be:

- internally focused: to improve or streamline processes or procedures within the organization's routine operations;
- externally or competitor focused: to assess the organization's performance in comparison to similar organizations;
- performance focused: to compare the organization's performance to the established industry best practices; or
- strategy focused: to assist with project analysis, implementation, and other planning initiatives of the organization.

Table 6.2

PERFORMANCE MEASUREMENT METHODS/FRAMEWORKS (MOST COMMON IN HEALTHCARE)

Framework/Method	Domains/Categories	Sample KPIs
BSC	Financial perspective	Accounts receivable Net income Operating profit margin Asset management
	Internal business process perspective	Staffing Inventory management Process efficiency Compliance and regulations
	Customer perspective	Patient experience/satisfaction Appointments and wait times Access to care Improved health outcomes
	Learning and growth perspective	Technological advancement Employee satisfaction Training and development Network right-sizing
TQM	Leadership	Leadership training Employee engagement Strategic planning Partnership development
	Service quality	Customer–supplier relationship Integrated systems Processes not people Continuous improvement
	Patient satisfaction	Courtesy and empathy Access and responsiveness Competence and reliability Communication/Understanding
P4P	Qualitative measures	Patient experience Patient health outcomes Employee engagement Productivity
	Quantitative measures	Financial impact/savings Accounts receivable efficiency
	Varying pay structures	Individual merit Team/group merit Commissions/bonuses Profit-sharing

BSC, balanced scorecard; KPIs, key performance indicators; P4P, pay for performance; TQM, total quality management.

Benchmarking as applied to healthcare impacts the organization and the providers of care as well as the population served. Many of the indicators are tied directly to the sector's regulations and compliance standards, and are compared to other organizations of similar size and purpose. Attributes used when determining a comparable healthcare organization or market include: type of practice, services provided, geographic location, capacity, and academics (teaching or nonteaching). Common healthcare benchmarks and comparative measurements are:

- resource management,
- patient outcomes,
- patient satisfaction,
- staffing ratios,
- employee satisfaction,
- employee turnover,
- patient mix,
- payer mix,
- number of readmissions,
- length of inpatient stay,
- appointment wait times, and
- patient safety.

These items are important for the survival of the organization as it strives to meet patient expectations as well as adhere to regulation and compliance standards.

STRATEGIC PLANNING AND PERFORMANCE MANAGEMENT

Once the organization has measured the correct KPIs and has identified the desired performance levels, leadership must plan the steps to achieve the desired level of performance and maintain it. Improved processes, systems design, and increased productivity are usually the intended outcomes, but getting there requires a plan with deliberate steps and milestones—a strategic plan. **Strategic planning** is the process of setting goals for your organization, then planning the steps and details required to achieve those goals. This process is particularly important in the healthcare sector, because of the rapid and often unforeseen changes in regulations and technology. As an industry, we welcome improvements and change for the betterment of our population's overall health, but it requires a great deal of versatility and adaptation. Healthcare organizations must implement changes all while maintaining routine operations and patient care. There are numerous models used for the strategic planning process, but they all include common elements connecting the goal(s) back to the organization's mission, vision, and values. The seven steps of the strategic planning process are shown in Figure 6.6, as implemented in a typical healthcare organization.

The first step in any strategic planning process is the clear communication of the organization's mission, vision, and values. This is the critically important process of ensuring that all stakeholders involved in the growth, sustainability, and planning processes are on the same page regarding the organization's direction. The next step is to identify the goals and associated actions required for the organization to achieve its mission. At this stage, all options

Figure 6.6

The strategic planning process

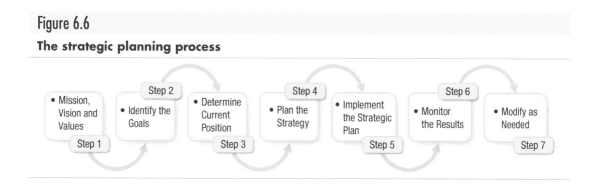

are presented, with the viability and practicality of these options assessed in the next step. The third step requires stakeholders to conduct an assessment of the organization's current position. The purpose here is to answer the question of whether the goals can be achieved given its current state. If the answer to this question is yes, then no major changes need to occur, and they can just build on the current state or functionality. If the answer to this question is no, changes need to occur, and a strategy needs to be developed. Step four of the strategic planning process is the creation of the strategic plan—what needs to happen to adequately position the organization for goal achievement. A well-thought-out plan must include all of the resources required to implement the strategy and ultimately achieve the goals. Human resources, financial resources, material and supply resources, external partners, and time frame must all be considered when drafting a strategic plan. After the plan is drafted and agreed upon by stakeholders, it is time for implementation, the fifth step in the process. This is the operationalizing of the strategic plan—doing the actual work required to update or change the organization to adequately support the mission, vision, and values, and reach the goals. The final two steps in the process are ongoing, as performance is monitored and modified as needed.

Change Management

Crafting a strategy is only part of the process by which an organization plans its path to achieve specific goals or transform to a future state. The implementation of the strategic plan must be well-thought out and systematically done, involving key stakeholders along the way. **Change management** is the process of transitioning the organization to meet its strategic goals or move into its future state by guiding everyone involved through the various stages of the change. Quite often, there will be technological changes or procedure changes, both of which may require staffing or workflow process changes. The scale and timing of this process takes coordination, as these changes not only impact current operations but future operations as well. Change management is truly a "team" approach, with employees throughout the organization doing their part to bring the updates or changes into view. Leadership (or those responsible for change management) must ensure that the following change management elements are in place:

- Identify the need for change (as evidenced by performance measurement or similar analysis).

- Communicate both the current state and the need for the change to employees and other relevant stakeholders.

- Clearly outline the change plan including all phases, stages, and KPIs for benchmarking, (ideally) in cooperation and discussion with stakeholders.

- Implement the change plan, with feedback from participants and benchmark review along the way.

- Finalize the change, evaluate the overall process, and manage the new processes and organizational changes going forward.

Critical to the success of change management is consensus within the organization. Leadership must strive to communicate effectively and get the buy-in of employees. Everyone involved must understand the shared need for the change, and understand what needs to be done to make the change successful. It requires commitment, willingness to change, and a clear view of the organizational benefits of the change for the various pieces to fall into place. The systems or process changes are important, but equally important are the understanding of and care for the employee impact. Change can be difficult, and some employees or other stakeholders may need help understanding what needs to be done, and the potential impacts on the organization. Whether the change impacts single or several departments or processes, it requires effective communication and management for successful implementation.

Performance Management

We typically think of performance management as a workflow review process between management and employee, but it can include so much more of the organization's operations and associated outcomes. **Performance management** can be defined as the process of controlling the activities that support the organization's mission, goals, and objectives. This process can be implemented at the macro-level, which manages performance at a consolidated level, or the micro-level, which manages performance at the employee level, including numerous teams, departments, and processes. While **performance measurement** identifies the indicators and standards by which to measure, performance *management*, as shown in Figure 6.7, is the guidance and hands-on adjustment of the processes needed to meet those standards. This process tends to create a culture of improvement, with all activities and priorities focused on the organization's mission and goals. In a sector as dynamic as healthcare, with rapidly changing measurements, procedures, and technologies, managing performance effectively is necessary for the adaptability and longevity of many healthcare organizations. Sound and effective performance management examines all phases and periods of operations—historical, current, and projected.

Figure 6.7

Performance management

Historical	Current	Change	Manage
Past Performance and Data Capture	Current Processes and Procedures	Implementation of Required Changes	Monitor and Manage Ongoing Performance

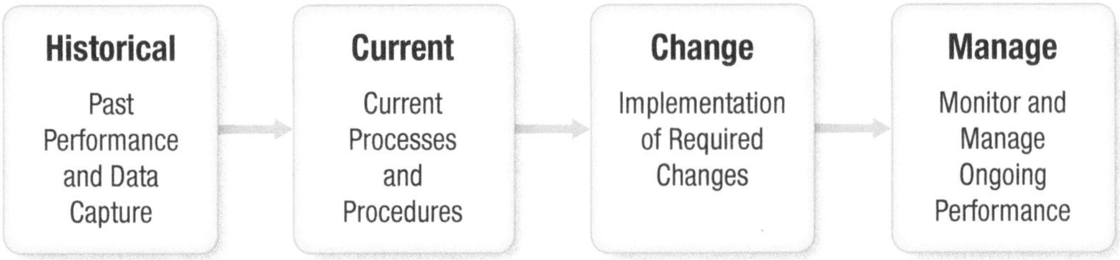

Data is the key to making the performance management process work. It requires the capture and analysis of data from both prior and current periods. The data analysis process will determine if the organization is operating as effectively and efficiently as required, or if change is in fact needed. Performance management encompasses patient as well as nonpatient operations, with all initiatives working toward achieving the organization's goals, objectives, and strategy for both the shorter and longer term.

CHAPTER SUMMARY

The healthcare organization's financial statements lay the foundation for real-time analysis and measurement. While the financial metrics are not the only ones considered in decision-making and strategic planning, they provide the context in which the organization must operate. Leadership and other stakeholders must realistically assess the organization's standing as well as its desired future state, combining the financial position with other KPIs selected for the performance measurement process. These KPIs often provide the source data for the strategic planning process, which is designed to facilitate the healthcare organization's mission support and achievement, continuous internal process improvement, increased competitiveness, and market or service expansion and growth. All of the concepts discussed in this chapter are connected to ultimately provide the best possible healthcare services and products to consumers.

KEY TERMS FOR REVIEW

assets	investing activities	profit margin
balance sheet	key performance indicators	profitability ratio
balanced scorecard	liabilities	ratio analysis
benchmarking	liquidity ratio	restricted assets
change in net assets	nonoperating revenue and	revenue
change management	expenses categories	statement of cash flows
debt ratio	operating activities	statement of owner's equity
expense	operating income	strategic planning
financing activities	pay for performance	total quality management
income ratio	performance management	unrestricted assets
income statement	performance measurement	

DISCUSSION QUESTIONS

1. What are the four financial statements and what elements are required for each?

2. Discuss how the various financial statements lend themselves to leadership's decision-making and strategic planning.

3. What are the steps in the performance measurement process? How might these steps be utilized for overall organizational improvement?

4. Define revenues and expenses. How do these impact an organization's financial position?

5. What is the BSC? How might the BSC be used in a traditional hospital or inpatient facility? Identify at least three indicators that would be measured in a hospital or inpatient setting.

6. How might the TQM framework be applied to nonclinical areas or departments?

7. Are performance measurement and performance management the same? Discuss the similarities and differences.

8. Define ratio analysis. Discuss how the concept of ratio analysis impacts decision-making within the healthcare organization.

9. Discuss how change management impacts strategic planning and performance management.

10. Define assets and liabilities. What role do they play in the interpretation of an organization's financial position?

PRACTICE PROBLEMS

Answers to this chapter's Practice Problems are available via Springer Publishing Connect™ by following the instructions on the opening page of this book and accessing Answers to Practice Problems on the Table of Contents.

1. Using the financial statements presented for Pantheon Health System throughout the chapter:
   a. Calculate the total margin (profit margin).
   b. Calculate the current ratio. Does the result appear favorable? Explain.
   c. Calculate days cash on hand. What does the result mean for Pantheon Health System's liquidity?

2. Organize the list of line items in Table 6.3 into a standard statement of operations (income statement) and calculate net operating income. Does the result indicate a profitable organization?

Table 6.3

STATEMENT OF OPERATIONS (INCOME STATEMENT)

Patient services revenue	$440,000
Bad debt	$30,000
Salaries and benefits	$125,000
Purchased clinical services	$90,000
Interest	$20,000
Investment income	$15,000
General administrative expenses	$70,000
Lease and rental payments	$50,000
Charitable contributions	$50,000
Depreciation	$60,000
Taxes	$25,000
Patient copays	$25,000
Other operating revenue	$15,000

3. Using what we know of balance sheet basics:

   a. Calculate the net asset value for each of the companies (listed a–c) in Table 6.4.

Table 6.4

NET ASSET TABLE

	Assets	Liabilities	Net Assets
Company A	$623,110	$598,311	?
Company B	$649,550	$569,911	?
Company C	$520,280	$461,455	?

   b. Then, using the net income calculated in Problem 2, calculate the return on assets for each of the companies in part a.

4. If the Community Hospital income statement reports $3,550,760 in revenues and $2,750,600 in expenses, with no additional nonoperating revenues or expenses, what is its operating income? If $5,000 of investment income and $1,500 of marketing materials were added to the income statement, what would be Community Hospital's operating income?

5. If the Community Hospital balance sheet reports $575,000 in total assets and $150,000 in net assets with no long-term liabilities reported, what are the hospital's current liabilities?

6. MediCo Pharmaceuticals reported net income for fiscal year 2022 (FY2022) of $8.3 million on total revenues of $45 million. Depreciation expense totaled $895,000.

   a. What were total expenses for FY2022?
   b. What were total cash expenses for FY2022? Assume that depreciation is a noncash expense.
   c. What is MediCo Pharmaceutical's estimated cash flow for FY2022?

7. Reorder the items in Table 6.5 to create a balance sheet with the correct categories/headings and placement.

Table 6.5

BALANCE SHEET

Accounts payable	$30,000
Long-term investments	$100,000
Supply chain inventory	$215,000
Accounts receivable	$75,000
Cash	$50,000
Long-term debt	$125,000
Property and equipment	$150,000
Other long-term liabilities	$15,000
Other assets	$45,000
Short-term debt	$40,000

CHAPTER 6 CASE: FINANCIAL STATEMENT ANALYSIS AND REVIEW

Using the financial statements presented in the chapter for Pantheon Health Systems, Subsidiaries, and Affiliates:

1. Identify at least three financial strengths and three financial weaknesses for the health system. Support your claims with specific information presented in the financial or operating data statements, and cite reasoning from your textbook.

2. Calculate the following profitability ratios for 2021 and 2022: (a) total margin and (b) the return on assets.

3. Calculate the following debt and asset management ratios for 2021 and 2022: (a) total asset turnover and (b) debt-to-equity ratio.

4. Discuss what's changed from one fiscal year to the next. How have these changes impacted the organization's financial standing?

REFERENCES

Financial Accounting Standards Board. (2022). *05 overview and background.* https://asc.fasb.org/1943274/2147481036

Healthcare Financial Management Association. (2021, September 13). *Accounting and financial reporting.* https://www.hfma.org/topics/landing-accounting-and-financial-reporting.html

Kaplan, R. S., & Norton, D. P. (1996). Using the balanced scorecard as a strategic management system. *Harvard Business Review*, 74(1), 75–85. https://hbr.org/2007/07/using-the-balanced-scorecard-as-a-strategic-management-system

Menaker, R., Witte, R. J., & France, T. J. (2020, March 12). *Principal principles: Critical accounting and financial concepts for healthcare leaders.* https://www.mgma.com/resources/financial-management/principal-principles-critical-accounting-and-fina

U.S. Department of Health and Human Services. (2021). FY 2022 annual performance plan and report—Executive summary: Performance management. https://www.hhs.gov/about/budget/fy2022/performance/performance-plan-executive-summary/index.html#performance

Healthcare Revenue Cycle Management

CHAPTER 7

Revenue Cycle Management: Health Insurance and Other Payment Mechanisms

OBJECTIVES

1. Describe and discuss the various government/public health insurance plans and the segment of the U.S. population covered by these plans.

2. Identify the types of commercial/private insurance plans and the differences between them.

3. Identify the drivers of healthcare cost and why health insurance is necessary to pay for healthcare services.

4. Discuss the Patient Protection and Affordable Care Act (PPACA) and the concept of healthcare reform.

5. Discuss the characteristics of insurance and the potential impacts on health insurance consumers.

INTRODUCTION

Our health and wellness are essential, with our shorter-term and longer-term outcomes dependent on the availability and affordability of healthcare services. There are healthcare options available to most, although accessibility and the ability to pay have proven to be challenging. In the United States, stakeholders have implemented several options for healthcare services in efforts to provide them for everyone, regardless of socioeconomic status. As the costs of medical care continue to rise, even well-established networks struggle to maintain reasonably priced coverage for a wide range of services. There are several key items that drive rising healthcare costs, some of which are simply a by-product of the provision of care. First, as a result of effective medicine and treatment, some are living longer and delaying retirement. This means a shift in senior-related illness coverage from traditional senior insurance plans to private insurance or employer group plans. Secondly, healthcare is a technology-driven industry fostering continuous improvement. With ongoing research and development, and continuous training to ensure highly competent healthcare professionals, increased costs are inevitable. In the United States, national or universal health insurance coverage is not a payment option. However, there are several categories of payers in place to assist with the costs of healthcare services. The categories of payers are designed to provide health insurance coverage for different populations within the U.S. citizenry, delineated by criteria such as age, illness, or income. While some providers accept most insurance plans, they may not accept all. This often requires consumers to find multiple payment mechanisms to get all of their healthcare needs met and covered. This chapter discusses the major types of healthcare insurers and payers, as well as the segments of the U.S. population they cover. We will begin our discussion with an overview of some key insurance terminology and define the basics of health insurance coverage.

WHAT IS HEALTH INSURANCE AND HOW DOES IT WORK?

Insurance, by definition, is a tool or agreement implemented between at least two parties to mitigate risk or financial loss. **Health insurance**, then, is the mechanism by which we cover health-related risks or losses. Health insurance is designed to cover a myriad of health-related expenses, including preventive care and treatment for existing illness, as well as maintenance for longer-term illnesses. Traditional health insurance covers not only hospital-based healthcare services, but outpatient, pharmaceutical, and specialist services. The person(s) covered by the health insurance policy is called the **insured** and the company responsible for the underwriting of the policy and financial coverage for services is the **insurer**. The insured and the insurer work together to ensure that the healthcare provider is reimbursed for services rendered. The health delivery collaborative process, beginning with the initial medical office visit and ending with claims submission, is shown in Figure 7.1.

Figure 7.1

Health insurance and the medical claim

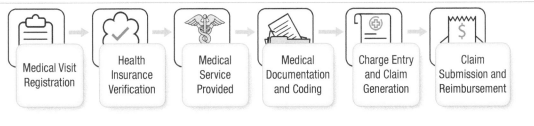

| Medical Visit Registration | Health Insurance Verification | Medical Service Provided | Medical Documentation and Coding | Charge Entry and Claim Generation | Claim Submission and Reimbursement |

The medical office visit, or the patient encounter, is the beginning of the insurance and **medical claims process**, with some services requiring preauthorization prior to the date of service. At the time of medical office visit registration, health insurance coverage for the anticipated services is verified. In many cases, the verification process is electronic, and is performed behind the scenes. For health insurance plans requiring preauthorization, case managers advise patients and healthcare providers on what services are covered by the current plan. While health condition dictates the medical services needed, these may not be covered by the health insurance plan (with payment required by the patient/insured). After insurance verification, medical services are provided and medical documentation for the visit is completed. Additional visits may be required, or referrals may be given for additional medical services, all requiring additional insurance verifications and preauthorizations. The medical provider's notes and documentation are then transcribed, and the necessary medical codes are assigned (this may happen simultaneously if the provider is using a tablet or in-room computer during the provision of medical services). Some healthcare organizations have transcriptionists and medical coders who specialize in the data entry and related coding of medical visit information to ensure accuracy and timeliness of billing. Code entry queues the associated charges as outlined in the organization's fee schedule or chargemaster, and the medical claim is produced. The medical claim is submitted to the insurance provider for review and payment for medical services. Payment of the claim is at the discretion of the insurer and may be denied based on a variety of factors such as missing patient or provider information, invalid or missing codes, billing for unauthorized services, or billing for services not covered by the insurance plan. In the event of a claims denial, the healthcare provider works to rapidly correct any errors and resubmit the claim. When all criteria have been met, and the insurer is satisfied with the documentation provided, the claim is approved and payment is remitted to the healthcare provider.

With the complexity and cost of medical services today, having medical insurance in some form is necessary. The types of insurance available to individuals and families may vary depending on circumstance and possibly location, but in most cases there are insurance providers to meet most needs. There are many insurance providers to choose from, ranging from publicly available plans through the government and states, to those offered by employers, each with its own eligibility requirements and covered health services. Individual health needs often dictate the level of insurance coverage needed as well as the specialization of the healthcare providers sought.

PATIENT PROTECTION AND AFFORDABLE CARE ACT

The **Patient Protection and Affordable Care Act** (PPACA, commonly referred to as the ACA) was implemented in 2010 and serves as a pivotal policy fostering healthcare reform in the United States. This comprehensive healthcare legislation mandated coverage and benefits for those who would have otherwise not had health insurance coverage at all. Some of the key changes enacted by the PPACA include the following:

   Dependents are covered by parents or policy holders until they are 26 years of age. This replaces previous legislation which made dependents ineligible at the age of 18 to 21, depending on the state.

   Insurers cannot deny coverage for insureds with preexisting conditions. Previously, some insurers would opt out of coverage for those with certain higher-risk, higher-cost health conditions to avoid incurring additional expense.

   Health insurance "marketplaces" or "exchanges" were created to assist with insurance application and registration. These electronic platforms made it possible for those seeking insurance coverage to "shop around" and find the best price for the level of coverage they needed.

   Expanded Medicaid programs provided healthcare insurance coverage for those previously excluded from eligibility. Prior to the implementation of the PPACA, adults at or below the **federal poverty level** (FPL) would not be eligible for healthcare coverage if they did not have children. The PPACA expanded coverage to include this population.

Although beneficial to those previously unable to afford health insurance, the legislation has not been without challenge. Some opposed to the passing of the legislation cite the increased financial burden to the states that expand to accommodate the additional beneficiaries. Health advocates argue that the longer-term effects of overall population health outweigh the financial risk, but political debates continue. To date, 40 states (including DC) have expanded their Medicaid coverage, providing approximately 35 million Americans with healthcare coverage (Kaiser Family Foundation [KFF], 2023) and their own versions on the insurance marketplace platforms. In addition to the changes made specifically for the Medicaid program, the PPACA included major adjustments to the FPL thresholds and qualifications for children younger than 19 years of age, pregnant women, and recipients of Supplemental Security Income (KFF, 2013). An uninsured penalty was also implemented under the PPACA, but is no longer upheld by the federal government and only continues in a few states. The administration of Medicaid is the most notable change implemented, but all facets of the healthcare sector and the insurers that provide coverage were impacted.

GOVERNMENT INSURANCE COVERAGE

Government insurance payers are often called public payers and are funded primarily through taxes (a combination of federal taxes and payroll taxes). Eligibility for coverage by these payers is relatively stringent, and beneficiaries must meet specific criteria set forth by each payer to qualify for insurance coverage. Coverage is provided by federal, state, and local agencies, or some combination of these, with each having standardized processes and deadlines for application. Theoretically, there are options for everyone not otherwise covered by commercial or private health insurance plans, with the goal of ensuring that everyone has some sort of insurance coverage for health needs and concerns. In some cases, beneficiaries qualify for coverage by multiple plans, but this may be dependent upon medical condition or longer-term prognosis. Government payers have essentially covered the entire uninsured U.S. population, with distinctions made by age, income, or illness. The availability of these plans is relatively widespread, but the process for application and overall qualification may still be a challenge for some. Medicare, Medicaid, the Children's Health Insurance Program (CHIP), the Veterans Health Administration (VHA), and TRICARE are the major government health insurance providers, each providing coverage for specific segments of the U.S. population. All are present in the healthcare sector we see today, with most providers accepting multiple insurers for reimbursement of healthcare services.

Medicare

Medicare was implemented in 1965 to cover healthcare expenses for persons 65 years of age or older (Centers for Medicare & Medicaid Services [CMS], n.d.). Eligibility requires individuals seeking coverage to be within 3 months of their 65th birthday and to have paid into the Medicare program via payroll taxes for the last 10 years. The **Centers for Medicare & Medicaid Services (CMS)** is the administrator for the Medicare benefit, providing guidelines and updates for the plan. Subsequent updates to the program added persons with long-term disabilities and end-stage renal disease (ESRD) to the list of covered individuals. Early Medicare plans only included two categories of care, but additional categories of care and coverage have been added in recent years. The program now covers four categories of care, identified as "Parts" A, B, C, and D, defined in Table 7.1. While all categories of Medicare are available for qualified individuals, all categories are not free of charge—which has proven to be a challenge to those recipients on a fixed income.

Medicare Part A is the traditional plan and is available free of charge to all who are eligible. Individuals must be enrolled in this basic plan before they are allowed to enroll into any of the other available Medicare part plans. Part A covers long-term care and hospital stays, which are

Table 7.1		

MEDICARE PROGRAM COVERAGE OPTIONS (PARTS)

Medicare Part	Coverage Category	Services Covered
Part A	Hospital coverage	Inpatient hospital stays, long-term care facilities, home healthcare services, and hospice
Part B	Medical coverage	Physicians' fees, outpatient services, and rehabilitation services (such as physical therapy and occupational therapy)
Part C	Medicare Advantage	Vision, hearing, dental, transportation, and other services not covered by Part A or Part B
Part D	Prescription coverage	Prescription drugs (for independent pharmacies or Medicare Advantage providers)

traditionally billed separately from physicians' fees. Medicare Part B, while available immediately upon eligibility for Part A, is not automatic and must be selected by the beneficiary, requiring them to pay a monthly premium for coverage. This category covers physicians' fees and outpatient services, with some services still requiring copays or deductibles. Both Parts C and D are optional plans, must be specifically selected, and are usually covered by private insurers servicing Medicare beneficiaries. The Medicare Advantage plans offered under Medicare Part C are structurally similar to the managed care plans offered by commercial and private insurers. Providers in this category often require copays for service, just as they do with non-Medicare insureds, and offer the same services. Part D covers prescription drugs as offered by independent pharmacies as well as those offered by Medicare Advantage providers. Parts C and D require enrollees to first enroll in Parts A and B. Current Medicare enrollment stands at approximately 64 million beneficiaries (CMS, 2021). There have been several legislative proposals introduced to foster Medicare reform in recent years, all of which are still heavily debated. The addition of hearing benefits (for coverage of hearing aids), increased coverage of telemedicine services, and reduced beneficiary copayments are among the changes being considered for the future of Medicare.

Medicaid

Like Medicare, **Medicaid** was implemented in 1965 to provide healthcare insurance coverage to those with limited income in accordance with the FPL. The FPL is an established guideline for individual and household income used to determine eligibility for government programs. Those below the threshold qualify for Medicaid, while those above the threshold typically would not. Current guidelines extend eligibility for those above the FPL to assist those who still have reasonable difficulty affording private insurance coverage. Individuals, families, pregnant women, and children within 133% of the FPL are eligible for Medicaid coverage. Some beneficiaries are categorized as "dual eligible," qualifying for both Medicare and Medicaid coverage due to disabilities and longer-term illnesses. Most Medicaid programs are administered like **managed care organizations (MCOs)**, with some medical providers choosing not to accept Medicaid as a form of reimbursement. Individual states administer Medicaid benefits, so the actual coverage varies according to what the states have implemented, although most of the funding for Medicaid programs comes from the federal government. Medicaid covers physician and hospital expenses, with some states offering additional benefits such as prescription drug and durable medical equipment coverage. While commercial insurance plans have been historically beyond financial reach for those with low income, Medicaid and the expanded marketplace and managed care options have made it possible for many to seek the healthcare they have needed.

Current Medicaid enrollment stands at approximately 84.3 million beneficiaries (CMS, 2022b), with many previously caught in the gray area: too much income for Medicaid, not enough income for private insurance. The PPACA expansion noted in the previous sections made health insurance coverage possible for many, although there is still a small portion of citizens still uninsured for a myriad of reasons. It is important to note that the financial assistance offered by some government programs is administered separately from the health insurance benefits of the program. Qualification for health insurance does not automatically mean qualification for financial assistance and vice versa. Children in families within this gray area or with adults who otherwise do not qualify for Medicaid benefits may be enrolled in CHIP.

Children's Health Insurance Program

The **Children's Health Insurance Program** (also known as CHIP) was implemented as law in 1997. The CHIP program is designed to provide health insurance coverage for children in families with income above the FPL guidelines, and those families that would otherwise be uninsured. Funding for CHIP is at the state level, but is supplemented by federal funding. CHIP currently has approximately 7 million children enrolled (CMS, 2022b). In recent years, some states have struggled to fund the program, causing short-term lapses in coverage. All have seemed to recover, with minimal to no major health incidents resulting from service denials. CHIP routinely covers annual wellness visits, prescription medications, imaging and laboratory services, and dental and vision care. While wellness visits are free, some services may require a minimal copay. In general, states saw a decrease in overall CHIP enrollment as PPACA legislation allowed more families to qualify for the Medicaid program. The Medicaid and CHIP programs are income dependent, with enrollment in the two programs seemingly always in flux. With the stringent income guidelines and required annual reevaluations comes the endless processing of paperwork as beneficiaries are deemed eligible or ineligible with very small changes in income. An increase or decrease of a few dollars in pay has proven to be enough to change an individual's or a family's Medicaid coverage. Although the healthcare exchanges and marketplace databases have reduced hard-copy paperwork in some instances, the revolving door of Medicaid is a large expense for some states. The PPACA set forth the minimum federal qualifications, but some states have chosen to cover additional portions of their population. Those needing coverage are encouraged to apply, even if they may not meet the initial income requirements.

Veterans Health Administration

The **Veterans Health Administration** (VHA) provides medical coverage for all U.S. veterans who served at least two consecutive/continuous years without a dishonorable discharge (U.S. Department of Veterans Affairs, 2022). Former military reservists or former National Guard members must have been called to active duty by a federal agency and have served the full ordered term. Medical coverage is provided for all who qualify, with some qualifying for additional coverage for vision, dental visits, and long-term care. Beneficiaries get to choose their location for care, and have the option of receiving care at other locations to meet all of their healthcare needs. Currently, approximately 9 million U.S. veterans are eligible to receive healthcare from the VHA, but many rely on commercial insurance plans for supplemental or even primary coverage (U.S. Department of Veterans Affairs, n.d.). Long wait times, excessive documentation, and limited resources make some seek commercial coverage instead of standard VHA coverage.

TRICARE

The **TRICARE** health insurance program insures active-duty service members, military retirees, and their families (TRICARE, 2022). The program is governed by the Defense Health Agency (DHA), with routine oversight provided by private health insurance industry contractors. The program was implemented as a replacement to the older Civilian Health and Medical Program of the Uniformed Services program (CHAMPUS), which was introduced in 1966. The TRICARE program essentially divides the coverage area into three regions: the East and West regions of the United States, as well as the overseas region, which covers beneficiaries in other countries globally (TRICARE, n.d.). Currently, there are approximately 10 million beneficiaries covered by the TRICARE program, which offers a wide selection of health plans to cover different military duty statuses and locations. Healthcare services are provided by an extensive network of military hospitals and providers, as well as civilian partners, which help comprise a highly integrated network.

Block Grants: A Little Extra Help

Block grants are larger sums of funding provided by the federal government to each state to fund a variety of state and local initiatives. The block grant disbursement mechanism was first introduced under the Johnson administration, with the aim of providing maximum flexibility to the implementing state and local governments (Finegold et al., 2004). The disbursement and utilization of this funding is left to the discretion of the receiving governments, with no guaranteed amounts for any one initiative. Block grants are very different from categorical grants, which award funding for a specified purpose, program, or initiative. The amount of federal aid awarded to state and local entities has fluctuated over time due to shifts in health priorities, with some programs faring better than others. The areas of training, education, social services, and employment have steadily decreased, while others such as community development and healthcare (preventive and treatment) have seen more robust funding increases. If the amount of federal funding has been decreased, the states will have to supplement the funding to ensure its residents' key health needs are met. Some of the largest block grants still in place include the Community Development Block Grant (CDBG), Social Services Block Grant (SSBC), and the Preventive Health and Health Services Block Grant (PHHS), which provides funding for a myriad of public health and community initiatives such as chronic illness screening and support, injury and domestic violence prevention, community health education, and emergency medical response (Centers for Disease Control and Prevention [CDC], n.d.). Block grants provide additional financial support to states annually to address the unique challenges that may exist among their populations. Many of these initiatives are underfunded or completely excluded from other types of healthcare funding. Block grants provide the additional funding needed for states to address concerns often overlooked by the major funding streams, which tend to focus on one part or segment of an issue.

PRIVATE/COMMERCIAL INSURANCE COVERAGE

Private insurance is health insurance coverage purchased by the beneficiary through employment or independently. As with government or public insurance coverage, private, commercial plans offer several tiers and types of plans to cover the health needs of a large population. The various plans cover a wide range of health scenarios and also vary in cost, with insurance premium payments withheld from an employee's pay or other account designated by the insured. The **insurance premium** is the total amount an insured pays for health insurance policy coverage annually. A **copayment** is the amount paid by the insured at the start each medical service visit. Copayment amounts vary by insurance plan and provider, with some being more costly than others. Emergency department visits, for example, tend to be higher cost than the general internal medicine visits, due to the additional services and diagnostic testing required. Copayments are required by each person seeking care, not just the policy holder. A **deductible** is the amount of money that must be paid by the insured before health insurance coverage is applied for healthcare services. Deductibles must be met individually as well as per family. The deductible rule is applied for the entire term of the policy (usually annually) and can vary in amount based on the plan. Higher deductible plans, which essentially offer less up-front coverage, are usually accompanied by lower premiums. Beneficiaries purchasing health insurance must decide on the appropriate level of coverage based on the specific needs of themselves and their dependents. Plans offered through employment are provided as "group" policies, with cost, coverage, and premium rates negotiated by the employer. Most employers have an "open enrollment" period where employees select their desired health plans or make changes to the plans they have previously selected. Employees may change health plan selections due to changes in premiums, medical conditions coverage, or life events (marriage, having a baby, adoption, etc.). Private/commercial insurance coverage, for many, is administered by an MCO that maintains a contracted provider network to manage healthcare costs, associated risks, and beneficiary volumes. Most MCOs provide a series of health insurance plans, with each having a slightly different set of requirements. Plans are typically differentiated by flexibility of care and cost to the consumer. As reflected in Figure 7.2, the most common managed care health plans have both similarities and differences, with the hard choices left to the beneficiary. Types of care needed and frequency of visits play a major role in the choice of plan, as do network options and copays. Let's discuss what each plan requires and what that means for consumers.

Health Maintenance Organizations

Health maintenance organizations (HMOs) are the most economical of the managed care plans and also the most restrictive. Under HMO guidelines, beneficiaries must select a **primary care physician** (or PCP) and coordinate all of their healthcare though this provider. Healthcare services other than doctor's office visits, such as imaging, laboratory work, or rehabilitative services, must be referred by your PCP and must be within the same network of contracted healthcare providers. These "in-network" providers have a contract or agreement with the insurance company to receive a predetermined reimbursement amount for each visit or service. The PCP coordinating this care also receives a predetermined amount for each routine medical office visit. This reimbursement is based on a per member per month (PMPM) reimbursement scale with no additional payments considered. An example of this would be a PCP with 100 assigned patients at a PMPM reimbursement rate of $50. The PCP would receive $5,000 per month in compensation for the assigned patients ($100 \times \$50$), no matter how many times they visit the doctor's office. A patient could visit just once and the PCP would receive $50 in reimbursement, or the patient could visit the PCP several times within the month and the PCP would still only be reimbursed $50. For this reason, some providers do not contract with HMO plans. HMOs and those participating in their networks offer the same medical care

Figure 7.2

Managed care organization plans

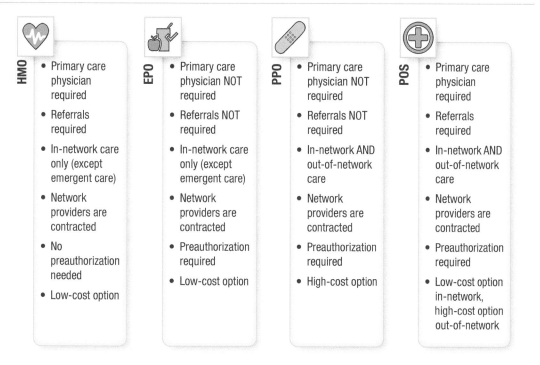

HMO
- Primary care physician required
- Referrals required
- In-network care only (except emergent care)
- Network providers are contracted
- No preauthorization needed
- Low-cost option

EPO
- Primary care physician NOT required
- Referrals NOT required
- In-network care only (except emergent care)
- Network providers are contracted
- Preauthorization required
- Low-cost option

PPO
- Primary care physician NOT required
- Referrals NOT required
- In-network AND out-of-network care
- Network providers are contracted
- Preauthorization required
- High-cost option

POS
- Primary care physician required
- Referrals required
- In-network AND out-of-network care
- Network providers are contracted
- Preauthorization required
- Low-cost option in-network, high-cost option out-of-network

EPO, exclusive provider organization; HMO, health maintenance organization; POS, point-of-service plan; PPO, preferred provider organization.

available with other plans, but other plans offer added coordination, referrals, and in some cases preauthorization.

Exclusive Provider Organizations

Exclusive provider organizations (EPOs) are similar to HMOs, with the added requirement of preauthorization for services. Although referrals are not required with this managed care option, services are still limited to in-network providers, except in an emergency care situation. Payment for any out-of-network care is the responsibility of the insured, with no coverage or financial assistance from the EPO insurance plan. For those that seek care within the network of contracted providers, this is a low-cost option.

Preferred Provider Organizations

Preferred provider organizations (PPOs) provide both in-network and out-of-network options, all of which require preauthorization from the insurance provider. Providers are contracted with the network, with the benefit amount and out-of-pocket amount varying per plan. PPOs are considered high-cost options because the plans typically have higher copayments and higher deductibles. By having higher out-of-pocket costs, premiums or payroll deductions are lower.

Point-of-Service Plans

Point-of-service plans (POSs) are very similar to PPOs, with increased out-of-pocket costs to the patient. All services under this plan require a copayment, and services must be preauthorized by the insurance provider to be considered for reimbursement. POSs only cover a portion of care as outlined at the time of enrollment, with the remaining portion of care being the responsibility of the insured. In-network healthcare services are usually covered at a higher rate, while expenses for out-of-network services will fall heavily on the patient. Both in-network and out-of-network services are offered.

Flexible Spending Accounts and Health Savings Accounts

Healthcare can be costly and, depending on an individual or family's health condition, the out-of-pocket amounts for care can be exorbitant. **Flexible spending accounts** (FSAs) and **health savings accounts** (HSAs) are a mechanism by which insureds can save money over time in preparation for larger healthcare expenses. FSAs are typically offered by an employer, with employees (usually the policy holder) given the opportunity to save a specific dollar amount or percentage from each paycheck in preparation for out-of-pocket expenses. The dollars saved can be used for any medical expense not typically covered by the existing insurance plan. FSAs are very popular for individuals or families with more complex health needs requiring more medical visits, since they may be faced with more copayments, prescriptions or refills, higher deductibles, or durable medical equipment. HSAs are savings plans designed to accompany high-deductible health insurance plans. Funds saved can be used for copayments and out-of-pocket expenses incurred prior to reaching the high annual deductible.

Risks for the Insurer

Moral hazard as applied to the healthcare sector is the overreliance on healthcare services due to the existence or possession of health insurance. In other words, insureds may seek healthcare services just because they have health insurance and would not have to pay for care. This directly impacts the risk incurred by the insurer that often results in additional preventive measures such as preauthorization, utilization management, and restrictive payment structures. Unlike other types of insurance (like automobile insurance or homeowner insurance), health insurance must provide coverage for all in a given population, no matter the risk or health condition. If a driver has had several accidents, the insurer could charge higher premiums for coverage of that person. If a home is located in a flood plain, the homeowner's insurance company could charge higher premiums for coverage in that location. In healthcare, however, insureds with illnesses at multiple acuity levels are required to receive the same premiums. An example of this would be coverage offered by an employer, where the employees are of varying ages and have varying illnesses. The rates offered through the employer would have to be the same for all employees, instead of being adjusted because of their individual health conditions. The uncertainty created by the grouping, or **pooling**, of unequal health conditions increases the risk assumed by the insurer. Another assumed risk by the healthcare sector and insurers is the concept of adverse selection. **Adverse selection** states that those who need healthcare insurance the most will secure it. This means that the insureds are much sicker, and the insurance provider will then pay for increased utilization and more costly healthcare services. Adverse selection is an unavoidable risk in health insurance because providing coverage for those who need it is exactly what it is designed to do.

ACCOUNTABLE CARE ORGANIZATIONS

As healthcare professionals continue to strive for the highest quality of care, various payment and care management mechanisms have been introduced. Along with the familiar Medicaid expansion implemented by the PPACA, the **accountable care organization** (ACO) is now a fixture in the healthcare management landscape. An ACO is an established network of providers dedicated to delivering the highest quality of care for patients as efficiently as possible. The ACO concept was first introduced as a quality and cost savings mechanism for the Medicare patient population, but has now been applied to all types of insurers (CMS, 2022a). Originally, ACOs were organized to participate in the Medicare shared savings program (MSSP), designed to foster coordination of healthcare service among providers. The organization of an ACO is completely voluntary and may reflect a variety of structures, ranging from a network of all PCPs to a network containing physicians, specialists, suppliers, and ancillary services. ACO members collaborate to provide coordinated healthcare, reducing waste and duplicative services and maximizing the quality of care for their patients. Savings from the coordinated care are shared by the ACO team members, in accordance to CMS payment guidelines (American Hospital Association, n.d.).

CHAPTER SUMMARY

The complexities of the healthcare sector are certainly evident in health insurance and all of its available options. We, as insureds, seek a variety of healthcare services, ranging from inpatient procedures to outpatient visits, all of which require reimbursement to be paid to the healthcare services provider. Associated expenses can be covered by the patient or by the insurance provider, but must be covered, nonetheless. As the cost of healthcare continues to rise, reliance on health insurance and available benefits will rise as well, not to mention the portions to be paid out-of-pocket. Health reform, as implemented by the PPACA and as evidenced by the expansion of managed care options, continues to seek ways to make care and expense manageable. Of course, the longer-term goal is to have everyone covered by some form of health insurance, positively impacting societal health outcomes.

KEY TERMS FOR REVIEW

accountable care organization

adverse selection

block grants

Centers for Medicare & Medicaid Services

Children's Health Insurance Program

copayment

deductible

exclusive provider organization

federal poverty level

flexible spending account

health insurance

health maintenance organization

health savings account

insurance premium

insured

insurer

managed care organization

Medicaid

medical claims process

Medicare

moral hazard

Patient Protection and Affordable Care Act (PPACA)

point-of-service plan

pooling

preferred provider organization

primary care physicians

TRICARE

Veterans Health Administration

DISCUSSION QUESTIONS

1. What is the role of the CMS? What insurance plans are governed by this agency?

2. What are the eligibility criteria for the government payers? Is it possible to qualify for more than one plan? Explain your answer.

3. Identify the major types of commercial managed care insurance plans. How do they differ?

4. Explain the difference between a copayment and a deductible.

5. Define the PPACA. What major impacts did this legislation have on health insurance coverage?

6. What is an ACO? How do patients benefit from an ACO structure?

7. Detail the medical claims submissions process.

8. Explain how data validity could impact the claims and reimbursement processes.

9. What are the two main risks faced by every insurer? Are there ways to mitigate these risks?

CHAPTER 7 CASE: WHO'S GOT YOU COVERED? CHOOSING THE RIGHT HEALTH INSURANCE PLAN

As the benefits administrator for your company, you are more than familiar with the available health insurance options. Over the past 5 years, you've explained the company's benefits package to both new and existing employees. Recently, however, you have experienced several life events that have made you look a little deeper into the plans you routinely recommend for colleagues. You've recently married and now you (and your new spouse) must compare benefits packages to see which makes the most sense. Additionally, you've expanded your family by adopting a child and becoming a caregiver for your older mother, both of whom require health insurance coverage. There are a lot of things to consider when making this decision, but the most relevant points are:

- Prior to marriage, your chosen health insurance plan was a basic HMO. The premium amount was minimal, so your household budget was only marginally impacted.

- Your spouse works for a larger company, which offers more health insurance options. The premium amounts are higher than what you are used to paying.

- Your adopted daughter previously had state-provided health insurance (CHIP) but will now need to be covered by the chosen family health insurance plan.

- Your mother is covered by Medicare but has recently been diagnosed with several longer-term illnesses.

As you begin to think through your situation, many unanswered questions come to mind. Making the right health insurance choice is critical for the overall health of your family, but unfortunately there seems to be no one-size-fits-all option here. You decide to discuss things with your spouse to be sure the right decisions are made for the family. The two of you must make some decisions on the following:

1. How would you determine which employer's health insurance plan to choose?

2. If both of you were in good health, does the health insurance plan chosen really matter? Explain your answer.

3. What would you do if your current provider is not a member of your spouse's insurance network, but it was a better network or plan than yours? Would you change providers or choose a different health insurance plan option? Discuss your choice.

4. Is premium a factor or does the network and offered benefits outweigh the impact of cost? Remember, you may be going from an individual plan to a family plan (to cover your daughter and newly dependent mother), which is a much higher premium and possibly more out-of-pocket costs.

5. Your mother has been diagnosed with several chronic illnesses, including ESRD. Along with her current Medicare coverage, what may be additional health insurance options?

REFERENCES

American Hospital Association (n.d.). *Accountable care organizations*. Retrieved February 21, 2023, from https://www.aha.org/accountable-care-organizations-acos/accountable-care-organizations

Centers for Disease Control and Prevention. (n.d.). *About the PHHS Block Grant Program*. U.S. Department of Health and Human Services. Retrieved February 21, 2023, from https://www.cdc.gov/phhsblockgrant/about.htm

Centers for Medicare & Medicaid Services. (n.d.). *History*. https://www.cms.gov/About-CMS/Agency-Information/History

Centers for Medicare & Medicaid Services. (2021, December 21). *CMS releases latest enrollment figures for Medicare, Medicaid, and Children's Health Insurance Program (CHIP)*. https://www.cms.gov/newsroom/news-alert/cms-releases-latest-enrollment-figures-medicare-medicaid-and-childrens-health-insurance-program-chip

Centers for Medicare & Medicaid Services. (2022a, December 15). *Accountable care organizations (ACOs)*. https://www.cms.gov/Medicare/Medicare-Fee-for-Service-Payment/ACO

Centers for Medicare & Medicaid Services. (2022b, October). *October 2022 Medicaid & CHIP enrollment data highlights*. https://www.medicaid.gov/medicaid/program-information/medicaid-and-chip-enrollment-data/report-highlights/index.html

Finegold, K., Wherry, L., & Schardin, S. (2004). Block grants: Historical overview and lessons learned. *New Federalism: Issues and Options for States*, A–63, 1–8. https://webarchive.urban.org/UploadedPDF/310991_A-63.pdf

Kaiser Family Foundation. (2013, April 25). *Summary of the Affordable Care Act*. https://www.kff.org/health-reform/fact-sheet/summary-of-the-affordable-care-act/

Kaiser Family Foundation. (2023, February 16). *Status of state Medicaid expansion decisions: Interactive map*. https://www.kff.org/medicaid/issue-brief/status-of-state-medicaid-expansion-decisions-interactive-map

TRICARE. (n.d.). *Regions*. U.S. Department of Defense, Defense Health Agency. https://www.tricare.mil/About/Regions

TRICARE. (2022, March 2). *Eligibility*. U.S. Department of Defense, Defense Health Agency. https://tricare.mil/Plans/Eligibility

U.S. Department of Veterans Affairs. (n.d.). *Veterans Health Administration*. https://www.va.gov/health/

U.S. Department of Veterans Affairs. (2022, November 14). *Eligibility for VA health care*. https://www.va.gov/health-care/eligibility

Revenue Cycle Management: Cost Estimation and Rate Calculations

OBJECTIVES

1. Define costs as incurred by health services organizations and as captured by the costs accounting process.
2. Discuss the differences in types of costs: direct, indirect, fixed, and variable.
3. Determine the key elements necessary for product pricing and rate setting.
4. Examine profitability and breakeven calculations with respect to changes in volume.
5. Define data capture and discuss its importance in the cost estimation process.

INTRODUCTION

The U.S. healthcare sector provides care in a multitude of ways, and therefore experiences a significant volume of patients. As noted in previous chapters, services provided may be inpatient, outpatient, virtual (via telehealth), prescription, medical equipment, and so forth, all with different units of measure included in the cost of care. When deriving the costs of care, all inputs to the provision of care—whether service or product—must be considered when determining how much expense the organization will incur in the production process. Cost estimation must be as complete and as accurate as possible, as it serves as the basis for subsequent rate calculations and the prices charged to the patients or consumers. To remain viable, healthcare organizations must be sure that the costs of doing business do not exceed the revenue generated by the business. Remaining profitable (or at least covering the base expenses) is important for longevity within the industry, as well as for maintaining the confidence and support of stakeholders. Activities performed by all areas and departments that contribute to the care delivery process must be included; therefore, the cost estimation, in most cases, must begin with the activity level to be sure all expenses are captured. Expenses related to patient care as well as standard operating expenses (human resources, finance, facilities, maintenance, etc.) must be included in costing to be sure they are included in the pricing decisions. Exactly how these items are covered requires a deeper dive into costing and the methods we typically use in the healthcare sector. This chapter examines the process of cost estimation and the impacts on rate calculations for a typical healthcare organization.

THE COST ACCOUNTING PROCESS AND DEFINING COSTS

Costs can be defined as the expenses incurred by an organization to produce a healthcare good or service (Berger, 2019; Menaker et al., 2020). The actual items included vary by organization and are dependent upon the human resources and material resources needed for the production process. The analysis of inputs, called **cost accounting**, is used in managerial accounting for decision-making purposes. There are several types of costs assessed for the decision-making process, which are categorized by their impact on the production process and the final product or healthcare service. Some costs are easier to assess than others, with many requiring a more detailed stepwise approach to cost estimation. All costs are important, however, and must be captured appropriately. The cost accounting process (shown in Figure 8.1) helps to accomplish this, with the process maintained for the longer term by using a dedicated software package.

Figure 8.1

The cost accounting process

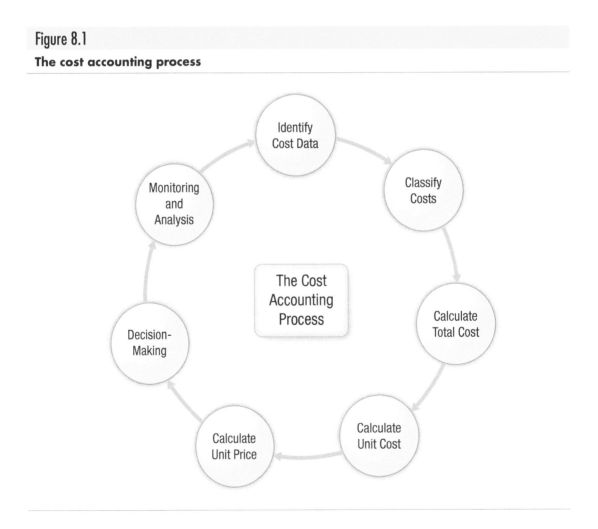

Classification of Costs: Direct Costs and Indirect Costs

Some costs have a definite, clear impact on the production of healthcare goods and services, while other costs are not as closely associated with the end product sold or consumed. **Direct costs** are costs immediately identified as key to the production of healthcare services, or to the task at hand. These are items that actually make the good or service possible. For example, clinicians make the office visit or medical procedure possible. **Indirect costs** are costs that the organization incurs that are not tied to the final healthcare good or service purchased or consumed, but still provide support to the process. Examples include delivery or supply chain materials and resources, housekeeping, and managerial and supervisory staff. While administrative functions like human resources and finance are indirect to patient care, they may be direct if tied to a specific administrative project, like bid and proposal drafting or contract negotiations for a health system. These indirect costs are considered "overhead," and are usually represented by a precalculated rate to be included in costing. The categorization of direct and indirect costs is dependent on the department and its output and unit of measure, with some departments being more direct than others. To determine if a cost should be considered direct or indirect, answer this question: Can this activity be traced back, or connected, to the production of a specific product or care for a specific patient or consumer? Reimbursement generally includes payment for direct costs and indirect costs, with indirect costs captured and calculated separately. Both types of costs are important and necessary for effective and efficient organization management, including both current operations and future planning. Table 8.1 provides examples of direct and indirect costs as they would typically appear in a standard health services organization.

Table 8.1

DIRECT AND INDIRECT COSTS WITH EXAMPLES

Department	Direct Cost Examples	Indirect Cost Examples
Physicians, nurses, clinical staff	Time and labor expense of hands-on care for a specific patient; single-use supplies/materials (syringes, bandages, etc.)	Clinical rounds or meetings regarding a patient's care; examination gloves; administrative supplies (charts/documentation, office supplies, etc.)
Laboratory services	Time and labor expense of performing lab testing for a specific patient; single-use supplies/materials (syringes, test tubes, testing reagents, etc.)	Laboratory instrumentation and sample testing machinery; equipment repairs and upgrades; administrative supplies (charts/documentation, office supplies, etc.)
Imaging services	Time and labor expense of performing an imaging procedure on a patient (MRI, chest x-ray, etc.); single-use supplies/materials (imaging film, contrast media, etc.)	Software purchases (for analysis); administrative supplies (charts/documentation, office supplies, etc.)
Human resources	N/A	All human resources functions are indirect; not attributable to patient care; captured in overhead
Pharmacy	Cost of the patient's medication (as charged by the pharmaceutical company)	While the pharmacist fills the prescriptions for each patient, the time and labor expense is not directly allocated to a specific patient
Housekeeping	N/A	All housekeeping functions are indirect; not attributable to patient care; captured in overhead
Finance	N/A	All finance department functions are indirect; not attributable to patient care; captured in overhead

It is important to be clear on what activities are directly connected to one patient's care and what activities are shared by all patients. Most patient care areas have some type of direct costs, even if those costs do not include labor expenses. Correct identification of costs is critical to the calculation of total cost and ultimately the product or healthcare service's total price.

Indirect costs, including overhead, must be allocated and properly assigned to the revenue-generating departments that incurred the indirect costs. Allocation, or in this case **cost allocation**, is the distribution of indirect costs to the revenue-generating areas. Items such as space leasing or rental, human resources, and finance departments support the entire organization, so indirect costs associated with these departments are typically allocated or distributed across all functional areas. Cost allocation requires the following key items:

- **cost pool:** the costs to be allocated, typically indirect costs or overhead costs
- **cost driver:** the basis for the allocation, the allocating department's unit of measure
- utilization of the department(s) receiving the allocation

An example of the cost allocation rate calculation: Pantheon Health System has an administrative division, which contains all of the salary and wage expenses for its leadership team. The administrative division serves all departments within the health system, but larger departments usually require more time. For the quarter, the administrative division has generated $50,000 in administrative services expense, which needs to be allocated to the revenue-generating departments to be included in the billing and reimbursement processes. The division provided 1,000 hours of services during the quarter.

BOX 8.1

Administrative Division: Cost Allocation Rate Calculation (Direct Allocation)

Cost pool (amount to be allocated)	= $50,000
Cost driver (basis for allocation: hours)	= 1,000
Cost allocation rate	= Cost Pool ÷ Cost Driver
	= $50,000 ÷ 1,000
	= $50 per hour

In the sample calculation shown in Box 8.1, the administrative division will allocate its services at a rate of $50 per hour. This hourly rate is then entered into the indirect/overhead allocation calculation for the various departments, based on their utilization. If the nursing department uses 50 hours of administrative services, the administrative division would directly allocate $2,500 ($50 × 50 hours) of its expense to the nursing department. Using this direct method, costs are allocated based on the receiving departments' utilization and the administrative division's cost driver, administrative services hours. If overhead costs are to be distributed equally no matter the utilization, the cost pool will then be divided by the number of receiving departments. If the allocation is to be calculated using a different driver, the costs distribution would be calculated according to the receiving department's contribution to that specific driver.

To illustrate this alternative allocation method, refer to the information presented in Box 8.2a as base data for Pantheon Health System's surgery division.

BOX 8.2a

Surgery Division: Cost Allocation Calculation (Base Data)

Surgical Department	Surgical Cases	Annual Revenue
Bariatric surgery	205	$10,100,000
Cardiovascular surgery	125	$16,500,000
Neurosurgery	248	$19,850,000
Orthopedic surgery	550	$13,688,500
Total	1,128	$60,138,500

In this example, the surgery division consists of four surgical departments: bariatric surgery, cardiovascular surgery, neurosurgery, and orthopedic surgery. If we refer back to the administrative division in Box 8.1, the cost pool, or amount to be allocated, is $50,000. Let us assume that the entire amount is to be allocated to the surgical division. If we changed the cost driver from administrative services hours to annual revenue contribution, we would have to use an alternative method for calculating the amount allocated to the various surgical departments, instead of the previously calculated allocation rate. Using the data given in Box 8.2a, we must first determine what percentage of the surgery division's total annual revenue is contributed by each surgical department. Then, we use each department's percentage to calculate how much of the $50,000 cost pool they will need to cover. The completed calculations are shown in Box 8.2b.

BOX 8.2b

Surgery Division: Cost Allocation Calculation (Annual Revenue Driver)

Surgical Department	Surgical Cases	Annual Revenue	Revenue %	Admin Allocation
Bariatric surgery	205	$10,100,000	16.79	$8,397
Cardiovascular surgery	125	$16,500,000	27.44	$13,718
Neurosurgery	248	$19,850,000	33.01	$16,504
Orthopedic surgery	550	$13,688,500	22.76	$11,381
Total	1,128	$60,138,500	100%	$50,000

The results show that neurosurgery contributes the largest percentage to the annual revenue, and therefore has a larger allocation of administrative services costs. To calculate the neurosurgery department's revenue contribution percentage: $19,850,000 ÷ $60,138,500 = .3301 or 33.01%. This percentage is then multiplied by the cost pool to determine how much of the administrative services expenses will be allocated to neurosurgery: $50,000 × .3301 = $16,505. The same calculation methods are applied to the other surgical departments, dividing the annual revenue for each by the total revenue amount, then multiplying the resulting percentage by the cost pool. Similarly, if the cost driver was the surgical cases, we would find each department's contribution to total surgical cases and use that percentage to allocate the cost pool.

Classification of Costs: Fixed Costs and Variable Costs

Along with determining if an incurred cost is direct or indirect, we must also assess the behavior of the cost in relation to the product or service being provided. In other words, we must determine if the costs of production or the costs of healthcare service delivery change when the volume changes. **Fixed costs** are costs that remain static with changes in volume—no increases or decreases for the shorter term. This usually includes expenses captured as overhead costs. Examples of fixed cost items are office space rental, overhead, utilities, and other expenses that are not directly impacted by patient volume. In longer-term planning, the overall fixed costs may be updated to reflect significant changes that impact total cost. Medical office space leasing is an example of a longer-term fixed cost subject to changes. If the lease term is 1 year and the price of leasing the space increases, that would provide the basis for increased fixed costs, not an increase of patient visits. Another example is utilities, which are usually independent of patient volume in the shorter term. The amount of electricity used to light a hospital room is not tied to the patient occupying the room. If the facility operates 100 rooms daily, the cost of utilities is relatively predictable and will not change if one patient is discharged and another is admitted. In the longer term, however, if the facility expands and now operates 150 rooms, the fixed cost amount would increase to reflect overall increased utilization.

   Variable costs, on the other hand, are dependent and change with variations in volume. Examples of variable costs in healthcare are medical supplies (single-use items such as bandages, syringes, gauze, etc.), medications, and associated supplies (IV tubing, IV bags, etc.) and laboratory reagents. These costs may be represented as the total variable cost or as a **variable cost rate**. Total variable costs would be a summation of variable costs provided for the different operational areas. The variable cost rate establishes a set cost per unit for each unit of volume, and then total variable cost is calculated. To illustrate this, let us use an example of phlebotomy laboratory testing. The laboratory has an established variable cost rate of $25 per patient test, which includes the required test tubes, pipettes, and testing solutions. The calculations of total variable costs (Box 8.3) for 250 patients (one test each) would be as noted.

BOX 8.3

Total Variable Costs Calculation

Volume (no. of laboratory tests):   250

Variable cost rate: $25.00

Total variable costs   = Volume × Variable Cost Rate

    = 250 × $25.00

    = $6,250.00

   For each additional laboratory test performed, the total variable costs will increase by $25.00. The variable cost rate is a "bundled" rate, which can be used in this instance because the items used for the laboratory test will be the same for each patient with no variation. This will allow the department to estimate its total expenses relatively quickly, barring any change in supply purchase price. As the department's supply purchase price changes, their variable cost rate may change as well. In cases where the laboratory tests may be variable because of patient differences (such as diagnosis or condition), a more detailed cost analysis must be done to capture the total variable costs. Unlike fixed costs that remain the same over a specified time period, variable costs may change more often due to changes in volume, supply price, or any other element included in the variable cost rate calculation. Tracking variable costs in relation to volume may provide important information regarding supply ordering and inventory (covered in Chapter 15).

Calculation of Total Costs

To adequately capture all costs for inclusion in the final pricing strategy, an organization must account for all costs involved in the creation of the healthcare product or service. This **total cost** will include items that are dependent on volume as well as those items that are not, and represents the organization's **underlying cost structure**. The underlying cost structure can be summarized using the following formula:

$$\text{Total Costs} = \text{Fixed Costs} + \text{Total Variable Costs}$$

Or

$$\text{Total Costs} = \text{Fixed Costs} + [(\text{Variable Costs Rate} \times \text{Volume})]$$

Remember, overhead does not fluctuate according to volume, and therefore must be included with the fixed costs in the underlying costs structure. The variable costs rate must be multiplied by the volume to accurately reflect the total variable costs. Let's examine the following scenario to get an idea of how total costs calculations would be considered in healthcare.

Scenario

Pantheon Health Systems is considering renting some of its unused office space to Lighthouse Medical, a small physicians group comprised of several primary care physicians and specialists. The space includes several smaller, private offices for patient consultation as well as several diagnostic imaging machines (MRI, CT, x-ray, ultrasound, etc.). As an additional service to Lighthouse, Pantheon has agreed to provide some basic administrative support for office management and billing for a fee. Before making the final decision and signing the lease agreement, Lighthouse would like to have a clear picture of the costs involved. As the lead financial analyst, you've been asked to prepare the basics of the lease agreement. The variables to include in the costs calculation are as follows:

- rent: $3,500 monthly
- utilities: $750 monthly
- administrative support: $30 hourly
- imaging: $25 per scan

Lighthouse considers its current business and anticipates no major changes in volume, which has historically been approximately 100 visits/scans monthly. Routine office visits would be of no additional cost, and the administrative expense should be based on a standard 40-hour work week. For this scenario, what is the underlying cost structure for this business arrangement?

Step 1: Calculate total fixed costs (independent of volume):

Fixed Costs = Rent + Utilities + Administrative Support

$$= \$3,500 + \$750 + (160 \text{ hours} \times \$30)$$

$$= \$3,500 + \$750 + \$4,800$$

$$= \$9,050 \text{ monthly fixed costs}$$

Step 2: Calculate total variable costs (dependent on volume):

Total Variable Costs = Variable Costs Rate × Volume

$$= \$25 \text{ per scan} \times 100 \text{ scans}$$

$$= \$2,500 \text{ monthly variable costs}$$

Step 3: Calculate total costs:

Total Costs = Fixed Costs + Total Variable Costs

$$= \$9,050 + \$2,500$$

$$= \$11,550 \text{ monthly total costs}$$

The business decision to be made by Lighthouse Medical is dependent on the financial goals of the group and how the total costs fit into their financial picture. Sustained volume and generated revenue are all determinants of this being a viable business arrangement, and knowing the total costs or underlying cost structure will assist Lighthouse in the decision-making process. This same process would have been done by Pantheon Health as they calculated the rental lease fees for those interested in renting the space. They would have possibly considered how much they currently pay for this space (as a portion of a mortgage or larger lease agreement) and how much they have to pay for sourcing the administrative services. This brings us to the next discussion, the difference between cost and price as relative to rate setting for healthcare organizations.

SPECIALIZED COSTING

Traditional costing may be relatively straightforward when categorized as direct to-patient care and as indirect administrative or operational costs captured at the department level. There are, however, other types of specialized costs that must be captured for inclusion and calculation of overall pricing. Some costs involve multiple departments or processes, which must be assessed and aggregated before moving to the pricing stage, providing service-level analysis. This service-level costing requires analysis of individual activities that comprise a process or the multiple processes that are required to represent a department's work. To further explain, we examine the concepts of activity-based costing and workload calculations.

Activity-Based Costing

Activity-based costing (ABC) is a costing approach which analyzes the individual units of work performed that contribute to the total cost of a process (Campanale et al., 2014; Menaker et al., 2020). Work performed includes required activities for the creation of a department's products or services. The reason many utilize the ABC method for more complex costing challenges is due to its detailed and precise results, which provide an in-depth look at tasks, processes, and workflows. It gives detail on the cost estimates for the smaller pieces of activity that make up the entire task. ABC is used for the allocation of indirect or administrative costs that need to be allocated to multiple patients or departments. The ABC process assists with determining an allocation rate for tasks at the activity level, even if the activities and rates within the process are different. Figure 8.2 shows the steps of ABC.

Figure 8.2

Activity-based costing

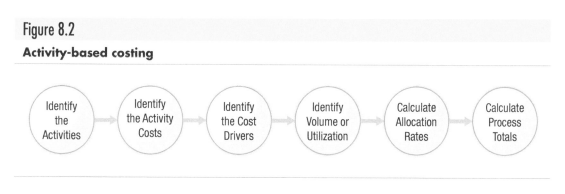

To demonstrate the ABC process, let's review the following scenario using Pantheon Health Systems and Lighthouse Medical from the previous example.

Scenario

Lighthouse Medical is leasing their office space from Pantheon Health Systems, but needs to know the costs of their service-level tasks to accurately price its imaging services and determine the allocation rate for providing services to other departments. Most patients that come in for imaging follow the same basic registration process, with the major difference of the visit being the type of screening performed. Lighthouse would like to use ABC to assess the costs of individual activities performed during each standard patient visit and determine the aggregate cost per CT and MRI imaging procedure.

Using the table of data in Box 8.4a, we can begin to identify the required items for our ABC calculation process:

Step 1: Identify activities: "Activity" column in Box 8.4.a.
Step 2: Identify activity costs: "Annual Costs" column in Box 8.4a reflects annual costs for each activity.
Step 3: Identify the cost drivers: "Cost Driver" column in Box 8.4a reflects the basis of measurement for each activity.
Step 4: Identify volume or utilization: "Activity Data" in Box 8.4a reflects the volume for each imaging test type.

For the remaining two steps, a series of basic calculations helps to calculate the allocation rates and cost per imaging procedure using the data provided in Box 8.4a (reflected in Box 8.4b).

BOX 8.4a

Lighthouse Medical ABC Calculation (Base Data)

Activity	Annual Costs	Cost Driver	Activity Data	
			CT Scan	MRI
Registration	$65,000	No. of tests	400	750
Procedure preparation	$80,000	No. of tests	400	750
Imaging procedures	$750,000	Minutes per test	15	30
Film prints	$85,000	Prints per test	3	6
Analysis and reporting	$80,000	Minutes per test	20	40

BOX 8.4b

Lighthouse Medical ABC Calculation (Activity Total and Allocation Rate)

Activity	Annual Costs	Cost Driver	Activity Data		Total		Allocation Rate	
			CT Scan	MRI				
Registration	$65,000	No. of tests	400	750	1,150	(Total no. of tests)	$56.52	(annual cost/total)
Procedure preparation	$80,000	No. of tests	400	750	1,150	(Total no. of tests)	$69.57	(annual cost/total)
Imaging procedures	$750,000	Minutes per test	15	30	28,500	(Minutes × no. of tests)	$26.32	(annual cost/total)
Film prints	$85,000	Prints per test	3	6	5,700	(Prints × no. of tests)	$14.91	(annual cost/total)
Analysis and reporting	$80,000	Minutes per test	20	40	38,000	(Minutes × no. of tests)	$2.11	(annual cost/total)
Total costs	$1,060,000						$169.43	

ABC, activity-based costing.

As we work toward an allocation rate for the department, we must first combine the volume data for the CT scans and the MRIs. To accomplish this, we use the cost driver as a guide for the calculation of total activity: so the "Registration" = 400 + 750 = 1,150 tests, and "Procedure preparation" (using the same cost driver) would be the same. The cost driver for these two activities is the number of tests, so we can simply add the tests together. Basically, according to our data table, one registration = one registration, and one procedure preparation = one procedure preparation, no matter the test type. To combine the imaging procedures for the two test types, the totals are calculated individually and then added together. The cost driver for this activity is the minutes per test, and since the minutes for each test type vary, we must calculate the totals individually first and then combine. The minutes for a CT scan are not equal to the minutes for an MRI, so we cannot combine these without first calculating total minutes for each. So, "Imaging procedures" = $(15 \times 400) + (30 \times 750) = 28,500$ minutes, where 15×400 (or 6,000 minutes) calculates the CT scan volume, and 30×750 (or 22,500 minutes) calculates the MRI volume. The same process is followed for the calculation of the "Film prints" = $(3 \times 400) + (6 \times 750) = 5,700$ prints and "Analysis and reporting" = $(20 \times 400) + (40 \times 750) = 38,000$ minutes.

For Step 5, the "Allocation Rates" are calculated by dividing the annual costs of each activity by the total volume of that activity, which will produce the average cost for one unit of the corresponding activity. Using the "Registration" activity as an example, we divide $65,000 in annual costs by 1,150 registrations, resulting in an allocation rate of $56.52 per registration. For Step 6, these allocation rates are then used to calculate total cost per procedure type. The activity data for each imaging procedure type is multiplied by the allocation rate, with all activities for each test summed for the total (shown in Box 8.4c).

BOX 8.4c

Lighthouse Medical ABC Calculation (Total Cost Per Imaging Procedure)

Activity	CT Total Cost	MRI Total Cost
Registration	$56.52	$56.52
Procedure preparation	$69.57	$69.57
Imaging procedures	$394.74	$789.47
Film prints	$44.74	$89.47
Analysis and reporting	$42.11	$84.21
	$607.68	$1,089.24

ABC, activity-based costing.

The "Registration" and "Procedure preparation" for each patient happens only once for each test, so the calculations for both test types reflect: $1 \times \$56.52 = \$56.52$, and $1 \times \$69.57 = \$69.57$ for these total costs. "Imaging procedure" total costs are calculated by multiplying the individual minutes by allocation rates, shown previously as $15 \times \$26.32 = \$394.80$ and $30 \times \$26.32 = \$789.60$, respectively. Totals for "Film prints" and "Analysis and reporting" are calculated similarly, with total costs for CT scans as $607.68 and MRIs as $1,089.24.

Workload Calculations

Another type of specialized cost estimation is the **workload calculation**, which is an estimate capturing anticipated labor expense for a project or process. This is a relatively straightforward process as long as the following key elements are known:

- tasks that comprise the project or process,
- completion time for each task,

> frequency and duration of the tasks/project, and

> pay rate of the employee completing the tasks.

Workload calculations are performed to assess new labor expenses when a new product or service is introduced, as well as incremental labor expenses when a service is modified or expanded. Workload calculations become extremely important for organizations with large numbers of employees, as well as for those with funding restrictions that require project or program-specific labor expenses. To demonstrate this, let us examine a basic workload calculation.

Scenario

An outpatient clinic is exploring the option of free walk-in diabetes screenings for residents in the neighborhood and would like to calculate the estimated labor expenses. The screenings would require a part-time RN who would perform the diabetes testing for 4 hours per day, Monday through Thursday (or 4 days per week working around any holidays), for the entire year. The RN has an hourly wage of $65, and medical supplies will be included in the clinic's operating budget, instead of separately. To do this workload calculation, since the screenings aren't timed individually, the estimate can be done using total screening hours.

Step 1: Screening hours per week = 4 hours per day × 4 days per week = 16 hours per week

Step 2: Screening hours per year = 16 hours per week × 52 weeks = 832 hours per year

Step 3: RN wages per year (all screenings) = $65 per hour × 832 hours = $54,080

This example shows the basic calculation for a part-time employee, but similar calculations would be used for full-time employees as well. Full-time labor expenses are often expressed in terms of **full-time equivalents** (FTEs), and may include additional items such as bonuses or fringe benefits. **Fringe benefits** are the items offered to employees in addition to salary and wages, such as health insurance coverage, memberships and subscriptions, free parking, or other items of value to the employee. Fringe benefits are often represented as a percentage of an employee's base salary, and will be classified as salary and wage expense. For example, if the RN in the previous scenario was a full-time employee with an annual salary of $54,080, the fringe benefit amount would be in addition to that salary. If the outpatient clinic offered fringe benefits of 33% in addition to the base salary, the calculation for the total (to be recorded in the accounting system as salary and wage expense) would be:

Base salary: $54,080

Fringe benefits (@ 33%): $54,080 × .33 = $17,846.40

Total RN compensation: $54,080 + $17,846.40 = $71,926.40

Similar calculations would be done for all employees deemed eligible for fringe benefits, with various offerings provided for different levels or types of employees. Capturing all associated benefits provides the organization with a clear picture of salary and wage expense, not only capturing everything incurred, but also helping to ensure adequate staffing levels for patient care and other required services. This is particularly important in clinical areas where clinician-to-patient ratios must be maintained, or in other areas such as clinical laboratories where workload and specimens must be processed within a given time frame.

RATE CALCULATIONS AND PRICE

Cost and price are not interchangeable, although both are very important to an organization's financial standing. As stated in the previous section, costs are the expenses incurred by an organization as they create or provide a healthcare good or service. **Price**, on the other hand, is the amount the organization will charge consumers or patients to utilize the services provided. The price includes the costs incurred, in addition to any profit margin the organization seeks to receive, as shown in Figure 8.3. This is the very reason it is critical for the organization to capture appropriate costs at all levels—any shortfall in cost capture means diminished profits or possibly diminished ability to cover any costs incurred.

Figure 8.3

The components of price

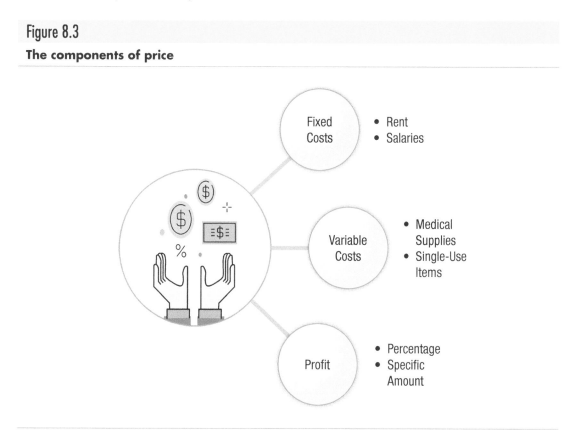

When determining the pricing structure, the goal is to at least cover the base costs, and in some cases a nominal profit amount is included. Volume drives the fluctuations in underlying cost structure as previously calculated, which will ultimately impact the price. Rate-setting is also heavily influenced by the reimbursement mechanisms established in a particular sector and the associated **patient mix**. Patient mix is the demographic breakdown or categorization of the patient population or community served. The categorization could be done according to medical diagnosis or type of insurance coverage (payer mix), both being an indicator of expense incurred as well as possible reimbursement (Healthcare Financial Management Association [HFMA], 2021; Widmer, 2016). (Reimbursement is outlined by the contractual agreements with insurers and other responsible parties, which we discuss in detail in Chapter 7.) We have discussed the fixed costs and variable costs components of price, so let us now examine the profit component of the pricing structure.

Profit, to be clear, does not always mean the surplus revenue that we think of in the typical sense. In the healthcare sector, this is usually the small amount of revenue dedicated to equipment maintenance and upgrades (Guo et al., 2016; HFMA, 2021). Approximately 75% of hospitals in the United States are not-for-profit (HFMA, 2021; Ramos-Hegwer, 2017), so the profit is a small amount with the dedicated purpose of asset management and new technologies. Reimbursement and the financial goals established by an organization are often contingent upon the contractual agreements in place with the various payers. The *payer mix* of the organization is the percentage of volume and associated reimbursement for the various contracted payers. Knowing the payer mix allows the organization to anticipate volume and revenue, establishing sound data for the pricing and rate-setting process.

Pricing Strategies and Profit Analysis

There are several pricing strategies that can be used to determine the price of healthcare services, differing by what is included and what is used as the basis for calculation. **Full-cost pricing** is establishing a price that covers direct fixed costs, direct variable costs, and overhead, which includes indirect expenses incurred that have been applied using the allocation process. **Marginal-cost pricing** is establishing a price that covers additional units of service, but not all costs incurred. In this pricing strategy, just the variable costs are covered (no fixed costs or overhead), making this a short-term approach (see Box 8.5).

BOX 8.5

Marginal Cost Calculation

Marginal Cost = Change in Costs/Change in Quantity Demanded

        Current number of ultrasounds = 1,000
        Current cost of ultrasounds = $125,000

        Future number of ultrasounds = 2,000
        Future cost of ultrasounds = $175,000

        Marginal cost = $50 per ultrasound

Without eventually employing a strategy that includes all fixed and variable items, the organization runs the risk of being in a loss position or not having the ability to cover its base costs, even without an anticipated profit amount. Longer-term marginal-cost pricing scenarios often include some form of **price shifting** to maintain financial footing. Price shifting is the process of charging higher pricing to one group of consumers to cover the financial shortfall of another group of consumers.

Breakeven is the baseline of most pricing strategies, which aims to ensure that all of the incurred costs are in fact covered. Breakeven can be calculated with a marginal profit amount (referred to as an **economic breakeven**) or with no profit included (**accounting breakeven**). A breakeven analysis answers the question: Have we established an adequate price that meets our financial goals? The calculations for breakeven include total costs elements as well as price and profit. This volume-driven formula provides a mechanism for detailed analysis of the included variables for informed pricing decisions and profit analysis. We can begin the profit analysis discussion by using the all-inclusive formula shown in Box 8.6.

BOX 8.6

Profitability and Breakeven Formula

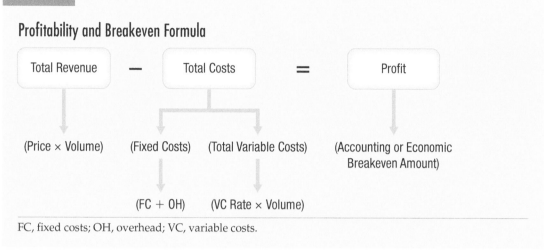

FC, fixed costs; OH, overhead; VC, variable costs.

Using this formula, decision makers can assess the current price as well as the desired profit for any segment of the organization. As the organization experiences fluctuations in volume, routine calculations can be done to assess the overall impact on price. To illustrate the profitability and breakeven analysis, let's revisit the Pantheon Health Systems and Lighthouse Medical scenario. Now that Lighthouse Medical knows how much their monthly expenses will be, they have to determine how much they'll charge patients for the office visit (includes scans), including a small profit amount to cover basic equipment upgrades, which they believe should be covered by $3,000. Using the same base data provided in the original scenario, the equation becomes:

$$(\text{Price} \times \text{Volume}) - (\text{Fixed Costs}) - (\text{Total Variable Costs}) = \text{Profit}$$

$$(\text{Price} \times 100) - (\$9{,}050) - (\$2{,}500) = \$3{,}000$$

Since all other elements are known, the variable we need to solve for is "Price." Following standard mathematical operations, we continue solving for "Price" by isolating the variable on one side of the equation:

$$(\text{Price} \times 100) - \$11{,}550 = \$3{,}000$$

$$\text{Price} \times 100 = \$14{,}550$$

$$\text{Price} = \$14{,}550 \div 100$$

$$\text{Price} = \$145.50 \text{ per office visit, including scan}$$

So, according to this calculation, Lighthouse should set the price at $145.50 per visit, if volume remains static at 100 patients monthly, and if they plan to earn $3,000 per month in profit (an economic breakeven). If they decide that they would just like to cover incurred costs and earn profit elsewhere in the business, then the profit side of the equation would equal zero (an accounting breakeven) and the price would be total costs divided by volume: $11,550 ÷ 100 = $115.50 per office visit, including scan.

While this example shows the typical pricing and profit analysis process, the rates for insurance reimbursement may differ (HFMA, 2021; Menaker et al., 2020). Government and public payers, for instance, have a predetermined reimbursement rate for their various medical services, no matter the costs incurred by the healthcare organization submitting the claim. Prices charged must be equitable, so established prices must be the same for all patients, meaning that other patients cannot be charged more to make up the decreased revenue from public payers. How do organizations adjust for the variations in revenue? They make adjustments to their payer mix. The sensible financial solution would be to have a higher number/percentage of patients covered by commercial insurance, which typically reimburses at a higher rate. Patients with government/public insurance would still be accepted (because the health and welfare of patients take priority over payment) but the organization may take fewer of these patients during the same financial period.

CAPITAL STRUCTURE AND CORPORATE COST OF CAPITAL

An organization's financial health is determined not only by its profitability, but by its risk and leveraged decision-making. While most seek to satisfy financial obligations using earned revenues and other assets, coverage may also come in the form of borrowing. **Risk** is the exposure to a negative financial outcome as influenced by financing decisions, particularly with borrowing or debt financing. The management decision for how to finance depends on the assets and the ability to generate revenue, as well as the possible return on equity (ROE) for borrowed funds. Ideally, there is an appropriate mix of equity and debt financing, which is assessed by calculating the ROE through dividing the net income by net assets. The **capital structure** is the determination of the ideal financing by comparing the ROE results for the anticipated equity financing percentage and the anticipated debt financing percentage. In some cases, debt can actually increase the ROE for an organization, so debt is not always a bad thing. Let's try an example for the capital structure analysis and ROE calculation.

Scenario

Community Health System (CHS) operates 365 days per year and generates $70,000,000 in annual revenues. The organization currently uses an all-equity approach to financing, has earnings (before interest and taxes) of $15,000,000, and holds $19,000,000 in assets. They would like to compare their current all-equity financing approach to a possible 60% debt financing approach. Use an interest rate of 7% and a tax rate of 33% in your calculations.

Capital Structure Analysis

Using one column for the equity financing calculations and a second column for the debt financing calculations:

Step 1: Create a balance sheet reflecting the financing options (like this example in Table 8.2).
   Here, the prepared balance sheet shows both approaches to financing: (a) the all-equity approach, which uses equity to secure assets; and (b) the debt approach, which uses 40% equity and 60% debt to secure the assets. For the equity approach, debt equals zero since nothing is borrowed, leaving the total equity (or net assets) equal to $19,000,000. For the debt approach, CHS would finance 60% of the asset value, or $19,000,000 × .60 = $11,400,000, leaving total equity (or net assets) of $7,600,000.

Table 8.2

BALANCE SHEET

	Equity Financing	Debt Financing (60%)
Assets	$19,000,000	$19,000,000
Debt	$ -	$11,400,000
Net assets	**$19,000,000**	**$7,600,000**

Step 2: Create an income statement reflecting the earnings, interest, and tax calculations (see Table 8.3).

Table 8.3

INCOME STATEMENT

	Equity Financing	Debt Financing (60%)
EBIT	$15,000,000	$15,000,000
Interest (7%)	$ -	$798,000
Taxable income	$15,000,000	$14,202,000
Taxes (33%)	$4,950,000	$4,686,660
Net income	**$10,050,000**	**$9,515,340**

EBIT, earnings before interest and taxes.

In this prepared income statement, the calculations begin with income (or as stated in this example, earnings before interest and taxes [EBIT]) of $15,000,000. Next is the subtraction of interest. Remember, interest is paid on the amount borrowed, NOT on the income amount, so the interest amount in the "Equity Financing" column is zero. The interest rate of 7% is applied to the amount borrowed: $11,400,000 × .07 = $798,000. Income/Earnings − interest = taxable income, leaving the entire $15,000,000 in the "Equity Financing" column and $14,202,000 in the "Debt Financing" column ($15,000,000 − $798,000). The tax rate of 33% is then applied to the taxable income, resulting in taxes of $4,950,000 and $4,686,660 for the "Equity Financing" and "Debt Financing" columns, respectively. Net income is the remaining income after the tax amounts have been subtracted: $10,050,000 net income for the equity financing option, and $9,515,340 net income for the debt financing option.

Step 3: Calculate the ROE for each financing option listed in Table 8.4.

Table 8.4

ROE CALCULATIONS

	Equity Financing	Debt Financing (60%)
Net income	$10,050,000	$9,515,340
Net assets	$19,000,000	$7,600,000
ROE	**.5289 or 52.89%**	**1.2520 or 125.20%**

ROE, return on equity.

In this final step of calculating the ROE, which divides the net income by net assets, the debt financing option yields a higher return for each dollar of equity. The interest paid on the borrowed amount serves to reduce the taxable income and taxes, providing a higher return. This translates to additional earnings to be utilized by the organization, or, in the case of a for-profit organization, additional earnings for the shareholders or owners.

When the organization has decided on its optimal equity and debt financing mix, they must then consider the cost of maintaining this capital structure. The **corporate cost of capital** (CCC) is then calculated using the debt and equity percentages and the required interest rate or rate of return for each. We can represent the CCC calculation by using this formula:

CCC = (Equity Percentage × Equity Cost) + [(Debt Percentage × Debt Cost) × (1 − Tax Rate)]

Where:

Equity Percentage (EqP) = the percentage of equity to be used in the financing decision,

Equity Cost (EqC) = the required rate/cost of financing using equity,

Debt Percentage (DtP) = the percentage of debt to be used in the financing decision,

Debt Cost (DtC) = the required rate/cost of financing using debt, and

Tax Rate (T) = the organization's tax rate

To demonstrate the CCC calculation, let's say CHS has decided on a capital structure of 60% equity and 40% debt. The cost of equity and debt are 15% and 9%, respectively, and CHS has a current tax rate of 23%.

$$CCC = \left(EqP \times EqC\right) + \left[\left(DtP \times DtC\right) \times \left(1 - T\right)\right]$$

$$CCC = \left(.60 \times 15\right) + \left[\left(.40 \times 9\right) \times \left(1 - .23\right)\right]$$

$$CCC = \left(.60 \times 15\right) + \left(3.6 \times .77\right)$$

$$CCC = 9 + 2.772$$

CCC = 11.772%

In this example, CHS's CCC is 11.772% for the financing mix or equity-to-debt ratio of 60/40. In an organization's financing mix, no matter which portion is greater, the equity percentage and the debt percentage must total 100%, representing the entire financing picture. As multiple CCCs are analyzed when comparing different corporate structures with varying weights of equity and debt, the lowest CCC is the best option.

When determining how to proceed with investments, the CCC is a key marker in the decision-making process. For an investment to be deemed profitable or worth the investment, it must meet the CCC, at minimum, but ideally surpass it with increased equity or profit. In most cases, expensive medical equipment and items used during routine operations meet this requirement if there is enough volume and subsequent revenue to justify the purchase. With new investments that have no historical utilization data, it may be more challenging to determine return.

DECISION-MAKING AND DATA CAPTURE

Cost estimation, as discussed in the previous sections, can provide an overview of an organization's expenditures or a detailed analysis of operations. In healthcare, cost estimation data is foundational and is essential to maintaining an effective and efficient sector, providing the best possible healthcare services. The challenge for some is determining what data to capture and, when recorded, how to interpret the data and transform it into actionable items. The process should begin with the organization's goals, mission, vision, and values, which guide all activities and desired outcomes. This may be different among organizations, but there are some items that are somewhat universal in healthcare. For proper management and decision-making, data capture should include information that assists with the following standard organizational functions:

- *Accounting:* This records all financial activity coming in and going out of the organization. This data helps decision makers to visualize what financial resources we have and how we are sending them. Accounting data includes revenues, expenses, assets, liabilities, and capital investments, as summarized and reported on the financial statements.

- *Budgeting and forecasting:* After the actual financial activity is recorded, decisions must be made on preparing for the future. Efforts to maintain the organization's operations (financial and patient care) must begin with proper planning. Using the accounting data, estimates for volume and utilization, revenues, and expenses can be made, ensuring adequate use and distribution of available resources.

- *Investments:* Data capture helps to determine what, how, and when to invest in projects and services by providing much-needed detail on available alternatives. Data for the "make or buy" decision, as well as the "expand or contract" decision, allows leadership to utilize available resources for the appropriate investments.

- *Patient and stakeholder experience:* The needs of stakeholders must be managed. Data capture through accounting methods and ABC provides decision makers with information at the transaction level for patients, clinicians, insurers, and other stakeholders, allowing for continuous improvement.

The healthcare sector must remain versatile as it changes to meet growing demand and unforeseen challenges such as the pandemic. Versatility and agility require the routine review of scope, products, and services to remain viable and competitive. Industry regulations such as those mandated by the Department of Health and Human Services or Centers for Medicare & Medicaid Services are outside of the healthcare organization's control, but must still be incorporated into the routine operating structure. Changing reimbursement mechanisms, such as the more recent value-based care models, require a deeper understanding of internal operations to inform strategic decision-making and ongoing analysis. Data capture is critical to the present and future success of healthcare organizations, and ultimately the changing healthcare landscape.

CHAPTER SUMMARY

Cost estimation is a very important part of an organization's financial operations, as it provides the baseline of pricing, reimbursement rates, budgeting, and financial planning. The process of cost accounting is necessary to accurately capture costs incurred while providing products and services to patients and other consumers. Volume and associated costs figure prominently in pricing and profit strategies, as providers and suppliers try to remain financially viable while providing the highest quality of care. Cost accounting and trend analysis establish the history of what the organization's performance has been, with breakeven and profitability analysis preparing a financial path forward. Sound cost estimation allows for budgeting accuracy, future planning, and the overall achievement of goals and objectives. Although there are numerous ways and software systems in place to perform the cost estimation function, the key is interpretation and planning using this data. Ideally, accurate cost estimation helps an organization to have effective longer-term planning, efficient resource utilization, meaningful stakeholder engagement, and improved profit margins.

KEY TERMS FOR REVIEW

accounting breakeven	direct costs	price
activity-based costing	economic breakeven	price shifting
capital structure	fixed costs	risk
corporate cost of capital	fringe benefits	total cost
cost accounting	full-cost pricing	underlying cost structure
cost allocation	full-time equivalents	variable cost rate
cost driver	indirect costs	variable costs
cost pool	marginal-cost pricing	workload calculation
costs	patient mix	

DISCUSSION QUESTIONS

1. What is the difference between cost and price?

2. What is the underlying cost structure?

3. What are the elements included in the underlying cost structure calculation, and why are they important to financial decision-making?

4. Define cost pool and cost driver as relative to cost allocation.

5. What is the difference between fixed costs and variable costs?

6. What is considered overhead and what types of items are included in it? Is overhead a fixed cost, direct cost, or indirect cost? Explain your selection.

7. Discuss the importance of data capture and how it helps with routine operations of the healthcare organization.

PRACTICE PROBLEMS

1. A new physical therapy office is being planned, which will be open during traditional operating hours and offer extended service hours as well. Total operating hours will be 16 hours a day, 5 days a week, as well as 6 hours on Saturdays. If you need to staff the registration desk at all times, how many FTEs will you need?

2. A department has four medical assistants, and they are due for a pay increase—a 7% increase to their annual salary. The increase is to be effective July 1st (the start of the new fiscal year), but the organization has had some financial challenges and has to postpone the increase. The raises will instead take effect on January 1st, and the medical assistants will be paid retroactively from the original effective date.

   a. If the medical assistants' annual salaries are $35,000, $40,000, $28,000, and $42,000, how much will the retroactive pay for each be when they are paid in January?

   b. Using the annual salaries from Part A, what is the fringe benefit amount for each medical assistant if the company's fringe rate is 30% of an employee's base salary?

3. Fill in the missing total costs and revenue items in Table 8.5.

Table 8.5

TOTAL COSTS AND REVENUES MISSING VALUES

	Revenues	Total Variable Costs	Fixed Costs	Total Costs	Profit
a.	$3,000	$2,400	?	$3,000	?
b.	?	$2,000	?	$2,600	$3,400
c.	$5,000	?	$1,600	?	$1,400

4. Community Hospital performs a myriad of radiology-based services and would like to review the department's fee schedule. The radiology department has fixed costs of $820,500, variable costs per radiology procedure of $55, and charges $190 for each procedure performed. Anticipated utilization is 11,000 procedures annually. There are currently no overhead costs allocated to the radiology department, and items such as utilities and housekeeping are paid at the hospital level.

   a. Are they charging enough to cover all expenses?
   b. What is the radiology department's current profit per procedure?
   c. What would the price per procedure be if the radiology department's desired profit was $600,000?

5. Using ABC techniques, calculate the allocation rate for each of the activities listed in Table 8.6. Then calculate the total cost of performing each test.

Table 8.6

ACTIVITY-BASED COSTING

Activity	Annual Costs	Cost Driver	Activity Data	
			Procedure A	Procedure B
Receive specimen	$5,000	No. of tests	1,000	500
Perform prescreens	$15,000	Minutes per test	5	3
Run all tests	$50,000	Minutes per test	10	10
Total costs	**$70,000**			

6. Your workplace has recently opened a new urgent care center and would like to assess its financial position to date. As the organization's new financial analyst, you are responsible for the analysis of the following data:

Number of walk-in visits: 13,500
Staffing/Salaries: $185,000
Utilities: $8,500

New building construction: $180,000
Medical supplies: $70,000
Contracted laboratory services: $25,000

Required patient document delivery to primary care physician: $5,000

   a. What is the urgent care center's variable cost rate?
   b. What is the total cost? If the utilization changed to 10,500 walk-in visits, what would the total cost be?
   c. If the urgent care center decided to increase the average cost per visit by 10%, what would the new average cost per procedure be (using the original stated utilization)?

7. City Finance Corporation is examining available options for its capital structure to determine which is the optimal structure. (a) Calculate the CCC for each of the structures in Table 8.7, then (b) identify which is the best/ideal structure.

Table 8.7

CAPITAL STRUCTURES FOR CORPORATE COST OF CAPITAL (CCC) COMPARISON

	Percent Debt	After Tax Cost of Debt	Cost of Equity	Tax Rate
A.	25%	8%	11%	0%
B.	53%	12%	23%	8.5%
C.	70%	7%	17%	7.1%
D.	22%	10%	12%	6.7%

8. The local research hospital offers a variety of procedures for early detection and treatment of various types of cancer. Each stage of cancer involves specific tests and treatments, but also has a varying number of patients. As the new senior financial analyst, you have to advise the executive team on pricing of services currently being offered. The chief financial officer (CFO) has mandated overhead of $225,000, a third of which is to be allocated to services noted in Table 8.8. Approximately $150,000 in profit is also directly contributed to these services. Use the data provided in Table 8.8 to create a fee schedule (list of prices) for services. Overhead and profit should be allocated proportionately to volume and revenue, respectively.

Table 8.8

COST ALLOCATION AND FEE SCHEDULE DATA

Services Offered	Annual Revenue	Variable Cost Per Procedure	Annual Direct Fixed Cost	Annual Number of Procedures
Stage screening	$250,000	$10	$50,000	5,000
Intro dosage	$100,000	$25	$30,000	2,500
Radiation	$500,000	$50	$15,000	2,000
Chemotherapy	$750,000	$75	$5,000	500
	$1,600,000		$100,000	10,000

CHAPTER 8 CASE: THE FINANCING NUMBERS GAME

The recent pandemic has forced several healthcare organizations to rethink how they do business, and Appalachian Cancer Research Center (ACRC) is no exception. ACRC is an established research and treatment facility located in the Blue Ridge Mountains. ACRC is considering an expansion opportunity, but must first fully analyze the organization's financial health before moving forward with the expansion. EBIT is $20,000,000, and the organization holds $18,000,000 in assets. As a newly hired financial analyst, it is now your responsibility to perform the necessary calculations and provide a final report to the executive team.

Prepare ACRC's financial statements, comparing its current all-equity financing approach to a possible 65% debt financing approach. Assume an interest rate of 9% and a tax rate of 32% for your calculations. For inclusion in the final report:

a. Create a balance sheet.
b. Create an income statement.
c. Calculate ROE.
d. Determine which financing option has the best ROE.

To further assess the expansion, ACRC would like to increase the services offered and needs to hire additional staff (for multiple departments) to do so. The organization needs additional clinical as well as administrative staff to make things work and to ensure the highest quality of care for the patients. The newest surgeon has been with the organization for just 9 months (with incurred salary expenses of $250,000) and the finance manager has been with the organization for 7 months (with incurred salary expenses of $75,000). To add an additional surgeon and an additional finance manager, leadership would like to estimate a few expenses. Calculate the following to help with the decision-making:

e. the estimated annual salary of a new surgeon,
f. the estimated annual salary of a new finance manager,
g. fringe benefits for each position, at a rate of 30%, and
h. onboarding and training sessions for each position, for a total of 40 hours each.
(Assume that the annual hours worked is 2,080 hours).

HEALTHCARE FINANCE COURSE PROJECT: COST ESTIMATION FOR PHASE I

The first phase of the course project begins with the creation of the SurgiFlex utilization data (Worksheet #1), introduced at the end of Chapter 5. The cost estimation portion of Phase I covers the concepts presented here in Chapter 8, and spans several worksheets which complete the Phase I calculations:

- Worksheet #2: SurgiFlex Salary and Wage Calculations
- Worksheet #3: SurgiFlex Revenue Calculations
- Worksheet #4: SurgiFlex Nonsalary Expense Calculations
- Worksheet #5: SurgiFlex Breakeven Calculations
- Worksheet #6: SurgiFlex Supply Vendor Analysis Calculations

Review the "Course Project: Phase I: SurgiFlex Robotic Surgery System Calculations" section of Chapter 16. With the exception of using the provided template for the creation of Worksheet #1, all other worksheets in the first phase are to be created by the student. All worksheets are to be connected to the SurgiFlex utilization data (Worksheet #1), as well as other relevant worksheet calculations in Phase I. Be sure to review the Microsoft Excel® Reference Guide located in the Appendices as needed.

REFERENCES

Berger, Z. (2019). Metrics of patient, public, consumer, and community engagement in healthcare systems: How should we define engagement, what are we measuring, and does it matter for patient care? *International Journal of Health Policy and Management*, 8(1), 49–50. https://doi.org/10.15171/ijhpm.2018.94

Campanale, C., Cinquini, L., & Tenucci, A. (2014). Time-driven activity-based costing to improve transparency and decision making in healthcare—A case study. *Qualitative Research in Accounting & Management*, 11(2), 165–186. https://doi.org/10.1108/QRAM-04-2014-0036

Guo, R., Berkshire, S. D., Fulton, L. V., & Hermanson, P. M. (2016). Use of evidence-based management in healthcare administration decision-making. *Leadership in Health Services*, 30(3), 330–342. https//doi.org/10.1108/LHS-07-2016-0033

Healthcare Financial Management Association. (2021). *Reducing the total cost of care*. https://www.hfma.org/industry-initiatives/research-trends.html

Menaker, R., Ritte, R. J., & France, T. J. (2020). *Principal principles: Critical accounting and financial concepts for healthcare leaders.* Medical Group Management Association. https://www.mgma.com/resources/financial-management/principal-principles-critical-accounting-and-fina

Ramos-Hegwer, L. (2017, May/June). The future of healthcare finance: Focusing your strategies amid uncertainty. *Healthcare Executive*, 32(3), 10–16.

Widmer, A. (2016). Of means and ends: The financialization and regulation of health care. *The Linacre Quarterly*, 83(4), 382–386. https://doi.org/10.1080/00243639.2016.1248168

CHAPTER 9

Revenue Cycle Management: Billing, Coding, and Collections

OBJECTIVES

1. Identify the different types of codes required for medical billing.
2. Identify the steps involved in the medical billing process.
3. Discuss the importance of the claims adjudication process.
4. Describe the importance of correct billing and transcription review.
5. Discuss the impacts of patient services revenue and reimbursement on the healthcare organization's overall financial position.

INTRODUCTION

Accounts payable and accounts receivable are both included in the **cash management process**. Effective cash management controls cash inflows as well as cash outflows, ultimately improving the organization's overall financial position. Ensuring sound cash management supports the strategic planning and longer-term investment potential of the healthcare organization. Cash management includes decisions that foster revenue generation and minimize expenses, while maintaining viability and liquidity for shorter-term purchases. Automation of services is a major piece of the cash management puzzle, which most providers have adopted in some form. Various software packages have been implemented to automate the billing, collections, and payment receipt portions of business, and to reduce processing time of hard-copy paper claims or bank deposits. On the accounts payable side, prompt payment of debts reduces late fees and additional charges, effectively managing cash outflows and keeping the inflow of goods and services stable. On the accounts receivable side, however, patient-related revenue requires considerably more effort. This chapter in our revenue cycle discussion focuses on the activities involved with patient billing and collections—the key to efficient reimbursement for healthcare services. This portion of the revenue cycle process must be meticulously managed to ensure that payment is received for all services rendered. There are checks and balances at multiple stages within the process, with guidelines established to ensure that the relevant information is captured, which usually varies by payer. Larger healthcare organizations have entire teams within the finance department dedicated to the **billing and coding process**, an integral part of revenue cycle management. Even in smaller organizations, considerable attention is given to ensure proper alignment of service delivery and the associated revenue recognition.

THE BILLING AND CODING PROCESS

Every type of patient healthcare service, whether an office visit, therapy session, or medical equipment fitting, finds itself at the beginning of the healthcare billing and collections process. The revenue cycle is the collective process of billing and reimbursement, as initiated by the provision of healthcare services. The steps involved in the billing process not only ensure efficient reimbursement, but also the effective collection of patient data used throughout the various functions and departments within the healthcare system. The data collected during the medical visit includes more than just the financial information used in the billing process. Key information such as current medical issue and overall health condition is captured, and just as importantly, each visit adds to the patient's longer-term medical history. The steps in the process may seem inconsequential, but those involved in the process surely understand the importance of each step. In Figure 9.1, we provide an overview of the billing and coding process, then examine some of the key operational indicators that drive collections.

Figure 9.1

The billing and coding process

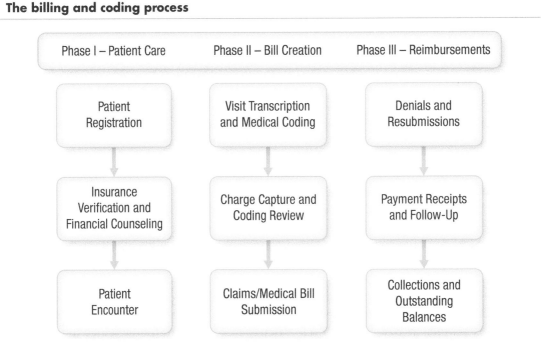

Where It Begins: Phase I: Patient Care

The billing and coding process begins with the focus of all healthcare organizations: the actual provision of patient care. The medical appointment is scheduled by the patient and the provider as they prepare to discuss the medical concerns at hand. When the patient arrives for the appointment and checks in, the billing and coding process begins. During this visit registration, the provider collects and verifies the patient's demographic information such as name, date of birth, residency, and reason for the visit. The patient often receives valuable information at this stage as well. Visit and treatment disclosures are provided, informing the patient of their rights, as well as what to expect during the medical visit.

With the registration of the patient comes the verification of insurance information. This step determines who will be responsible for the payment for medical services delivered. If the patient has insurance coverage, the insurance company is contacted to approve the visit. Depending on the type of insurance plan, the medical visit may have required preauthorization or preapproval for the medical care by the insurance company or by the primary care physician. If the patient does not have insurance coverage, the registration representative may engage in financial counseling to assess the availability of financial resources for the patient. In most cases, healthcare would be unattainable without medical insurance of some kind. Government and public insurance options are reviewed, to see if the patient qualifies for coverage by one of these plans. With the expansion of Medicaid under the Affordable Care Act, several affordable options were made available for those that would normally be unqualified for insurance coverage. Reasons for this could be unemployment or underemployment, no coverage options by employers, or the possible need for secondary or supplemental coverage. Self-pay, or out-of-pocket payments by the patient, is usually the last option, due to the costliness of medical care. Payment plans and other payment agreements can be put in place if no insurance coverage options are available. Establishing financial responsibility is very important at this stage, as the insurance companies note and assess risk, and the patient, if responsible, will pay or make payment arrangements. If a copayment is required by the insurance company, the patient pays this at registration prior to the start of the medical visit.

The most important step in the patient care phase is the actual **patient encounter**, or the medical office visit. Here, the medical provider provides the consultation and care as required by the patient's condition or medical concerns. This session not only provides medical treatment, but serves as an information session for the provider and patient. The provider will ask clarifying questions to gather context for the medical concerns, while the patient will ask clarifying questions on the reasons for the condition or possibly the post-visit next steps. Treatment as deemed appropriate by the clinician is rendered, and the patient will receive any post-visit instructions. Medications, prescriptions, and referrals for additional medical care or specialty services are also provided at the conclusion of the medical visit.

Phase II: Medical Bill and Claims Creation

After the provider has held the patient consultation, the medical notes must be transcribed to the patient's official medical record. To achieve this, medical professionals use a variety of methods: transcribing professionals, who actually type the information for addition to the medical record, or transcription software packages, which rely on the voice recording of the provider's visit notes. Both of these methods are effective and the choice of which to use depends solely on the preference of the medical provider. Traditionally, medical providers maintained a hard-copy patient chart that contained all of the information regarding the patient's medical history and associated treatments. With the implementation of the **Health Information Technology for Economic and Clinical Health (HITECH) Act** of 2009 and the **American Recovery and Reinvestment Act** (ARRA), medical providers were required (and incentivized) to convert their hard-copy records to electronic digital formats. The **electronic medical record** (EMR) was created from this legislation and is now a standard fixture in the transcription and documentation process. Some organizations have adopted the **electronic health record** (EHR), which is an EMR with a broader scope. While the EMR contains the medical information for a patient at that specific provider's location, the EHR is a comprehensive record that contains the patient's medical history from all providers, specialists, and services. After the official visit details have been transcribed, the components of the medical visit are assigned the appropriate medical code for billing purposes.

There are several types of required medical codes, organized in a few important ways: by diagnosis, by procedure, or by payer-specific codes. The first required code in the medical billing process is the *International Classification of Diseases (ICD)-10 code*. The *ICD* coding system identifies the patient's diagnosis or reason for the medical consultation as required for all healthcare payers, and is maintained by the World Health Organization (WHO). *ICD* codes are indeed international and are used worldwide in various formats as dictated by the country. Currently, the 10th revision is used in the United States, although an *ICD-11* iteration was approved by WHO in 2019 and released in early 2022. The *ICD* codes change as the healthcare industry streamlines the identification of existing illnesses and discovers new ones.

The **Current Procedural Terminology (CPT) code** is the second required billing code. This code, created and standardized by the American Medical Association (AMA), supports the *ICD* code by identifying the treatment and procedures for the identified diagnosis (AMA, n.d.). This, too, is a required medical code for all healthcare payers, although it was originally created for programs administered by the Centers for Medicare & Medicaid Services (CMS). There are several categories of CPT codes that help medical professionals capture and analyze various data, specifically specialized medical procedures, performance measurement and management metrics, and emerging technologies or new healthcare services. The third code present on the medical bill, if applicable, is the **Healthcare Common Procedure Coding System (HCPCS) code**, which is also administrated by the CMS (CMS, 2023a). HCPCS codes support the CPT code by providing the next level of documentation and coding for the medical diagnosis and related procedure or treatment. This code denotes the use of personal medical supplies, services, and equipment (such as wheelchairs, crutches, ambulance/medical transportation, etc.) not typically captured in other codes. This code may not be required for all patient visits. While WHO maintains the *ICD* standards, which are utilized globally, CPT and HCPCS codes are updated by the AMA and the CMS, allowing for more frequent revisions.

The codes that appear on the medical bill (as reflected in Table 9.1) must align for the **medical claim** to be accepted by the insurance provider. The treatment provided must be the correct treatment for the diagnosis as well as the level of **acuity** (severity of illness). Every CPT and HCPCS code must be aligned with a valid *ICD-10* code and must be the correct treatment

Table 9.1

BILLING CODE SNAPSHOT

Medical Billing Code	Question Answered
ICD-10 code	What is the patient's medical diagnosis? What is the reason for the medical visit?
CPT code	What treatment or service was provided for the identified diagnosis or medical condition?
HCPCS code	What are the supplies or devices needed for treatment of the identified diagnosis or medical condition?

CPT, Current Procedural Terminology; HCPCS, Healthcare Common Procedure Coding System; *ICD, International Classification of Diseases*.

for that particular diagnosis, even if there are multiple issues addressed in the same medical consultation. For example: If a patient has a medical visit for an ear infection and also has the physician examine a swollen knee, the medical bill will include an *ICD-10* code for both conditions. The corresponding CPT codes must be appropriate to each of these conditions, possibly an ear irrigation procedure for the ear infection and a cortisone injection for the knee swelling. These codes are often used in conjunction with **diagnosis-related groups**, or DRGs, to calculate a provider's inpatient and outpatient surgery reimbursement (CMS, 2023b). DRG codes are applied at the end of a patient's hospital stay, assigning a value to the provider's resources used for that inpatient stay. The DRGs' value is driven by the severity of illness, with sicker patients needing more care and resources. Each DRG code represents a fixed reimbursement amount, no matter the costs incurred by the provider. The **chargemaster** is the organization's list of established services and procedures used to bill payers. The procedures and corresponding codes represented in the patient's EMR and associated claim must be present in the chargemaster.

Prior to the submission of the claim to the insurer, there is an internal review process performed by the provider to ensure or at least improve the accuracy of the claim. The claims review process, referred to as **claims scrubbing**, is designed to identify any errors or missing information that may result in the rejection or the denial of a claim. The scrubbing process also checks for regulatory compliance, which includes the required diagnosis and treatment codes, as well as any formatting requirements set forth by the insurer. When the claims have been scrubbed and are deemed free of error, they are referred to as **clean claims**, and are ready for submission. When all medical visit activities and charges have been captured, and the medical billing codes have been reviewed, the medical claim or request for payment is submitted to the insurance provider. This is usually an automated process, as most claims today are submitted electronically to expedite the process and accommodate large volumes of claims submissions. The type of claim information required, and format of the data, is specific to each type of payer, with most using software packages designed for their specific billing process and data requirements. Even though not immediately responsible for the payment of services, the patient still receives a summary of the healthcare service visit, called the **explanation of benefits**, or EOB. The EOB provides the same summary information as the medical insurance claim (such as diagnosis and treatment), as well as the charges for service and amounts to be covered by the insurance plan. Any amount not reimbursed by the insurer will be the responsibility of the insured if no additional insurance or secondary payer is in place. There is also a **superbill** created, which is a detailed list of the patient's diagnosis, treatments, supplies, provider charges, and any other costs directly related to the patient visit. The superbill is not a claim and is used by patients intending to bill the insurer directly.

Phase III: Reimbursements

After the claims have been submitted, the accounts receivable team monitors the submitted claims and receipts to ensure that revenues are received in a timely fashion. This will include the management of payment denials and claims resubmissions. There are several possible reasons for **claims denial**, which may include missing preauthorization or primary care physician referral, incorrect or misaligned coding, or duplicative billing. All of these reasons would require corrections on the provider side of the process and resubmission of the medical claim. Billing errors can be costly, causing missed revenue for denials or penalties for erroneous coding and resubmissions, so follow-up throughout the process is critical. Upon receipt of payment from the insurance provider, balances are usually billed to a secondary payer, or, in the event of no additional insurance options, the patient. The collections process for any outstanding charges varies in duration at the discretion of the healthcare provider. Patients are usually contacted to make payment arrangements for the bill balance, agreeing to a payment schedule that is feasible according to their financial situation. Payments that are not received by the insurer or the patient are absorbed, or "written off," by the provider if not received within 90 to 120 days. A **write-off** is the process of eliminating a recorded debt or amount owed due to noncollection. For an item to be written off, the entire collections process has to be exhausted with no other viable collections options available. This is often captured on the financial statements as "bad debt" or "doubtful accounts," and includes items that the organization no longer expects payment on. Additional processes are in place to ensure that the reimbursement phase goes as smoothly as possible. The claims process is critical to the reimbursement phase for maintaining the financial viability of the healthcare organization, and surely deserves further exploration here.

CLAIMS ADJUDICATION PROCESS

The healthcare claims process can be complex and lengthy depending on the insurer and overall timing of the healthcare provider's coding and submission. The term **adjudication** means to judge or decide a final ruling based on evidence presented. Healthcare claims adjudication, then, is the judgment or decision made by the insurer regarding the final payment of the provider's healthcare claim. Submission of claims can be done electronically or manually, with both types of submission subject to the same review process. There are several steps in the adjudication process outlined in Figure 9.2, requiring both the insurer and provider (and often the patient) to discuss and agree to the final terms of payment.

The first step in the **claims adjudication process** is the initial claims review. During this initial review, which is usually done electronically, the submitted claim is checked for spelling errors in the patient's or provider's data, or the medical diagnosis and treatment data. This very basic review is designed to ensure that the most important data that filters through and impacts all other decisions is correct. If any initial review data is incorrect or missing, the claim is rejected and sent back to the provider for corrections and resubmission. The automatic review is often done electronically, like step one, but checks for the next level of errors. It is important to note that a **claims rejection** and a **claims denial** are not the same. A claim can be rejected based on the initial review, with the intention of receiving corrections and moving forward with the remaining steps in the claims adjudication process. A claims denial is the denial of payment, after all submitted documentation has been reviewed in the context of policy coverage and medical necessity. This second step validates the patient's actual policy coverage for the items listed on the medical claim. Examples for denial at this stage are (a) lapsed eligibility, where the policy has expired; (b) no insurance benefit or coverage for the visit or treatment; or (c) the visit or treatment was not preauthorized as required by the health insurance policy. Duplicate claims or duplicate treatment data entry are also caught during this second review. The clinical review is a claims review that examines the medical aspects of the claim. This review is performed by a medical doctor or RN who examines the claim for medical necessity, appropriateness of treatment, and treatment-specific preauthorizations. Questions or concerns during this phase always involve the provider, who is ultimately responsible for treatment options presented to the patient and how the agreed upon treatment is performed. The clinical discussion may include a great deal of medical jargon and may also rely on medical standards as set forth by the industry, neither of which are decisions made by the insured or patient. Step four in the claims adjudication process, the payment decision, is

Figure 9.2

The claims adjudication process

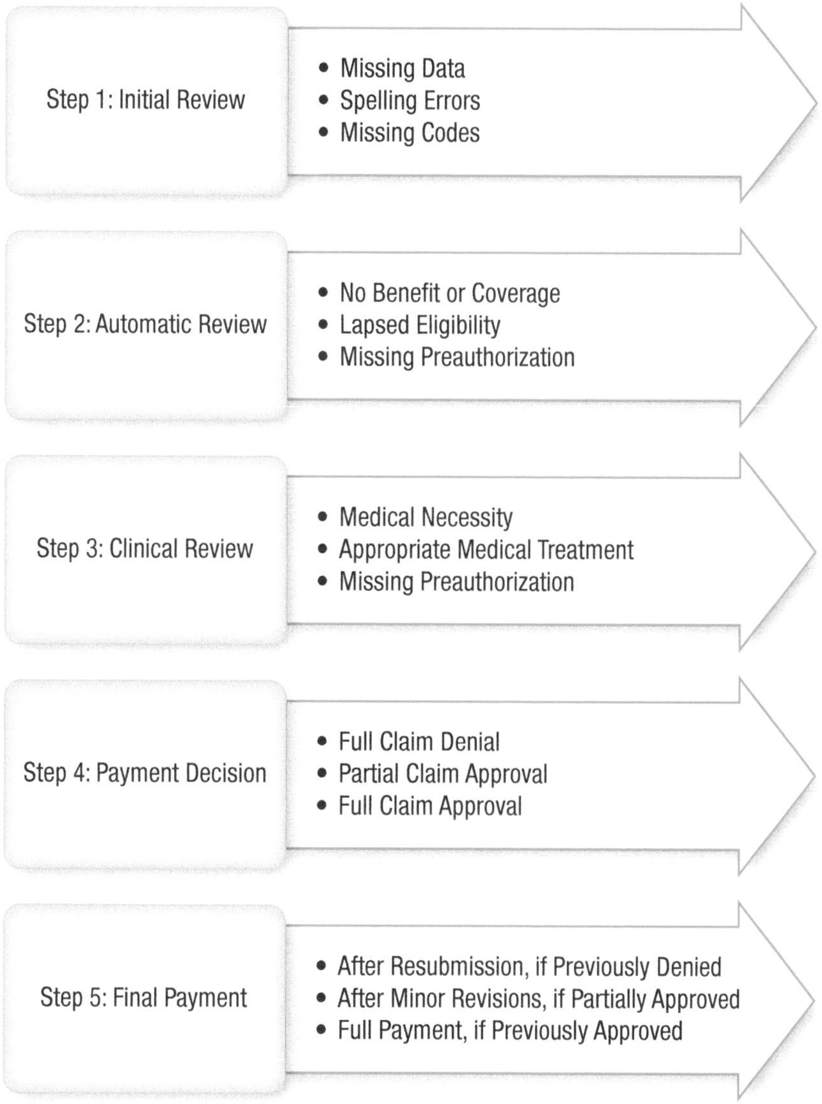

Step 1: Initial Review	• Missing Data • Spelling Errors • Missing Codes
Step 2: Automatic Review	• No Benefit or Coverage • Lapsed Eligibility • Missing Preauthorization
Step 3: Clinical Review	• Medical Necessity • Appropriate Medical Treatment • Missing Preauthorization
Step 4: Payment Decision	• Full Claim Denial • Partial Claim Approval • Full Claim Approval
Step 5: Final Payment	• After Resubmission, if Previously Denied • After Minor Revisions, if Partially Approved • Full Payment, if Previously Approved

based on the outcomes of the previous three stages of review. If the visit and treatment were deemed medically unnecessary or were uncovered by the health insurance policy, the claim would be fully denied. In this situation, payment would most likely become the responsibility of the secondary insurance plans or the patient. For payment decisions of partial approval, the insurer may pay the portion of the claim that is covered and medically necessary, but would not reimburse the provider for items on the claim deemed invalid. The uncovered portion of the claim would then become the responsibility of a secondary insurer, or become an out-of-pocket obligation for the patient. The patient could then make payment arrangements with the provider, or use a superbill to seek additional reimbursement where possible. Fully approved claims are processed for payment, sending the full reimbursement amount to the provider or the organization's finance department where it is applied to the correct patient services revenue accounts.

The claims adjudication process is a very important phase of the revenue cycle process, as it often dictates how quickly funds will be received by the healthcare provider. The goal is to receive the incoming payments as quickly as possible to meet other financial obligations. Many organizations realize that sound revenue cycle management is a well-thought-out and choreographed process requiring considerable planning and effort on the front end. Patient pathway reviews and internal workload analyses are just two of the factors influencing the timeliness of claims submission and payment receipts, but many other options are explored. A few key management focal points can improve just about any process, ensuring that things run as efficiently as possible:

- improve/upgrade technology
- improve/streamline patient access
- documented denials management process
- performance measurement and analysis

Sound revenue cycle management processes rely on software programs specifically designed to address revenue-related issues. Smaller organizations may find software purchases or upgrades cost prohibitive, but, depending on the size and utilization of the services offered, it may be worth the investment. Systems designed for claims review can catch errors in patient demographic or provider information before submission to the insurance company, allowing for corrections on the front end and reducing rejections and delays later in the process. Technological advancements can also be used in the improvement of patient access. Some organizations did this during the height of the pandemic, as patients still needed to be seen. Medical practices and facilities with larger volumes automated the check-in and registration process by using mobile applications and fillable forms for submission. This made it possible to minimize contact time and lobby crowding during a time when social distancing was required. Telemedicine also became a mainstay for some organizations, not only for the continuity of care for patients, but for the reduced staffing needed for check-in and registration. Just as technology drives more efficient operations and patient access, it can also assist with the management of the organization's claims, denials, and resubmissions. As the revenue cycle management process is key to the viability of the organization, it must be honed to run smoothly even for challenging situations, such as claims denials. A documented denials management process should help to (a) quickly identify the underlying reason for the claims denial, (b) correct the current instance of the error and prevent future occurrences of the same issue, and (c) resubmit revised claims in a timely manner. Ideally, the number of denials should decrease over time as the organization makes corrections or adjustments to its internal processes, improving the acceptance rates and decreasing the overall claims adjudication time caused by delays and resubmissions. When systems are running at optimal (or at least improved) efficiency, performance measurement and analysis should be done to further fine-tune the revenue cycle. An electronic system can help the organization monitor its revenue functions over time, to recognize internal issues that may need to be addressed, as well as patterns of behavior exhibited by payers. While all issues will not be within the organization's realm of control for change, the organization can adjust its practices, or possibly its contracting and payer agreements, to address claims processing and payment trends.

COLLECTIONS AND RECEIVABLES MANAGEMENT

Outstanding payments, as with claims processing delays and denials, can cause major problems with revenue cycle management, leading to longer-term accounts payable issues and revenue loss. Ideally, an organization will have a documented collections process to receive payments as quickly as possible and to effectively manage any outstanding balances. Given delays in billing and coding or claims processing, payers may accumulate large outstanding balances that must be routinely reviewed to ensure timely collections and revenue recognition. Two of the most common indicators used for the collections process are the collections aging schedule and **patient accounts receivable** (PAR). The **collections aging schedule** reflects accounts receivable balances in intervals, according to the timing of payments. Aging schedules can vary by organization but typically cover a period of at least 90 to 120 days. By maintaining and reviewing aging schedules, the organization can estimate revenue for a given period, which allows for adjustments and planning. It also identifies issues with accounts or payers, which may possibly require adjustments to contracting or collection terms. PAR (measured in days) is the average time for collection of outstanding reimbursement for services already rendered, using the organization's aging schedule as an element in its calculation. This indicator works with the aging schedule to provide insight on a payer's reimbursement history, identifying trends and concerns. To illustrate this, consider the following scenario.

The local hospital uses the intervals listed in Exhibit 9.1a for the aging schedule of all accounts: 0 to 30 days, 31 to 60 days, 61 to 90 days, and 91 to 120 days. Its major third-party payer has outstanding receivables of $75,000. If the payer historically pays 70% of submitted claims within 30 days and the remaining 30% equally in the remaining months, (a) what does the payer's aging schedule look like, and (b) what is the payer's PAR in days?

EXHIBIT 9.1a. Aging Schedule

Aging Interval	Percentage Paid	Amount Paid
0–30	70%	$52,500
31–60	10%	$7,500
61–90	10%	$7,500
91–120	10%	$7,500
	100%	**$75,000**

In the aging schedule shown in Exhibit 9.1a, four intervals are noted with the corresponding payment percentages. This particular payer remits most of its outstanding balance in the first month of collections, which is considered timely. The organization fares well with this payer's account because it receives enough of the outstanding balance during the first month to possibly avoid delays in its own accounts payable process or lost revenue. The total percentage paid, and the total amount paid, must reflect the entire outstanding balance for the payer, in this case, $75,000. The percentage paid during any specific interval will vary by payer and reflect its own payment history. The PAR indicator is typically represented in days and provides information on the average number of days it takes for the provider to receive payments from a particular insurer or payer. This average calculation will be different for each account or payer, since the percentage paid during each aging interval varies by account. PAR uses the percentage paid and the respective aging schedule interval to calculate the average days until payment receipt. Using the information presented in Exhibit 9.1a, the PAR is calculated as shown in Exhibit 9.1b.

EXHIBIT 9.1b. Patient Accounts Receivable Calculation

Aging Interval	Percentage Paid	Amount Paid	PAR Per Interval
0–30	70%	$52,500	$(.70) \times (30 \text{ days}) = 21 \text{ days}$
31–60	10%	$7,500	$(.10) \times (60 \text{ days}) = 6 \text{ days}$
61–90	10%	$7,500	$(.10) \times (90 \text{ days}) = 9 \text{ days}$
91–120	10%	$7,500	$(.10) \times (120 \text{ days}) = 12 \text{ days}$
	100%	**$75,000**	**Total PAR = 48 days**

PAR = Percentage Paid × Aging Interval

The PAR in the scenario shown in Exhibit 9.1b totals 48 days, which means, on average, it takes 48 days for this payer to reimburse the provider. This PAR result would shift if they had a history of paying late or toward the later intervals of the aging schedule. For example, if 70% of the receivables owed were to be paid in the fourth interval (91–120 days), with the remaining 30% split equally among the first three intervals (10% for each interval), the calculation would then change to: $(.10 \times 30 \text{ days}) + (.10 \times 60 \text{ days}) + (.10 \times 90 \text{ days}) + (.70 \times 120 \text{ days}) = 102$ days. Late payments such as this could be a major accounts receivable challenge for the local hospital. A late payment scenario such as this would prompt more routine follow-up from the accounts receivable team as they work with the payer on sending payments in a timelier manner. In general, organizations devote considerable effort toward receiving payments sooner rather than later, giving them more control over cash inflows and revenue recovery. If the claims volume is large and outside of the scope of the organization's staffing capabilities, the billing and collections functions may be outsourced to a **clearinghouse**, which specializes in quick electronic review, correction, and submission of medical claims. Clearinghouses are used by both larger providers and large payers, with large volumes of claims submitted and reviewed daily.

The aging and accounts receivable analyses performed in the previous text are in fact applied to all of an organization's accounts, but are also applied to the organization as a whole. Instead of using one account or payer's outstanding balance and aging schedule, you would use the organization's total receivables balance (total amount of patient revenue billed) and the aging schedule. This calculation can be performed monthly or annually to reflect the reporting period that the organization is processing. The previous scenario examined the local hospital's collection for one account in the shorter term, so to illustrate the organization-level calculation, we will perform an annual calculation for the following scenario.

The local hospital uses the following four intervals for the aging schedule of all accounts: 0 to 30 days, 31 to 60 days, 61 to 90 days, and 91 to 120 days. The hospital operates every day of the calendar year (365 days) and on average generates $17.5 million in patient revenue annually. If the hospital typically receives payments per aging interval of 30%, 25%, 30%, and 15%, respectively, determine the following: (a) What does the hospital's aging schedule look like? (b) What is the hospital's PAR in days? and (c) What is the hospital's receivables balance or outstanding patient revenue at the PAR point?

EXHIBIT 9.2a. Organization-Level Aging and Patient Accounts Receivable Calculations

Aging Interval	Percentage Paid	Amount Paid	PAR Per Interval
0–30	30%	$5,250,000	(.30) × (30 days) = 9 days
31–60	25%	$4,375,000	(.25) × (60 days) = 15 days
61–90	30%	$5,250,000	(.30) × (90 days) = 27 days
91–120	15%	$2,625,000	(.15) × (120 days) = 18 days
	100%	**$17,500,000**	**Total PAR = 69 days**

PAR, patient accounts receivable.

As noted in Exhibit 9.2a, all of the patient revenue is received within 120 days as reflected in the aging schedule. This appears perfectly acceptable until examined in the broader context of the PAR days. It may also signal challenges with the payer, which may impact future payments. The PAR calculation shows that, on average, it takes 69 days for the local hospital to receive its outstanding revenues, which means that payments are not received until more than 2 months after medical services have been rendered. Depending on the hospital's financial position, this 2-month payment delay could result in challenges with payroll or vendor payments if this revenue were to be the source of funding for those accounts. Remember, PAR is a weighted average, so in most cases there are some accounts that pay earlier in the aging schedule, and there are some patient revenue accounts outstanding after 69 days (which is also evident in the aging schedule, as a portion of the patient revenue is received in the fourth interval). To calculate the outstanding patient revenue or **receivables balance** at the PAR point, which is represented in days, we must first determine exactly how much patient revenue the hospital has received by the 69th day in the aging schedule. To calculate this, we must first represent the annual patient revenue in terms of days. Exhibit 9.2b shows how to calculate the outstanding patient revenue.

EXHIBIT 9.2b. Outstanding Patient Revenue/Receivables Balance

Annual patient revenue:	$17,500,000
Operating days annually:	365
Patient revenue per day:	**$47,945**

Receivables balance = Patient Revenue Per Day × PAR
Receivables balance = $47,945 × 69
Receivables balance = $3,308,205

PAR, patient accounts receivable.

Using the information provided in the scenario shown in Exhibit 9.2b, we can divide the annual patient revenue by the number of operating days to get revenue per day, shown as $47,945 (rounded). Operating days will vary by organization, and may be dependent upon the organization's business model, location, or services provided. To then calculate the receivables balance, you multiply the daily patient revenue by the PAR calculated in Exhibit 9.2a to get

$3,308,205. This means that on the 69th day of the aging schedule, the payer has remitted all but $3,308,205 of the owed patient revenue. Ideally, receivables would be paid within a 30-day time frame or within the first interval, but the real-time average falls between 30 and 60 days. Assessing the accounts payable standing of the organization as a consolidated figure allows the organization to assess its collections process and possibly adjust if needed, if the receivables are coming in toward the end of the aging schedule, as we see in this situation. Of course, the first step would be to drill down to see if a specific account or a specific payer is having a major impact on the process as a whole, then go from there. Having control over this process makes the difference in an organization's ability to regulate its revenue as well as the current and future plans dependent upon it. Let's take a closer look at the broader impacts of accounts receivable management.

IMPACTS OF ACCOUNTS RECEIVABLE MANAGEMENT

The accounts receivable process is more than just invoicing payers and patients and receiving payments. In most healthcare organizations, patient services revenue directly supports other projects, programs, or initiatives. Delays in collection or payment receipts could result in delays in other important items, which could also mean additional incurred costs for the organization. Proper accounts receivable management provides detail on payers' reimbursement history, which includes information on claims acceptance rates, claims rejection and denial rates, and the timeliness of payments. Analysis of the organization's "payer mix" shows the breakdown of payers by type (government/public, commercial, self-pay/patient-pay, etc.), which is used to estimate reimbursement and adjust collections efforts accordingly. Calculating payer mix is done similarly to the aging and PAR calculations shown in the previous sections, with payer percentages added to the calculation.

EXHIBIT 9.3a. Payer Mix Calculation

Payer (Individual)	Accounts Receivable Amount	Accounts Receivable Percentage
Medicare	$3,750,000	15%
Medicaid	$1,250,000	5%
Blue Cross	$10,000,000	40%
Aetna	$7,500,000	30%
Patient pay	$2,500,000	10%
	$25,000,000	**100%**

In Exhibit 9.3a, the payer mix calculation reflects each payer's portion of the total accounts receivable amount of $25 million. Two commercial plans, Blue Cross and Aetna, account for 70% of the organization's accounts receivable, with the remaining 30% shared between the Medicare, Medicaid, and patient pay payer types. This provides a high-level summary of activity, showing the payers with the highest billed amounts that may require focused claims review, submission, and follow-up efforts. The next step in the payer analysis process would be to drill down on the specific payers or payer types to assess the aging detail relative to the accounts receivable amounts noted.

Analyzing each payer's payments by aging interval allows us to see their payment history and estimate when our payments will be received. In this example (Exhibit 9.3b), we see that 48.75% of all outstanding receivables will be received within 30 days, 25.50% will be received within 31 to 60 days, 16% within 61 to 90 days, and the remaining 9.75% will be received within the 91 to 120 days' time frame. With more than half of the outstanding receivables paid after the initial 30 days, claims follow-up and collections efforts would be focused on expediting the receipt of the later payments. Individual payer payments show that within the first aging interval, Medicare pays 25% of its outstanding balance ($937,500/$3,750,000), Medicaid pays 10% ($125,000/$1,250,000), Blue Cross pays 65% ($6,500,000/$10,000,000), Aetna pays 60% ($4,500,000/$7,500,000), and patient pay/self-pay accounts pay 5% ($125,000/$2,500,000). Payer type or payer category analysis would consolidate the individual payers into government or public payer (Medicare and Medicaid), commercial payer (Blue Cross and Aetna), and patient pay categories. The consolidated receivables payments for the 0- to 30-day interval reflect government/public payer payments of $1,062,500 (the summation of the Medicare and Medicaid figures from Exhibit 9.3b), which is approximately 21.25% of the category's outstanding receivables ($1,062,500/$5,000,000), with the commercial and patient pay categories reflecting 62.86% and 5.00% of payments, respectively, using the same calculation methodology. All of the various types of analyses provide the needed data for sound accounts receivable management. It is important to note that all incurred expenses may not be reimbursed by the insurer. Depending on the type of medical insurance plan and documented coverage, only a portion of the healthcare claim may be eligible for repayment, with the remaining amount becoming the responsibility of the patient. These "allowable" charges are predetermined, so the provider can estimate how much service reimbursement will be.

EXHIBIT 9.3b. Payer Mix With Aging Detail

Payer (Individual)	Amounts Paid by Aging Interval				
	0–30	31–60	61–90	91–120	Total Paid
Medicare	$937,5000	$1,875,000	$750,000	$187,500	$3,750,000
Medicaid	$125,000	$125,000	$750,000	$250,000	$1,250,000
Blue Cross	$6,500,000	$2,000,000	$1,000,000	$500,000	$10,000,000
Aetna	$4,500,000	$1,875,000	$750,000	$375,000	$7,500,000
Patient pay	$125,000	$500,000	$750,000	$1,125,000	$2,500,000
	$12,187,500	$6,375,000	$4,000,000	$2,437,500	$25,000,000
Total paid by aging interval	48.75%	25.50%	16.00%	9.75%	100.00%

CHAPTER SUMMARY

The billing and coding process in healthcare financial operations is an integral part of the organization's viability in both the shorter and longer term. It is more than just bringing in the money—it is securing resources for current as well as future routine operations and strategic initiatives. The broader concept of revenue cycle management is rooted in the successful implementation and oversight of accounts receivable guidelines and processes, which drive overall financial health. While the adjudication process is outside of the organization's realm of control, the review, corrections, and follow-up of the associated billing and medical claims are internal processes requiring constant monitoring and improvements. Most billing and collections functions are performed electronically, allowing the provider and the payer to have detailed recordkeeping as well as more efficient processing. The patient experience and quality patient care are the main focus of our healthcare sector, but profitability, even if only minimal, must remain an important part of the healthcare organization's strategic plan.

KEY TERMS FOR REVIEW

acuity

adjudication

American Recovery and Reinvestment Act

billing and coding process

cash management process

chargemaster

claims adjudication process

claims denial

claims rejection

claims scrubbing

clean claims

clearinghouse

collections aging schedule

Current Procedural Terminology (CPT) code

diagnosis-related group

electronic health record

electronic medical record

explanation of benefits

Healthcare Common Procedure Coding System (HCPCS) code

Health Information Technology for Economic and Clinical Health (HITECH) Act

International Classification of Diseases (ICD)-10 code

medical claim

patient accounts receivable

patient encounter

receivables balance

superbill

write-off

DISCUSSION QUESTIONS

1. What is an *ICD-10* code? What information does it provide in the context of patient care and medical billing documentation?

2. What are CPT codes and HCPCS codes? What information do they provide in the context of patient care and medical billing documentation?

3. How are the codes discussed in this chapter related, and how do they influence the reimbursement of healthcare services? Who has the responsibility of updating the codes?

4. Define the steps in the healthcare claims adjudication process. How can a provider take steps to ensure that the adjudication process goes smoothly with minimal delays?

5. Discuss how the ARRA and HITECH Act legislation have impacted the healthcare revenue cycle management process. Are the impacts identified an improvement to the process, or a hindrance? Explain your answer.

6. When it comes to PARs management, the more oversight the better. The most efficient processes include timely claims submissions as well as dedicated revenue recovery efforts. Describe how challenges with PARs could impact the routine operations in healthcare organizations of varying sizes or capacities.

7. Define the term "chargemaster" and discuss how the chargemaster affects the billing and collections process.

8. What is an aging schedule? What role does the aging schedule play in the billing and collections process?

9. Why is payer mix important when assessing a healthcare organization's financial position and financial health? Can an organization's payer mix be adjusted or changed? Explain.

10. What is the PARs balance and how is it connected to the payer mix?

PRACTICE PROBLEMS

Answers to this chapter's Practice Problems are available via Springer Publishing Connect™ by following the instructions on the opening page of this book and accessing Answers to Practice Problems on the Table of Contents.

1. Mountain Medical Center (MMC) has an aging schedule with the aging intervals and corresponding payment amounts shown in Box 9.1. Complete the aging schedule to reflect the percentages of the total amount paid for each interval.

BOX 9.1

Mountain Medical Center Aging Schedule

Aging Interval	Amount Paid	Percentage Paid
0–30	$12,100,000	?
31–60	$5,500,000	?
61–90	$3,300,000	?
91–120	$1,100,000	?
	$22,000,000	

2. Using MMC's completed aging schedule from Problem 1, which contains four intervals, calculate the PAR (PAR, in days). On average, how long does it take for MMC to receive patient revenue reimbursement for all intervals?

3. As the lead accounts receivable representative for your healthcare organization, you are tasked with the assessment of patient revenue accounts. Currently, 35% of insurers reimburse on the 30th day, 50% reimburse on the 60th day, and the remaining 15% on the 90th day.

a. Calculate the PAR for the organization.
b. Calculate the amounts paid at each interval if the overall value of the patient revenue accounts is $13.5 million.

c. If the organization operates 365 days per year, what is the outstanding patient revenue or receivables balance for the organization, using the PAR and revenue amounts noted in parts a and b? If the collections efforts were increased and 30% of the second interval receivables was paid within 30 days, what would be the adjusted PAR?

4. Calculate the payer mix for each of the payers given in Box 9.2. Which payer has the largest percentage of the accounts receivable balance?

BOX 9.2

Payer Mix Calculation

Payer Name	Accounts Receivable Amount	Accounts Receivable Percentage
Medicare	$6,385,500	?
Medicaid	$2,128,500	?
Blue Cross	$17,028,000	?
Aetna	$12,771,000	?
Patient pay	$4,257,000	?
	$42,570,000	100%

5. Using the accounts receivable data in Problem 4, determine the percentage of the accounts receivable balance for each payer type (government/public, commercial/private, and patient pay/self-pay).

6. Expanding upon the payer and accounts receivable data in Problem 4, create an aging schedule with the following four aging intervals: 0 to 30 days, 31 to 60 days, 61 to 90 days, and 91 to 120 days. To calculate the paid amounts for each interval, assume that each payer pays 45% of their outstanding balance in the first interval, 30% of their outstanding balance in the second interval, 15% of their outstanding balance in the third interval, and the remaining 10% of their outstanding balance in the fourth interval.

7. Using the aging schedule created in Problem 6, calculate the PAR for each payer. If the collections efforts were increased and 10% of the second interval receivables was paid within 30 days, what would be the adjusted PAR?

CHAPTER 9 CASE: FOLLOW THE MONEY: A SCENARIO FOR ACCOUNTS RECEIVABLE MANAGEMENT

Mountain Medical Center (MMC) is a large community facility offering a wide range of services for both adults and children. Inpatient, outpatient, and emergent care are available, as well as phlebotomy, pharmacy, and rehabilitation services. With the exception of a few niche medical specialists, MMC relies on its in-house resources for all of the services provided. There are no other large healthcare providers in the area, and most of the private practice clinicians have contracted medical privileges with MMC. Staffing within the organization is robust, with clinical teams delineated by specialty and patient population (adult or pediatrics). All payer types are accepted for healthcare service coverage, with payment plans or reduced fees available for self-pay and lower income patients. Logistically, MMC has very few challenges with scheduling, patient wait times, or general workflow.

As with many healthcare organizations, the recent pandemic has uncovered or exacerbated underlying issues with revenue cycle management. Rising costs of supplies and equipment have led to increased expenditures and accounts payable, all of which have been covered by the current revenue structure. While MMC has been able to meet its debt obligations, the finance department leadership has noticed a reduction in revenue that may impact the organization's bottom line. Before additional fiscal challenges arise, they decide to analyze the current billing and collections functions to ensure efficiency and identify areas for improvement. Specifically, they intend to review the current chargemaster, the internal claims review process, and the current payer mix to determine if changes or updates need to be made.

As one of the finance directors, you must consider the billing and collection functions at the operations level (ensuring efficient and effective processes), as well as at the organizational level (ensuring alignment with the revenue targets and longer-term goals). Staffing levels have not been an issue and all processes are properly documented, so you decide to assess the actual implementation of the billing procedures and chargemaster-related regulatory requirements. After this front-end analysis, which reviews the activities leading up to claims submission, the aging and accounts receivable amounts will be reviewed by the payer to identify issues with reimbursement. To begin, you must review MMC's chargemaster (Box 9.3) and aging schedule (Box 9.4) for the current fiscal year.

BOX 9.3

Mountain Medical Center Chargemaster

Mountain Medical Center				Mountain Medical Center			
Revenue Code	Charge Description	SVC Type	Current Charge	Revenue Code	Charge Description	SVC Type	Current Charge
0110	Room and board (three nights)	IP	$4,785.38	0400	Imaging (PET, ultrasound, x-ray)	OP	$375.00
0240	Ancillary services	IP	$2,500.00	0410	Respiratory therapy (30 minutes)	OP	$125.00
0250	Pharmacy (per prescription)	OP	$175.00	0420	Physical therapy (30 minutes)	OP	$150.00
0260	IV therapy services	IP	$685.00	0430	Occupational therapy (30 minutes)	OP	$125.00
0270	Medical/ Surgical supplies	IP	$215.55	0440	Speech therapy (30 minutes)	OP	$125.00
0271	Outpatient supplies	OP	$125.00	0445	Inpatient therapy (per session)	IP	$175.00

(continued)

BOX 9.3

Mountain Medical Center Chargemaster (*continued*)

Mountain Medical Center				Mountain Medical Center			
Revenue Code	Charge Description	SVC Type	Current Charge	Revenue Code	Charge Description	SVC Type	Current Charge
0272	Sterile supplies	IP	$260.80	0450	Emergency department	OP	$3,500.00
0274	Prosthetics and orthotics	OP	$1,750.50	0470	Audiology	OP	$395.00
0280	Oncology	IP	$3,267.90	0480	Cardiology (admissions)	IP	$5,200.00
0290	Durable medical equipment (DME)	OP	$2,000.00	0510	Outpatient specialty clinic	OP	$575.00
0294	DME supplies and medications	OP	$500.00	0513	Psychiatric clinic	OP	$395.00
0301	Chemistry laboratory (per test)	IP	$215.00	0515	Pediatric clinic	OP	$395.00
0304	Dialysis laboratory (per test)	IP	$195.00	0526	Urgent care	OP	$325.00
0307	Urology laboratory (per test)	IP	$175.00	0610	MRI	OP	$375.00
0310	Pathology laboratory (per test)	IP	$205.00	0722	Labor and delivery	IP	$5,450.75
0320	Radiology	IP	$395.00	0730	EKG/EEG	OP	$410.00
0350	CAT scan	OP	$375.00	0750	Gastroenterology	OP	$750.00
0360	Operating room services	IP	$5,500.00	0771	Vaccine clinic (per dose)	OP	$75.00
0370	Anesthesia	IP	$1,575.00	0900	Behavioral health (outpatient)	OP	$575.00

IP, inpatient; OP, outpatient; SVC, service.

BOX 9.4

Mountain Medical Center Aging Schedule

Payer Name	Amounts Paid by Aging Interval				Total Receivables
	0–30	31–60	61–90	91–120	
Medicare	$10,215,000	$20,430,000	$8,172,000	$2,043,000	$40,860,000
Medicaid	$2,036,000	$2,036,000	$12,216,000	$4,072,000	$20,360,000
Blue Cross Blue Shield	$78,650,000	$24,200,000	$12,100,000	$6,050,000	$121,000,000
United Healthcare	$48,366,000	$20,152,500	$8,061,000	$4,030,500	$80,610,000
Patient pay	$1,574,500	$6,298,000	$9,447,000	$14,170,500	$31,490,000
	$140,841,500	$73,116,500	$49,996,000	$30,366,000	$294,320,000

You begin your analysis by assessing your chargemaster inpatient and outpatient figures, benchmarking against the current national averages. This type of benchmarking will allow the organization to possibly adjust the chargemaster. This helps to answer the question, "Are we charging enough, or are we leaving money on the table?"

1. According to the AMA and the Department of Health and Human Services data, the average nightly cost of inpatient room and board is $2,465. How does MMC compare to this? Should the MMC nightly rate be increased or decreased to fall within the range of the national average?

2. The national average for all outpatient services is $500. How does MMC compare to this? Should the MMC average outpatient cost be increased or decreased to fall within the range of the national average?

3. If the combined outpatient rehabilitative therapy services see 500 patients annually, each with a standard session of 30 minutes, what is the estimated revenue if the patient volume is shared equally (rehabilitative therapy services include respiratory, physical, occupational, and speech therapies)?

4. MMC has received approval from the state's rate-setting organization to increase the average charge for diagnostic laboratory services by 10%. What would be the new/updated per-test rates for these services (diagnostic laboratory services include chemistry, dialysis, urology, and pathology laboratories)?

5. Nationally, approximately 15% of all emergency department cases require operating room services. (This estimate holds true for MMC's ED and OR as well.) The medical director of the ED has increased capacity by 30% by adding additional administrative and clinical staff. What would be the estimated revenue increase for the ED and OR if the original ED case volume was 27,375 annually and each patient required the following services in addition to the department's base services:

Emergency Department	Operating Room Services
• Ancillary services	• Anesthesia
• Imaging (PET, ultrasound, x-ray)	• EKG/EEG
• Outpatient supplies	• Medical/Surgical supplies
• Pharmacy (per prescription)	• MRI
• Vaccine clinic (three doses)	• Room and board (two nights)

The next step in the analysis is to review the organization's aging and payer data to determine the potential impacts on revenue. Using the previously noted aging schedule:

6. What is the percentage of total accounts receivable paid for each aging interval? What might the resulting percentages indicate in the context of billing collections and follow-up?

7. For the aging interval with the largest accounts receivable paid, which payer contributes the most? What is the payer's percentage contribution to the total amount collected for that aging interval?

8. When analyzing accounts receivable by individual payer, what is the payer mix? Which individual payer contributes the most to the accounts receivable?

9. When analyzing accounts receivable by payer category, which payer category contributes the most to the accounts receivable (and associated revenue)? (Assume that the payer categories are government/public, commercial, and patient pay/self-pay.)

10. Suggest at least three (3) improvements for both the chargemaster and the billing and collections/aging process. Overall, how does MMC appear to be doing with this very important function of the revenue cycle management process?

HEALTHCARE FINANCE COURSE PROJECT: PAYER MIX FOR PHASE I

The concepts and calculations presented here in Chapter 9 should be used as a model for creating the SurgiFlex Revenue Calculations worksheet (Worksheet #3) in Phase I of the course project. The payer mix for the payers in the project are responsible for specific revenue or reimbursement amounts for each of the surgical cases reflected on the SurgiFlex Operating Data worksheet (Worksheet #1). Review the "Course Project: Phase I: SurgiFlex Robotic Surgery System Calculations" section of Chapter 16. Be sure to also review the Microsoft Excel® Reference Guide located in the Appendices as needed.

REFERENCES

American Medical Association. (n.d.). *CPT overview and code approval*. Retrieved February 22, 2023, from https://www.ama-assn.org/practice-management/cpt/cpt-overview-and-code-approval

Centers for Medicare & Medicaid Services. (2023a, February 1). *HCPCS—general information*. U.S. Department of Health and Human Services. https://www.cms.gov/Medicare/Coding/MedHCPCSGenInfo

Centers for Medicare & Medicaid Services. (2023b, February 7). *MS-DRG classifications and software*. U.S. Department of Health and Human Services. https://www.cms.gov/Medicare/Medicare-Fee-for-Service-Payment/AcuteInpatientPPS/MS-DRG-Classifications-and-Software

Reimbursement Mechanisms and Revenue Recognition

OBJECTIVES

1. Understand the connection between service delivery, claims submissions, and reimbursement.
2. Identify the various mechanisms used for healthcare provider reimbursement.
3. Discuss how reimbursement translates to revenue, and its impact on the organization's bottom line.
4. Discuss the impacts of the various reimbursement mechanisms and the broader influence on rising healthcare costs.

INTRODUCTION

This last chapter in our revenue cycle section (Module III) explores reimbursement mechanisms and revenue recognition strategies most common in the healthcare sector. The various providers discussed in earlier chapters have similarities as well as differences when it comes to incurred costs and reimbursement. All seek timely payments, as reimbursement supports any number of shorter-term and longer-term organizational goals, but the mechanisms used to secure those payments depend on insurer contracts and agreements. Some insurers will compensate the healthcare provider based on the expenses incurred or the resources used while providing care, while others have a set amount of reimbursement for each service, no matter the cost incurred by the provider. Some insurance plans factor deductibles and copayments into the provider reimbursement structure, while other plans cover the entire requested reimbursement amount. No matter the reimbursement mechanism chosen, timely revenue recognition is critical to the sustainability of the healthcare organization. Expenses must be correctly captured and billed within the parameters of the payer agreement. We have discussed cost estimation and healthcare claims submission in previous chapters, which leads us to our current discussion on how much providers will be paid for the services rendered to their patients. A **reimbursement mechanism** is the term for the payment methodology that guides the reimbursement process for a given payer and provider. Several reimbursement mechanisms exist, each with its own requirements, benefits, and challenges.

FEE FOR SERVICE

Fee-for-service (FFS) reimbursement is a payment structure that reimburses the healthcare organization or provider for services performed, without regard to quality or service value. In other words, the more services rendered, the more revenue received, as these services are unbundled and paid for individually. Providers can bill and seek reimbursement for each unit of service: per office visit, per examination, per procedure, per test, and so forth. In an FFS arrangement, the provider has minimal risk of lost revenue, with all incurred and allowed costs eligible for reimbursement. Often called "volume-based" reimbursement, healthcare providers have control over how many services are provided, and therefore have direct control over how much revenue is received. Medical procedures and treatments must still be medically necessary for the particular diagnosis, but there may be little regulation on the number of services performed if done by different providers. With this payment model, overall healthcare costs are increased due to overutilization, duplicative services, or inefficiency of processes. The phenomenon of "defensive medicine" may also be a factor here, as providers exercise due diligence and perform testing or assessments that may have already been done by another provider to avoid possible claims of mistreatment or malpractice. While some types of reimbursement under the FFS model allow for incremental charges or revenue, other types serve to restrict the amounts charged and billed by providers.

There are three basic categories of payment under this reimbursement structure: cost-based (retrospective) reimbursement, charge-based reimbursement, and prospective reimbursement. **Cost-based reimbursement** pays the medical provider for costs incurred during the provision of healthcare goods and services. This is a form of retrospective payment, based on the historical series of events. Items covered in this category of payment must be considered direct costs and be necessary for patient care, allowable as defined in the contractual agreement. Cost-based reimbursement considers costs incurred for each episode of care, and is not typically bound by the provider's published chargemaster or fee schedule. If costs are incurred beyond the published rates, they will be reimbursed if determined to be directly related to care and medically necessary. This is a positive for the patient or insured, as this methodology typically leaves very little to be covered by the patient. Cost-based reimbursement, in some cases, incentivizes providers to increase patient visit volume or the number of services provided to a patient, all for the purpose of additional revenue instead of quality or medical necessity. **Charge-based reimbursement** pays the medical provider for services rendered according to the provider's established rates or fee schedule. In this situation, a provider is only paid up to the published rate, leaving any costs incurred above it out of the total reimbursed amount. Since providers will have to absorb the additional expense, many strive to keep costs within the published fee schedule amounts. As a result of healthcare reform, some payers reimburse at discounted rates as prescribed by managed care plans, which have the intended focus of coordination of care. These discounted rates can also impose financial risk for the provider if the incurred costs go beyond the discounted rate. **Prospective reimbursement** is a method that pays the provider before healthcare services are actually rendered. The reimbursement is based on expected costs and is predetermined by the payer. The predetermined amount can be paid in one of several ways: per-procedure payments, per-diagnosis payments, per-diem payments, and bundled payments. Per-procedure reimbursement provides payment for each procedure performed and documented. This method requires that each procedure be documented separately, which means a longer list of items and documentation for longer, more complex inpatient stays. Providers and payers traditionally use this method for outpatient procedures, which tend to be lower in severity and have fewer individual procedures. Per-diagnosis reimbursement pays the provider according to the patient's diagnosis and the typical care that accompanies it. Nothing outside or above the prescribed care will be reimbursed, and all pre-care and post-care is included in the established per-diagnosis rate. **Per-diem** reimbursement pays the provider a set amount for each inpatient day, no matter the services rendered to the patient. There are no itemized charges and no additional reimbursement. All per-diem rates are not the same, however, and they may differ by department or medical unit within an inpatient facility or differ by type of care. Bundled payments provide one lump-sum payment to the provider or facility for all services rendered. This payment method does not consider itemized charges or individual documentation, but instead pays one amount for all services provided by all departments and providers, no matter the primary diagnosis or length of stay. While retrospective payments provide opportunities for increased reimbursement, charge-based and prospective payment methods may limit the amount of reimbursement providers receive and may decrease the number of services offered to the patient.

CAPITATION/CAPITATED PAYMENTS

Reimbursement and payments for healthcare services are often outlined by the contractual agreement between the payer and provider, and in some cases are applied broadly to a patient population. **Capitation** pays a provider a predetermined amount for each patient seen, no matter how many services are provided. These are often referred to as "global payments," and are applied to a provider's entire population of assigned patients. Capitated payments are commonly used in managed care organizational structures such as health maintenance organizations (HMOs), which are intended to maximize care and control costs. With this type of payment structure, the provision of healthcare services is managed to minimize risk and exorbitant incurred expenses. Care is usually restricted to in-network providers or those with existing contractual agreements, with primary and preventive care being the focus. Services rendered outside of these must be referred by the assigned primary care physician (PCP) and approved by the insurance company.

When PCPs are contracted with an insurer under a capitated agreement, they are assigned a specified number of members. This patient population will utilize this provider as the primary contact for all medical care. The PCP receives a single payment for each assigned member during the contract period. Capitated payments are typically paid monthly and are referred to as the PMPM payment, or "**per member per month**." A basic example of PMPM would be a PCP who has 100 assigned patients. If the capitated agreement with the insurer states that the PMPM is $25, then the provider's monthly payment would be $100 \times \$25 = \$2,500$. Most insurers include routine preventive and diagnostic services in the PMPM payment, such as immunizations, laboratory testing, and imaging; however, some capitated agreements reimburse for services outside of primary care separately. Specialists may have their own capitated payment agreements or may be contracted at discounted FFS rates for a given population. Larger or more complex healthcare organizations, such as hospitals, have a PMPM structure that reflects the various services and types of care offered, resulting in a multilevel reimbursement calculation. Inpatient services, outpatient services, and specialized medical areas would have a PMPM calculation based on the number of patients they see annually. The calculations for each are done separately due to differing annual volumes, then consolidated for an estimated total PMPM from one provider. For organizations with multiple services or multiple PMPMs, frequency of each service and the total population are now included in the calculation. **Frequency** is the number of patient visits, or the number of procedures performed in a particular medical category annually. Many organizations capture this using the number of medical claims submitted for the specific procedure or type of care. The **total population** as referenced in the PMPM discussion is the total number of patient visits, or the number of procedures performed across all categories of care. These two items are used to calculate the **utility rate**, or service utilization, to be used for the PMPM calculation. The PMPM for each service is then calculated by multiplying the utility rate by the cost per visit/procedure or unit cost, and dividing the result by 12 to reflect the monthly payment. To illustrate the PMPM calculation, let's refer to the information provided in Exhibit 10.1a.

EXHIBIT 10.1a. Hospital PMPM Calculation

Utility Rate = Annual Frequency / Total Population
PMPM = (Utility Rate × Unit Cost) / 12
Total Population = 1,000

Service Category	Annual Frequency	Unit Cost	Total PMPM
Inpatient Services			
Medical-surgical	625	$1,000	$52.08
Maternity	75	$1,000	$6.25
Mental health	100	$400	$3.33
Subtotal			$61.66
Outpatient Services			
Outpatient surgery	230	$1,500	$28.75
Lab/x-ray	500	$300	$12.50
Emergency dept.	800	$300	$20.00
Subtotal			$61.25
Total (All)			**$122.91**

PMPM, per member per month.

The hospital in Exhibit 10.1a offers both inpatient and outpatient services, with both categories of care containing services or procedures of varying frequencies and unit costs. The total population metric is 1,000 patients, which means for every 1,000 patients/procedures, x-number of patients (frequency) will utilize that service. In a scenario such as this, the PMPM must be calculated individually for each service, then subtotaled for each category. As we examine our first service calculation, medical-surgical, we get the following PMPM:

Utility Rate = Annual Frequency / Total Population = 625 / 1,000 = .625

PMPM = (Utility Rate × Unit Cost) / 12 = (.625 × $1,000) / 12 = $52.08

Performing the same calculation for the other inpatient services, the inpatient PMPM result is $61.66. When added to the outpatient services PMPM, the total amount to be reimbursed to the hospital for all services is $122.91. Of course, there are many other services offered by most hospitals, but this serves as a basic example of how capitated reimbursements are calculated.

Depending on the insurance plan, all of the PMPM reimbursement could be the responsibility of the insurer, or a portion of the amount due could be the responsibility of the patient. The patient portion would be recognized as the "**copay**" amount, with the remainder of the PMPM due from the insurer. Let's expand our PMPM example to include a patient copay amount and the remainder/balance to be paid by the insurer, which is shown in Exhibit 10.1b.

EXHIBIT 10.1b. Hospital PMPM Calculation With Patient Copay

Utility Rate = Annual Frequency / Total Population
PMPM = (Utility Rate × Unit Cost) / 12
Total Population = 1,000

Total Reimbursed PMPM

Received From Patients

Balance Due From Insurer

Service Category	Annual Frequency	Unit Cost	Total PMPM	Copay Frequency	Copay Unit Cost	Copay PMPM	Net PMPM
Inpatient Services							
Medical-surgical	625	$1,000	$52.08	0	$-	0	$52.08
Maternity	75	$1,000	$6.25	0	$-	0	$6.25
Mental health	100	$400	$3.33	0	$-	0	$3.33
Subtotal			$61.66			$0.00	$61.66
Outpatient Services							
Outpatient surgery	230	$1,500	$28.75	0		0	$28.75
Lab/x-ray	500	$300	$12.50	0		0	$12.50
Emergency dept.	800	$300	$20.00	600	$75.00	$3.75	$16.25
Subtotal			$61.25			$3.75	$57.50
Total (All)			**$122.91**			**$3.75**	**$119.16**

PMPM, per member per month.

To calculate the PMPM for patient copays, we use the same calculation as the total PMPM. We incorporate the copay frequency and copay unit cost, which is the patient's out-of-pocket amount. The total population of 1,000 patients remains the same. Our example only reflects a copay for emergency department (ED) services, so the rest of the copay items are zero. Interpreting the copay frequency and unit cost for every thousand ED patients, 600 of them will have a copay of $75.00.

Utility Rate = Annual Frequency / Total Population = 600 / 1,000 = .60

PMPM = (Utility Rate × Unit Cost) / 12 = (.60 × $75.00) / 12 = $3.75

With the patient copay PMPM subtracted from the total PMPM due, the remaining insurer obligation is $119.16. The copay frequency is a subset of the total frequency, so in the case of the ED, 600 out of 800, or 75% of the patients, will have a copayment due at the time of service. PMPM reimbursement is based on a specified number of monthly patient visits or procedures, so services rendered beyond the contracted volume are unpaid. This poses a great deal of risk to providers, as repeat visits or additional medical services may result in lost revenue. Revenue restricted by volume, as is the case with capitated payments, could potentially limit the services offered to patients with insurance plans such as HMOs, impacting the overall quality of care provided. Some providers may also limit the number of HMO plans they contract with, or they may not accept PMPM-based reimbursement at all. To ensure the best quality of care at an optimal price, many insurers are seeking to adopt value-based and other alternative payment methods as modern approaches to reimbursement.

ALTERNATIVE REIMBURSEMENT MODELS

Although controlling the cost of healthcare goods and services continues to be a challenge, the goal of ensuring quality patient care and positive health outcomes has garnered the attention of payers and clinicians alike. Traditional reimbursement mechanisms such as FFS and capitation may unintentionally prioritize the financial aspects of healthcare, with the patient experience remaining at the status quo. More recent payment strategies, however, prioritize patient health outcomes and incentivize providers for meeting established wellness and cost-savings goals. Early plans were implemented to foster improvements for the Medicare population of beneficiaries, but today's alternative reimbursement models have been applied to almost every type of payer, with intended value to both providers and patients. Shared savings among providers and payers is among the list of benefits, as is high value-coordinated healthcare for patients. There are many similarities in reimbursement methods, and some are tailored to specific healthcare conditions, but each has a defined role within the healthcare sector's broader vision of value-based care. In alternative models, quality of care drives the reimbursement process instead of visit or procedure volume, resulting in improved outcomes at a lower cost.

Bundled (Episode-Based) Payments

Duplicative services or unnecessary treatments contribute greatly to healthcare expenditures, as increased patient volumes have traditionally been used to increase provider revenue. Regulating volume by reinforcing value has been one approach to minimizing overproduction of healthcare services. **Bundled payments** (also referred to as episode-based payments) are designed to reimburse a provider with a predetermined lump-sum payment, covering one specific episode of care, usually identified by diagnosis-related groups (DRGs). Pretreatment consultations, testing and assessments, and posttreatment follow-up are included in the episode of care, instead of being compensated separately. The agreement can also include multiple providers and facilities if the diagnosis or medical treatment warrants care from more than one specialty. The goal of this reimbursement strategy is to deliver high-quality, effective healthcare services from the provider, as well as establish a standard treatment plan for all of the provider's patients with the same diagnosis. Ideally, shared accountability among providers will reduce waste and foster cost savings.

As shown in Figure 10.1, bundled payments do not outline a reimbursement amount for each service rendered, just a lump-sum payment for the entire episode of care. The PCP and all of the other specialists and facilities contracted with a payer under a bundled payment structure have agreed to this predetermined amount. If costs for the episode of care are less than the reimbursed amount, the providers keep this amount as savings. If the costs exceed the reimbursed amount, however, the providers must absorb the additional costs at a loss. Episode-based payments incentivize providers to closely manage costs, in order to ensure effective and efficient healthcare provision. Detailed claims, medical records, and financial records must

Figure 10.1
Bundled payment reimbursement

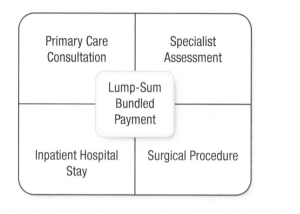

Healthcare Service	Bundled Payment	Traditional Payment
Primary Care Consultation		$ 100.00
Specialist Assessment		$ 125.00
Surgical Procedure		$ 5,000.00
Inpatient Hospital Stay		$ 7,500.00
	$ 12,725.00	$ 12,725.00

still be maintained to prevent cost cutting at the expense of patient care. Some value-based reimbursement structures actually limit the amount of savings to prevent this from occurring.

Savings and Risk-Sharing Payment Plans

As value-based reimbursement plans become more prevalent across the healthcare sector, providers of all types are seeking to manage quality and costs of care. High-quality healthcare at the lowest possible cost is the focal point, with shared savings and shared risks incorporated into the overall structure of the value-based agreements. **Accountable care organizations** (ACOs) are groups of providers and facilities that work together to coordinate the healthcare for an assigned population of patients. This coordination of healthcare services includes preventive care, treatment of current illnesses and post-acute care, and reductions in care-based hospital readmissions and ED visits. Payments to ACOs could be bundled episode-based payments, production-based payments, or incentive-based payments, all predicated on achieving positive health outcomes and high standards of care. The ACO structure was originally created to care for Medicare beneficiaries, but has since been adapted to address the needs and populations of Medicaid and commercial insurance plans as well. The **Medicare shared savings program** (MSSP) was the program that created ACOs under the Patient Protection and Affordable Care Act (PPACA) legislation as a mechanism to foster improved medical outcomes for Medicare beneficiaries and reduce the overall cost of care. This program encouraged the voluntary formation of ACOs and offered several savings and risk-sharing options for providers to choose from. Under the MSSP, each ACO would be responsible for the care coordination of at least 5,000 Medicare beneficiaries, and would be reimbursed under one of two available tracks: the basic track or the enhanced track. Basic track reimbursement allows for up to 50% shared savings if costs are below the established targets, and up to 40% shared risk if the costs are above the established targets. The enhanced track allows for up to 75% shared savings and up to 75% shared risk, both based on established targets. Although able to choose their level of risk and reward, ACOs not meeting the required quality of care standards are not eligible for shared savings or reimbursement of any kind. This quality requirement realigns the focus from financial metrics to quality and population health metrics, as intended by value-based reimbursement strategies.

Pay-for-Performance Plans

With improved health outcomes and quality at the forefront, some reimbursement structures measure adherence to established quality metrics and standards over time as a means of determining payments. **Pay-for-performance** reimbursement plans (also called P4P or value-based purchasing) use the established metrics as the benchmarks to incentivize and penalize providers' trended performance. Measurable items include more than just care efficiency and reductions in cost, as patient safety, patient experience, and clinical processes are also considered. P4P payments are typically distributed from a savings pool or bonus pool if all requirements have been met. As with ACOs and other alternative reimbursement models, no payment or bonus is distributed if the performance standards or continuous improvement requirements have not been met.

Although P4P is used by organizations in all sectors and industries, the most detailed and expansive P4P programs have been implemented by the Centers for Medicare & Medicaid Services (CMS) as mechanisms to increase healthcare quality for Medicare and Medicaid populations. These value-based programs were created to address the healthcare needs and concerns of specific subpopulations within the largest two public/government payers, offering incentives tied to performance and quality, like other value-based plans. The most common CMS P4P value-based programs, rooted in the healthcare Triple Aim (improved patient experience, improved population health, and reduced cost of care), are aligned with other CMS quality initiatives, and include programs featured in Table 10.1.

Another key piece of legislation that guides public health program administration is the **Medicare Access and Children's Health Insurance Program (CHIP) Reauthorization Act** (MACRA). MACRA implemented financial incentives for providers with the creation of the Quality Payment Program, which was designed to improve the quality of patient care for Medicare and CHIP beneficiaries. There are two paths or participation options for the Quality Payment Program: a merit-based option and an alternative payment option. The first option, the Merit-Based Incentive Payment System (MIPS), provides clinician payments based on reported performance for established quality measures to include Medicare Part B claims assessment, clinical data registry requirements, and clinical quality measures, to name a few. The second option, Advanced Alternative Payment Models (APMs), incentivizes providers for participation in payment programs designed to improve quality and contain costs. Incentive payments can be based on traditional costs savings methods or based on all-payer option savings, with a percentage of savings distributed to providers. While these programs and the benchmarks are well defined, there are some programs that offer flexibility and modification based on medical judgment and evidence-based clinical management. The **Delivery System Reform Incentive Payment Program** (DSRIP) is an initiative that offers such flexibility for the Medicaid program. Under DSRIP, providers can change the patient's care plan to improve their individual health outcomes. The program goal is to reduce the number of readmissions and ED visits overall, while improving the Medicaid (and, in some cases, the CHIP) population's health. This Medicaid redesign waiver supports the states' guidance on measurable outcome metrics and milestones, changes to clinical practice and management, and cost-saving strategies and supplemental

Table 10.1

CMS P4P AND VALUE-BASED PROGRAMS

Program Name	Program Description
End-Stage Renal Disease Quality Incentive Program (ESRD QIP)	Measures quality of services of renal dialysis facilities; achievement of established benchmarks, quality improvement, clinical measures
Hospital-Acquired Conditions Reduction Program (HAC)	Monitors (negative) change in medical condition as directly related to the inpatient stay; adherence to safety standards to reduce falls/fractures, pressure sores (positioning), facility-borne infections
Home Health Value-Based Purchasing (HHVBP)	Examined preparedness and appropriateness of the patient's home health setting; coordinated care of patients, communication with patient and caregivers, and team discussions
Hospital Readmissions Reduction Program (HRRP)	Evaluates coordination of care and discharge planning; improved communication to reduce unplanned readmissions
Skilled Nursing Facility Value-Based Purchasing (SNFVBP)	Assesses SNF readmissions, SNF-associated infections, and nurse staffing; improved overall care to Medicare beneficiaries
Hospital Value-Based Purchasing Program (VBP)	Measures quality of care for the inpatient setting; quality of care, patient experience, implementing evidence-based care standards, patient safety, cost reduction, efficiency, and care effectiveness
Value Modifier Program (VM)	Adjusts payments to all clinicians/care providers based on quality of care and costs of care; overall improvements to clinical outcomes

CMS, Centers for Medicare & Medicaid Services; P4P, pay for performance; SNF, skilled nursing facility.

payments to Medicaid providers. As the initial DSRIP programs expire under initial federal legislation, some states are implementing their own unique version of the program to continue its important Medicaid improvement programs and initiatives.

REVENUE RECOGNITION METHODOLOGIES

Reimbursement mechanisms exist in many forms, providing payments from multiple payers for any number of healthcare products and services. Estimating revenue for budgeting and longer-term strategic planning is equally as important as accurate expense capture. Revenue, as defined in Chapter 4, is the income generated by the provision of healthcare goods and services, but the determination must be made on whether or not the generated amount is enough to cover expenses as well as fund future initiatives. In terms of revenue recognition, the more detailed an organization's expense data collection is, the better. There may be dozens of payer contracts to manage, with each having its own definitions of services and performance standards, as well as reimbursement structures and payment schedules. Payment schedules outline the types of medical services and products covered and the dollar amount or calculation of reimbursement of each outlined service. Reimbursement methodologies in contracts could include all or any combination of the following parameters:

- discounted fee-schedule payments
- reimbursement as a percentage of total charges

- bundled or episode-based payments
- capitated PMPM payments
- per-diem (for inpatient cases) payments
- stop-loss guidelines (for rate or price changes)

All of these have the potential to alter revenue recognition expectations, making cost and charge capture even more important. Sound revenue recognition is dependent on the accuracy and completeness of payer contract negotiations and contract inclusions, including performance and utilization requirements; billing, collections, and claims processing; and accounts receivable management and receivables posting. Although most of the contract parameters, rules, and payment logic is programmed to process automatically, the system needs to be flexible enough, and the financial professionals must be adept enough, to make changes and updates to the payment framework when needed. Standard FFS contract agreements reimburse for allowable charges for costs incurred while providing medical care, so no changes need to be made for this straightforward methodology. The variations in reimbursement and calculations for the previously noted methodologies often require more attention, especially if they are in the same contract, working in unison. The revenue for a specific population of patients could look very different, depending on the reimbursement methodology applied. To illustrate the differences in revenue recognized under different reimbursement methodologies, let's examine the following scenario and the seven-part solution set.

Scenario

A PCP provides healthcare services for a population of 500 patients with varying insurance payers, health conditions, and demographic backgrounds. The PCP has multiple payer contracts, each with its own performance requirements and payment schedule. Currently, 55% of this patient population are insured by commercial insurance, 30% by Medicare, and 15% by Medicaid. All of the contracted insurers have a managed care component, a standard fee schedule reimbursement component, and alternative payment provisions. The PCP incurs the following expenses while providing healthcare to patients: $100 for each office visit, $15 for each screening/test, and $35 for office administration and overhead, totaling $150 for each office visit.

First, calculate the number of patients with each insurance type to use in the various revenue calculations.

- commercial: 55% of 500 = 275 patients
- Medicare: 30% of 500 = 150 patients
- Medicaid: 15% of 500 = 75 patients

Part 1—FFS Calculation: Approximately 20% of commercial insurance patients have FFS insurance coverage. What would be the reimbursed amount if each of these patients had one office visit?

FFS Payment = Rate × Volume

FFS Payment = $150 × 55 Patients (275 × .20)

FFS Payment = $8,250

Part 2—Discounted FFS Calculation: Using the same commercial insurance population with FFS coverage, a payer with a discounted fee schedule arrangement of 15% would have the following reimbursement amount:

FFS Payment = Rate × Volume

FFS Payment = ($150 − 15% discount) × 55 Patients

FFS Payment = $127.50 × 55 Patients

FFS Payment = $7,012.50

Part 3—Total Charge Percentage Payments: This would be similar to the discounted FFS agreement, with the percentage applied to total charges instead of individual fee schedule items. The percentage to be paid may vary depending on payer agreement. As an example, assume that the CMS agrees to reimburse the provider for all Medicare and Medicaid patients at 60% of total charges. The reimbursement calculation for this would be:

Medicare + Medicaid patients = 225 Patients

Total Charges = Rate × Volume

Total Charges = $150 × 225 Patients

Total Charges = $33,750

Percentage Payment = $33,750 × .60

Percentage Payment = $20,250

Part 4—Bundled Payment Calculation (Episode-Based Payments): Bundled or episode-based payments are lump-sum payments made to the provider for all care surrounding one diagnosis or medical issue. To illustrate, assume that the Medicare patients assigned to this provider are now required to undergo an additional screening, a physical therapy session, and a follow-up assessment with the provider if they meet certain conditions. These added medical requirements increase the total charges and amount due by approximately $125, and, when added to the initial office visit, total $275. The CMS agrees to a bundled payment of $275 for all Medicare beneficiaries assigned to the provider to cover all associated costs of care, no matter the health condition. If only 20% of the Medicare patients require the additional services, what would the provider's reimbursement be?

Medicare Patients Assigned = 150 Patients

Medicare Patients Requiring Additional Services: 150 × .20 = 30

If reimbursement covered patients without the additional services at the standard rate of $150 and only the patients with additional services at the bundled rate:

Standard Payment = 120 (without additional services) × $150 = $18,000

Bundled Payment = 30 (with additional services) × $275 (bundled rate) = $8,250

Total Split Payment = $26,250

If reimbursement covered all Medicare patients at the bundled rate:

Total Bundled Payment = 150 × $275 = $41,250

In this situation, the provider earns profit with the bundled payment when applied to all Medicare beneficiaries in the amount of $15,000 ($41,250 – $26,250). If unforeseen expenses were to arise, causing incurred expenses to exceed the total bundled payment amount, the provider would be in a loss position for this group of patients. An example here could be added patient transportation. If the provider now had to arrange medical transport for all Medicare patients at a cost of $50 per patient, the expense incurred would exceed the total bundled payment received.

Incurred Expense per Patient = $275 + $50 = $325

Amount Needed (full reimbursement) = 150 × $325 = $48,750

Total Bundled Payment = 150 × $275 = $41,250

Loss for Provider = $7,500 ($48,750 – $41,250)

Part 5—Capitated Payment Calculation: A capitated payment is a set payment per enrollee or beneficiary, paid to the provider during the contracted time frame. This is most commonly done with managed care insurance plans that have strict coverage, requiring all healthcare services to be provided in-network (contracted providers and facilities). To illustrate this, let's assume that one of the commercial payers with this provider agrees to a capitated payment of $150 for each patient enrolled in its plan, covering the provider's standard office visit expense. This commercial payer covers approximately one-third of all commercial patients. The capitated payment is to be paid monthly, with no additional reimbursement to be made (PMPM). If half of the payer's commercial population has two office visits for each of 3 months, what does this mean for the provider's total reimbursement?

Commercial Patients Covered by Payer = 275 × .33 = 91 Patients (rounded)

Commercial Patients PMPM Payment = $150 × 91 Patients = $13,650

Commercial Patients With Two Visits = 91/2 = 46 Patients (rounded)

Additional Visits = 46 × 3 = 138 (one visit per member is already included in the standard PMPM)

Additional Visit Expense = $150 × 138 visits = $20,700

In this situation, the additional visit expense is unrecognized revenue, a loss for the provider, since the PMPM amount applies no matter how many times a beneficiary visits the provider. The PMPM amount pays for one visit per enrollee, and that's it.

Part 6—Per-Diem Payments: This type of payment is usually applied to inpatient hospital stays or residential/long-term care overnight settings. With per-diem rates, the facility is paid one predetermined, contracted amount for all services provided; this includes clinicians and facilities charges, such as room and board. This is very similar to the bundled, episode-based reimbursement for providers applied to the inpatient setting and related services. If standard daily inpatient costs for a patient under a typical FFS arrangement would be itemized as shown in the text that follows, what would be the FFS reimbursement in comparison to a per-diem rate of $4,000 for a three-night stay in a private room?

Physician fees: $1,500 per day

Room and board: $3,000 per day

Imaging services: $100 per day

Pharmacy services: $50 per day

Total Itemized FFS Charges/Reimbursement: $4,650×3 days=$13,950

Total Per-Diem Reimbursement=$4,000×3 days=$12,000

In this example, the physician and facilities have a total loss of $1,950, because the per-diem rate only covers $4,000 per day. If the patient were to have a semi-private hospital room, sharing the space with another patient and cutting the room and board expense in half, the FFS amount would be decreased by $1,500, making up some of the loss. Other factors such as fewer imaging and pharmacy services could also decrease the total amount due, and further reduce the loss from the limited per-diem rate.

Part 7—Stop-Loss and Rate Change Contract Inclusions: The purpose of **stop-loss provisions** in contracts is to control the amount of increased expense a payer would have to cover. Stop-loss clauses can be implemented as limits to excess charges or as limits to rate increases. The impact of the rate increase can be illustrated as:

Contracted Reimbursement Rate=75% of Billed Charges

Contracted Rate Increase (Maximum)=5%

Provider Rate Increase=10%

New/Increased Reimbursement Rate=(1+Contracted Rate Increase / 1+Provider Rate Increase)×Contracted Reimbursement Rate

New/Increased Reimbursement Rate=(1.05 / 1.10)×.75

New/Increased Reimbursement Rate=.9545×.75=.7159 or 71.59%

Medical Service or Procedure Billed Price=$1,500

Medical Service or Procedure Increased Price (10%)=$1,650

Contracted Reimbursement Rate Payment=$1,125 ($1,500×75%)

Increased Reimbursement Rate Payment=$1,181.25 ($1,650×71.59%)

The increased reimbursement rate payment reflects a 5% increase as outlined in the contract from the original contracted payment amount of $1,125 ($1,125 × 1.05%=$1,181.25). The payer is only responsible for up to 5% of the provider's increased expenses. Anything above this amount must be absorbed by the provider. This prompts providers to closely control costs and to stay within the range of the contracted increase, ideally while provided the best quality healthcare.

Another type of quality-based reimbursement utilized by healthcare providers and payers is the **resource-based relative value scale** (RBRVS). This method of reimbursement was originally designed for determining the amount of reimbursement for Medicare providers, but has been adopted for other providers as well. The RBRVS assigns a specified number of **relative value units** (or RVUs) to each Current Procedural Terminology (CPT) code and the healthcare provider's related expenses. RVUs for physician reimbursement include three categories of costs: the physician's direct labor costs, which capture the actual hands-on time based on the severity of illness; the physician's overhead costs, which capture practice-related indirect expenses; and the physician's malpractice costs, which apply a portion of the insurance coverage to each patient. RVUs must be provided on medical claims submitted for reimbursement, along with the other required codes (*International Classification of Diseases, 10th Revision* [*ICD-10*]; CPT; Healthcare Common Procedure Coding System [HCPCS]; etc.). When calculating the provider's reimbursement, payers apply two additional metrics to the total RVUs: the Geographic Practice Cost Indices (GPCI) and the RVU conversion factor. The GPCI adjust the total RVUs to account for differences in the provider's regional economy. An example of this would be adjustments for average office staff salaries or office space rental (both included in overhead), which are considerably higher in certain regions like Seattle, California, or New York. As with the base RVUs, the GPCI accounts for the three categories of costs incurred by each provider. When the RVUs have been adjusted using the GPCI, they are then multiplied by the RVU conversion factor for calculation of total payment. The conversion factor is determined annually by the CMS, and is used to convert the RVUs to dollars. This process essentially crosswalks a healthcare provider's standard fee schedule, which is based on CPT codes, to an RVU-based fee schedule for quality-based payments.

In Figure 10.2, the three types of RVU and the three types of GPCI represent the three categories of physician-incurred costs: labor costs (represented as RVU^1/GPCI^1 in Figure 10.2 and the following example), overhead expense (represented as RVU^2/GPCI^2), and malpractice expense (represented as RVU^3 and GPCI^3). To illustrate the calculation, let's review the following example.

A general practice physician located in Long Beach, California, is preparing a claim for submission to the CMS. The CPT code for the patient's visit is 99213—Low Intensity Outpatient Office Visit. For this CPT, the RVU guidelines indicate the following:

RVU^1 (Work/Labor) = 1.3, GPCI^1 = 1.048

RVU^2 (Overhead/Practice Expense) = 1.75, GPCI^2 = 1.25

RVU^3 (Malpractice Insurance) = 0.09, GPCI^3 = 0.75

Total RVUs = $(1.3 \times 1.048) + (1.75 \times 1.25) + (0.09 \times 0.75) = 3.6174$

Figure 10.2

RBRVS/RVU payment calculation

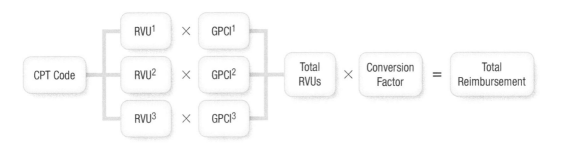

Note: The three types of RVU and the three types of GPCI represent the three categories of physician-incurred costs: labor costs (represented as RVU^1/GPCI^1), overhead expense (represented as RVU^2/GPCI^2), and malpractice expense (represented as RVU^3 and GPCI^3).

CPT, Current Procedural Terminology; GPCI, Geographic Practice Cost Indices; RBRVS, resource-based relative value scale; RVU, relative value units.

Multiplying the total RVUs by the conversion factor of $33.5983, total reimbursement for this patient visit is $121.54 (rounded).

The RVUs and GPCI values will vary according to provider, specialty, location, and patient acuity, but the process of calculating total RVUs and reimbursement remains the same. If the provider renders a service that does not currently have an assigned CPT code, the service is not reimbursable. Commonly unreimbursed items include activities such as relationship management and academic functions performed by many providers but not considered quantifiable or directly related to a patient's medical care. Relationship management would include distribution of patient satisfaction surveys, or any activity designed to enhance the patient experience. Academic functions would primarily be a focus at a teaching or research institution, but would include any activities related to teaching or mentoring clinical students and residents, as well as continuing education efforts like learning a new procedure for patient treatment.

REIMBURSEMENT AS REVENUE: WHAT PULLS IT ALL TOGETHER?

So far, we've discussed the various methods by which a healthcare organization is reimbursed for services rendered and goods produced. How does this translate to revenue for the organization? Reimbursement is the payment for costs incurred—in the case of healthcare providers, labor or supply costs associated with the provision of care. Revenue is defined as income from operating activities, and often includes reimbursement from health insurers or other payment sources, as contractually agreed.

CHAPTER SUMMARY

Revenue recognition and reimbursement represent just a portion of an organization's revenue cycle management process, which all begins with patient registration. Attention to the revenue cycle ensures that the organization is operationally able to provide healthcare services to its targeted population of patients, for both the shorter term and longer term. The payment end of the revenue cycle includes communication from all parties involved–patients, providers, and payers— to ensure timely, medically necessary treatment; effective and efficient follow-up; and contract-appropriate reimbursement. Challenges such as patient access and claims denials continue to plague many providers, with both having a tremendous impact on the healthcare organization's financial health and viability. As discussed in this chapter, there are many methods for reimbursement, each requiring different information, inputs, or values. The key to maximizing reimbursement is efficient internal processes, accurate and complete data collection, timely claims submissions, and dedicated patient accounts receivable and reconciliation efforts. In most cases, providers have multiple reimbursement contracts and are therefore required to meet multiple sets of performance standards or claims data requirements. While this can seem redundant, it is important for ensuring quality patient care, while doing so as efficiently and effectively as possible.

KEY TERMS FOR REVIEW

accountable care organization	capitation	copay
bundled payments	charge-based reimbursement	cost-based reimbursement

Delivery System Reform Incentive Payment Program

fee-for-service reimbursement

frequency

Medicare Access and Children's Health Insurance Program (CHIP) Reauthorization Act

Medicare shared savings program

pay for performance

per diem

per member per month

prospective reimbursement

reimbursement mechanism

relative value units

resource-based relative value scale

stop-loss provision

total population

utility rate

DISCUSSION QUESTIONS

1. Discuss how accurate claims submission could impact provider reimbursement.
2. If a provider has multiple reimbursement contracts, what would you suggest as best-practice strategies for effective revenue cycle management to ensure timely payment receipts? Define an ACO, and detail how this payment methodology could benefit all patient populations, not just the Medicare population it was initially intended for.
3. Identify some potential positive and potential negative impacts of capitated payments, including PMPM reimbursement. Does the capitated reimbursement methodology benefit the provider? The patient? The payer?
4. What is the MACRA legislation, and how does it affect healthcare reimbursement?
5. If the payer contract includes a stop-loss provision, what does this mean for provider reimbursement?
6. Although quality healthcare is the goal, are volume-based reimbursement mechanisms less effective in terms of patient care than quality-based reimbursement mechanisms?
7. In your opinion, will quality-based reimbursement mechanisms reduce the overall growth rate of healthcare costs? Explain your opinion.

PRACTICE PROBLEMS

Answers to this chapter's Practice Problems are available via Springer Publishing Connect™ by following the instructions on the opening page of this book and accessing Answers to Practice Problems on the Table of Contents.

1. Calculate the discounted fee schedule reimbursement if the payer is responsible for reimbursement at 65% of the billed charges in the following list.

    Medical consultation/office visit (standard): $80.00

    Phlebotomy panel (standard): $50.00

    Prescription refills (2): $10.00 each

    Vaccines (2): $25.00 each

    If the provider receives a $20 copayment from the patient, what is the remaining amount due from the insurance payer?

2. Community Hospital has just initiated a contract with an HMO and wants to be sure of its estimated reimbursement. Hospital leadership decides to use last year's patient volume as an indicator of this year's potential patient volume, since no major increases in patient visits or procedures are expected. Using the information provided in Table 10.2, complete the PMPM calculation for Community Hospital.

Table 10.2

COMMUNITY HOSPITAL PMPM CALCULATION

Service Category	Annual Frequency	Unit Cost	Total PMPM	Copay Frequency	Copay Unit Cost	Copay PMPM	Net PMPM
Inpatient Services							
Medical	1,000	$1,150					
Surgical	700	$1,695					
ICU/NICU	175	$2,300					
Maternity	100	$1,500					
Mental health	60	$1,150					
Subtotal							
Outpatient Services							
Outpatient clinics	1,500	$500		750	$15.00		
Ambulatory surgery	375	$1,000		50	$150.00		
Lab/x-ray	500	$75		-	$-		
Pharmacy services	900	$30		800	$10.00		
Emergency dept.	3,000	$725		1,000	$75.00		
Subtotal							
Total (All)							

PMPM, per member per month.

3. A provider charges $125 for a standard office visit, but uncovers several expenses that have been inadvertently left out of their rate calculation. They decide to increase their office visit charge to $150 to cover the additional incurred costs. If the health insurance payer has a 10% stop-loss clause in the contract agreement with the provider, what will be the payer's new reimbursement rate?

4. A provider has a total patient population of 500 patients, covered by three different health insurance payers. Each payer uses a different reimbursement methodology, and the provider would like to calculate total reimbursement for their patient population. The provider intends to use the following data in their calculation:

    Medicare patients: 35% of the provider's patient population

    Medicaid: 20% of the provider's patient population

    Blue Cross Blue Shield (BCBS): 45% of the provider's patient population.

    Medicare uses an RVU calculation for reimbursement, Medicaid uses a discounted FFS calculation for reimbursement, and BCBS uses bundled payment amounts for reimbursement.

The basic fees schedule items the provider would like to charge/bill for include the following services and associated prices:

- Medium intensity office visit (CPT code—99214): $100.00

- Imaging services (x-rays, scans, etc.): $75.00

- Pharmacy services/refills: $25.00

- Transportation and in-home follow-up: $50.00

What would the provider's total reimbursement be for all 500 patients, if:

- Total RVUs are 3.915 and the conversion factor is $33.29?

- Medicaid's contract states reimbursement at 60% discount?

- BCBS pays $212.50 for episode-based/bundled care?

5. In a P4P reimbursement model, a provider has to meet specific performance guidelines to qualify for the varying levels of reimbursement and shared savings. If the provider is to be awarded $20 for each 3% decrease in hospital readmission rates and earns 1% of every $100 saved in inpatient costs, what is the provider's total reimbursement if the number of readmissions went from 290 to 205, saving approximately $45,000?

6. An insurance payer reimburses $100 for each mammogram performed at an imaging center, with no initial copay required from patients. Some patients require a second 3-D imaging procedure, but this is not reimbursed by the insurer. The second imaging costs $125 and has a required patient copay of $10. If the total mammogram imaging population is 250, and 15% of them require the second imaging service, how much is the financial loss for the imaging center?

7. ACOs manage both shorter-term and longer-term outcomes for an assigned patient population, as defined by the insurance provider. You are one of five providers assigned to the Medicare population in your area, which totals approximately 3,750 beneficiaries. Over the course of 6 months, the ACO has managed to increase diabetes and hypertension screenings by 25% and 20%, respectively. Baseline screenings were 50% for diabetes and 40% for hypertension, with total savings of $30,000 in acute care savings. If your P4P agreement states that your shared savings is calculated as .05% per dollar saved if 2,500 patients get diabetes screenings plus $1 for each additional patient screened, and .03% per dollar saved if 1,750 patients get hypertension screenings plus $1 for each additional patient screened, what is the total amount of savings to be shared by the five providers?

CHAPTER 10 CASE: PICKING UP THE TAB: ESTIMATING REVENUE FOR HEALTHCARE SERVICES

You have recently been promoted to the chief financial officer position for Pinnacle Health Inc., a major healthcare system providing services for a wide range of medical needs. The health system has been around for quite some time, and has locations spanning several counties within your state. Over the past few years, increased legislation has changed the financial landscape of the healthcare industry, requiring a more thorough analysis of your organization's operations. You decide to examine your patient mix as well as your payer mix to see if adjustments need to be made or if revenue can be increased. To begin your analysis, you summarize and review the demographic, insurance, and financial data for the community, as shown in summary tables Box 10.1 (demographic data), Box 10.2 (insurance coverage data), and Box 10.3 (aging by payer).

BOX 10.1

Pinnacle Health Inc. Demographic Data

County/City Locations	Current Population	Resident Race				Resident Age Range					
		Black	Latinx	White	Other	0–17	18–24	25–40	41–55	55–64	65+
Archer County											
Bluefield	12,375	3,094	2,475	6,188	619	495	4,084	3,713	3,094	743	248
Mountville	17,850	1,785	1,250	14,280	536	1,250	2,678	5,355	3,570	4,463	536
Roland City	10,244	5,122	2,561	2,049	512	205	410	3,073	2,254	2,561	1,741
	40,469										
Mercer County											
Ellena	45,525	22,763	9,105	9,105	4,553	3,642	4,553	9,105	13,658	5,463	9,105
Endsburg	29,128	2,913	2,039	23,302	874	583	1,165	8,738	6,408	8,738	3,495
Johnsboro	30,127	15,064	7,532	6,025	1,506	2,410	3,013	6,025	9,038	3,615	6,025
	104,780										
Potter County											
Minerva	77,000	53,130	15,400	7,700	770	6,160	7,700	15,400	23,100	9,240	15,400
Orchestra	49,110	4,911	3,438	39,288	1,473	3,929	4,911	9,822	14,733	5,893	9,822
Spheres	60,000	25,800	13,200	18,000	3,000	1,200	2,400	18,000	13,200	15,000	10,200
	186,110										
Total Population	**331,359**										

BOX 10.2

Pinnacle Health Inc. Community Insurance Coverage Data

County	Health Insurance Coverage (as Percentage of County Population)				
	Medicare	Medicaid (incl. CHIP)	Dual Eligible	Commercial/ Employer	Patient Pay/ Uninsured
Archer County	6.24%	17.09%	0.47%	72.17%	4.03%
Mercer County	17.78%	18.76%	0.86%	55.53%	7.07%
Potter County	19.03%	14.19%	1.58%	62.19%	3.01%

CHIP, Children's Health Insurance Program.

BOX 10.3

Pinnacle Health Inc. Aging Schedule by Payer

Payer (Individual)	Amounts Paid by Aging Interval				
	0–30	31–60	61–90	91–120	Total Paid
Medicare	$3,850,019	$2,156,270	$1,036,024	$375,017	$7,417,330
Medicaid	$1,031,296	$1,466,298	$728,028	$187,542	$3,413,164
Dual eligible	$149,642	$143,794	$840,034	$250,038	$1,383,508
Commercial	$7,150,028	$2,863,513	$3,920,012	$750,036	$14,683,589
Patient pay/unsured	$137,521	$575,022	$727,440	$1,125,019	$2,565,002
	$12,318,506	$7,204,897	$7,251,538	$2,687,652	$29,462,593

1. What percentage of the total community is represented by each county?

2. If the total billed amount is allocated to each county based on the percentage identified in Question 1, how much would each county be responsible for, by payer?

3. Historically, the 25 to 40 age range and the 41 to 55 age range make up 80% of the commercial insurance coverage as noted in Boxes 10.1 and 10.2. If this still stands true, which county would have the greatest contribution to the commercial billing amount?

4. Using the Medicare percentage per county, calculate the number of persons insured by Medicare in each county. Repeat the calculation for all payers shown in Boxes 10.1 and 10.2.

5. Using the number of persons insured by Medicare from Question 4 as the number of discharges, calculate total Medicare revenue per discharge. Repeat the calculation for all payers shown in Boxes 10.1 and 10.2.

6. In efforts to increase commercial payer revenue, Pinnacle Health has signed contracts with two additional commercial payers. The first payer intends to only cover residents of Archer County and plans to offer the HMO option. If the first payer offers a PMPM of $100 per enrolled resident, and approximately 7% of the county's Medicaid residents will switch to the HMO's coverage, how much additional revenue will be recognized?

7. The second payer intends to only cover Potter County residents and reimburse at 75% of billed charges. If 13% of the county's Medicaid residents will switch to this new insurance plan, what will be the additional revenue recognized if the commercial revenue per discharge is used as the baseline?

HEALTHCARE FINANCE COURSE PROJECT: REVENUE ANALYSIS FOR PHASE I

The concepts as presented in Chapter 10 can be used in conjunction with the payer mix calculations from Chapter 9. As revenue is recognized in the context of payer mix and utilization, changes can be made to the payer mix, contracting terms, or utilization to impact the organization's recognized revenue. Review the "Course Project: Phase I: SurgiFlex Robotic Surgery System Calculations" section of Chapter 16. Be sure to review the Microsoft Excel® Reference Guide located in the Appendices as needed.

Budgeting and Operations

CHAPTER 11

The Budgeting Process

OBJECTIVES

1. Identify the steps/stages of the budgeting process.
2. Define the term "operating budget" and discuss how it differs from the capital budget.
3. List the approaches to budgeting and detail the differences between the approaches.
4. Discuss the considerations and challenges that may impact the budgeting process.

INTRODUCTION

The first three modules of this textbook provide background on the healthcare finance function and detail how we quantify the business of healthcare. This first chapter of Module IV begins our discussion on how we use what we have quantified to move the organization forward. A part of what keeps healthcare organizations viable and competitive is the ability to manage current operations effectively and efficiently, as well as the ability to properly plan for the organization's future. Although the type and focus of an organization may differ, there is one element of planning that all must include in the governance and leadership process: the budget. There are many items included in the standard budget, which has several approaches for data collection, data compilation, and budget completion. The chosen approach is at the discretion of the organization, but just as with accounting processes and recordkeeping, budgeting methods and inclusions must adhere to established regulatory requirements. This chapter explores the various approaches to budgeting and the practical uses in planning for the shorter-term and longer-term organizational outcomes.

THE BASICS OF BUDGETING

Healthcare organizations utilize detailed internal processes to capture expenses incurred during the provision of services, as well as the resulting generated revenues. The intended goal of this data collection is to ensure the highest quality healthcare at the lowest possible cost. This goal is not just for current operations, but for the future state of the organization as well. A **budget** (also called the **operating budget**) is an organization's estimation of future revenues, expenses, and profits as realized through projected patient visit volume or patient encounters. As with any core accounting and finance process, the budget is designed to cover one specific time frame, usually the fiscal year (FY), and covers all operating areas of the organization. The basic budget is often referred to as the operating budget because it includes routine operating items *and* does not contain larger capital expenditures and projects. The operating budget helps to guide the financial performance of the organization and establish measurable metrics by which to gauge that performance. Revenue, expenses, and profit are analyzed independently before being consolidated into the final budget, creating a revenue budget and expense budget, both driven by volume projections. To begin the organization's operations analysis and prepare for the rest of the **budgeting process**, the organization creates the **statistics budget** containing the projected volume of activities and output. Volume projections are based on an organization's actual performance, with adjustments made to include anticipated increases or decreases to standard operations. This projection then serves as the basis for budgeted revenue, budgeted expenses, and the resulting profit estimations for the upcoming FY.

The **revenue budget** projects the organization's revenues based on the projected patient volume or healthcare product sales. The fee schedule and pricing will be included as stated and/or published for the year; reimbursement will be included as contracted or negotiated (by the insurers) for the year. For example, if there are no anticipated changes in reimbursement rates or pricing, the current rates will be used to estimate the budgeted revenue. On the other hand, if the organization plans to renegotiate its payer contracts, the updated reimbursement rates will be used for the budgeted revenue. The revenue budget also includes estimations on patient mix and payer mix, as directly related to specific payers and reimbursement. The **expense budget** estimates the organization's expenses as they will be incurred during the budgeted time frame. This includes routine, nonrevenue-related expenses such as utilities and office space rental, as well as revenue-related expenses such as direct clinician payroll and medical supplies. As with the revenue budget, the expense budget is prepared based upon the projected volume and anticipated costs as they will be during the upcoming operating period. One of the biggest drivers here is labor costs and the proper allocation of necessary human resources. Permanent staffing is ideal and the most predictable, but with clinical operations there is always the potential for purchased or contracted labor, which drives payroll dollars up. **Profit estimations** are derived from the remaining revenue after all expenses have been covered, in addition to any adjustments required to reach leadership-identified profit targets. Profit estimations may also require changes to the revenue or expense budgets, as they both contribute to the overall profit outcomes for the organization. If the organization has determined a specific target percentage or dollar amount, volume as well as the associated revenues and expenses must be updated to reflect what must be done to meet that target. Working together with the volume projections, the revenue budget, and the expense budget, profit estimations help answer the following questions about the organization's future:

- What healthcare products and services will we produce?
- What will be the volume of the healthcare products and services we produce?
- What resources (human and material) will be needed for production?
- What will be the prices for the items we produce?
- Will we ultimately have enough resources to satisfy the requirements for production inputs and meet the financial goals of the organization?

The budget and the budgeting process quantify all these questions and essentially create an operating plan for the budgeted year. All areas within the organization are included in this budgeted plan, with some areas playing a unique role in the budgeting process. Now that we have reviewed the basics of the budget, let us dig a little deeper into the budgeting process and the various responsibilities required to make it all work.

THE BUDGETING PROCESS: WHO DOES WHAT?

The budgeting process and those involved may vary a bit by organization, but there are key elements that are required for budgeting no matter the organization. All budgets are comprised of subunits or subbudgets, with all of the various pieces comprising the whole. Each subunit or department must determine their department-specific inputs, work processes, and outputs, and, when consolidated with all other subunits, create the budget for the entire organization. The calculation of the budgeted items may differ by department, but the output for consolidation must include volume, revenue (if revenue is generated from the department's activities), and expense. The budgeting process at the micro-level and macro-level includes the steps identified in Figure 11.1.

Figure 11.1
The budgeting process

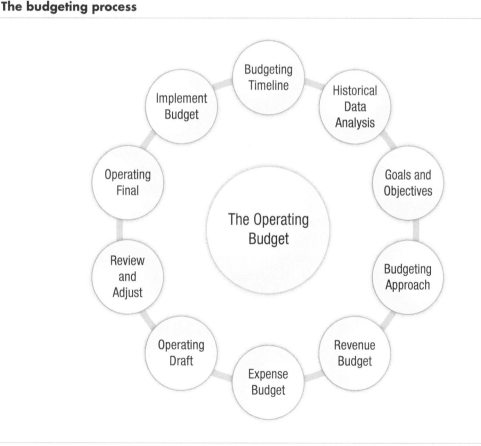

The first step in the budgeting process is to establish the *budgeting timeline*. The timeline is the allotted time frame, beginning to end, that the organization has to complete all budgeting activities. This period could span 3 to 6 months or more, with the time frame determined and communicated by the finance department (or organization-level preparers). Planning, development, and assessment are all included in the timeline, and all happen simultaneously across departments within the organization. The communication of the various due dates is critical to efficient process management, leading up to budget completion and implementation. The timeline and the budgeting process requirements are the responsibility of each department or unit head, or a designated financial representative (in smaller organizations, for example). *Historical data analysis* is the next step in the budgeting process. Each functional area must review their prior actual performance to determine what changes need to be made. This information is typically distributed by the finance department, or responsible for data collection within the organization (an example would be the quality management or the performance measurement and management departments that some organizations have). Historical data is the actual work performed during prior periods that has contributed to the department's revenue, expenses, or both. Changes may reflect the need to meet a specific production or revenue target or to simply optimize their internal processes and overall performance. Review of prior performance, although required for the budgeting process, is part of the longer-term performance management and planning strategies (detailed in Chapter 13). Once the data analysis is completed, the budget changes as well as the desired outputs and outcomes for the upcoming FY are aligned with the broader *goals and objectives*. The department will have its own targets, goals, and objectives, but (ideally) all of the departments will have a part in achieving the organization's overarching goals and objectives. This may include meeting previously established internal benchmarks, meeting the needs of the patients or community served, or improving specific tasks for achievement of goals at the organizational level.

Budgeting Approaches

There are several approaches to budgeting, which are determined by several organizational factors. The governance structure, type of product or service produced, and age of the organization are just a few factors influencing the **budgeting approach** chosen by the leadership team and finance department. Once the budgeting timeline is communicated throughout, the governance structure of the organization determines the flow of information for the rest of the budgeting process. **Top-down budgeting** happens when the executive team informs the functional areas of exactly what their budget will be, based on leadership's assessment of historical data, goals, and objectives. This flow of information leaves very little influence in the hands of the front-line leadership who may be more knowledgeable on the daily operations and directly responsible for outcomes. Top-down budgeting is not as common in larger, more complex healthcare organizations, where there are numerous services offered and populations served. **Bottom-up budgeting** happens when the flow of budgeting information is communicated from front-line leadership to the executive team. This flow of information captures the nuances, special circumstances, and operational challenges that those without direct responsibility would be unaware of. This is the most common method of communication within complex healthcare organizations, as all involved in the process strive to capture all relevant information in the budgeting process. After the flow of information is determined for the budgeting process, the data collection and budget calculation method must be chosen. The calculation method is determined by the function of the department and its contribution to the organization's total financial picture. Departments are identified as cost centers or revenue centers, and their budgeting information is collected and calculated accordingly. A **cost center** incurs expenses and adds to the organization's total liability but does not generate revenue. Cost centers are often unrelated to patient care but are necessary for the operation of the healthcare organization. Departments that fall within the cost center category include strictly administrative departments and those that support patient care without a direct connection to that care. Human resources, finance, housekeeping, and facilities management are examples of cost centers, as they incur expenses (through labor and supplies) but do not generate any kind of revenue. Cost centers will create an expense budget but will not have a revenue budget. A **revenue center** (also called a profit center) incurs expenses, but it also generates revenue for the organization. This revenue can be patient care-related revenue or other operating revenue, like the hospital gift shop, cafeteria, or parking garage. Departments that deliver direct patient care such as those with inpatient admissions or outpatient visits are examples of revenue centers, incurring labor and supply expense as well as generating patient services revenue. These departments will create a revenue budget and an expense budget.

We know that all departments within the healthcare organization participate in the budgeting process, even if not directly responsible for patient care. The function of the department often determines the budgeting approach, as does the way by which the function is performed. There may be several budgeting approaches within a healthcare organization, with all being valid choices for their respective areas. Some of the more common budgeting approaches and general descriptions are shown in Table 11.1.

Table 11.1

COMMON APPROACHES TO BUDGETING

Budgeting Approach	Description
Activity-based budgeting	Assesses individual activities within a work process or department
Fixed budgeting	No adjustments for volume changes, pricing changes, increased expenses, seasonality, and so forth
Flexible budgeting	Adjusts for changes in volume, pricing, expenses, seasonality, and so forth
Incremental (baseline) budgeting	Adjusts the budget from a prior period by a specific amount or percentage
Program budgeting	Assesses the inputs, outputs, and outcomes of an entire program, capturing data across departments
Rolling (forecast) budgeting	Reevaluates and adjusts the budgeted figures quarterly
Service-line budgeting	Analyzes service-line level data for workflow analysis
Zero-based budgeting	Requires justification for all budgeted items, without the basis of historical data

Activity-based budgeting is a very detailed approach to budgeting, which includes the analysis and costing of individual activities. This approach is most prevalent in departments that have multiple methods of performing a specific task or process. A phlebotomy laboratory is an example of such a department that has several ways of performing "blood work" or phlebotomy screenings. Screenings or tests performed can include glucose testing, enzyme testing, or cholesterol testing, with each type of screening requiring different steps in the testing process. This ties directly into the activity-based costing method as covered in Chapter 8 of this text. Revisiting the Lighthouse Medical example used to illustrate activity-based costing, the cost estimates for CT and MRI imaging were calculated for five activities (see Boxes 8.4a–c). For activity-based budgeting, each of the five activities would first be analyzed individually, with the historical data for each serving as the foundation for the budgeted projections. Then, the budgeted amounts for the individual activities would be totaled for each type of imaging.

The **fixed budgeting** approach is "static," meaning there is no change or adjustment to the established budgeted figure. This is particularly problematic in a sector such as healthcare that must be flexible enough to adapt to changes in patient volume and industry regulations. The rigidness of the fixed budgeting approach has proven to be quite unrealistic in many healthcare organizations, as this approach translates to inevitable cost overruns and unrecognized revenue. The **flexible budgeting** approach is just the opposite of the fixed budgeting approach, as it considers changes to patient volume, pricing, and expense updates, as well as seasonality. This approach to budgeting allows the organization to adjust operations based on expected conditions, increased patient volume (requiring additional staffing and associated labor expense), or updated reimbursement legislation (requiring changes to the chargemaster and subsequent payer reimbursement).

EXHIBIT 11.1. Fixed Budget and Flexible Budget

Department	Previous FY Actuals (3yr Avg)	Current Budget (Fixed)	Current Budget (Flexible)
Inpatient surgery	$17,500,000	$17,500,000	$19,250,000
Outpatient surgery	$10,150,500	$10,150,500	$11,165,550
Ancillary services	$6,550,175	$6,550,175	$7,205,193
	$34,200,675	$34,200,675	$37,620,743

If a healthcare organization analyzes its historical data for the past 3 years and anticipates a 10% increase, the budget can be prepared as fixed or flexible. As shown in Exhibit 11.1, the fixed budget for inpatient surgery, outpatient surgery, and ancillary services uses the previous 3 years' average, with no adjustment to anticipated changes in operations. The flexible budget, however, includes the 10% increase in its budget projections. The decision to exclude the anticipated change could have multiple implications impacting the budget and longer-term performance:

- If this were revenue dollars, the exclusion of the 10% would result in understated revenue, which could mean missed funding opportunities for resources or projects.

- If this were expense dollars, the exclusion of the 10% would result in cost overruns, which could mean a negative budgeting impact or unnecessary cost control measures.

- If this were a volume estimate instead of dollars, the exclusion of the 10% would result in understated revenues and expenses, which could mean unrecognized revenue, inadequate staffing, or materials/supply shortage possibly limiting care.

The **incremental budgeting** approach, although not as restrictive as fixed budgeting, tends to limit the amount of financial flexibility of the healthcare organization. With the incremental approach, the previous year's budget is used as the foundation or baseline and is then increased by a specific dollar amount or percentage. The increase could be an amount implemented to reach a specific target, to reflect market pricing, or to adjust for inflation. The increase is applied to the baseline once, with no further adjustment for volume or other operational changes. So, if leadership determines that a 7% increase from actual performance is to be applied, it would be applied once with no additional increases or decreases in response to actual performance. Using the dollar amounts shown in Exhibit 11.1 as a baseline, we would then increase the actuals for each department by 7%, making the budgeted amounts for inpatient surgery, outpatient surgery, and ancillary services $18,725,000, $10,861,035 and $7,008,687, respectively. The results with this type of budgeting are like the fixed budgeting results, with expense overruns and unrecognized revenue.

Rolling budgeting, or the rolling forecast, begins with the basic flexible budgeting approach, but is routinely updated as changes are considered. For example, if the flexible budget includes an anticipated increase to department revenues in the second quarter of the FY and that increase in revenue is different than what was budgeted, the rolling budget will make the adjustment at the end of the first quarter, essentially updating the projections for the future quarters. The rolling budget is typically updated quarterly but can be updated monthly, and always extends out to include projections for a full year; this allows the healthcare organization maximum flexibility when calculating its budget.

EXHIBIT 11.2. Rolling Budget

Department	(Original) Annual Budget				Annual
	Quarter 1	Quarter 2	Quarter 3	Quarter 4	Total
General inpatient	$15,375,891	$16,144,686	$16,951,920	$17,799,516	$66,272,013
Intensive care inpatient	$19,425,850	$20,397,143	$21,417,000	$22,487,850	$83,727,843
Emergency department	$17,295,650	$18,160,433	$19,068,454	$20,021,877	$74,546,414
	$52,097,391	$54,702,262	$57,437,374	$60,309,243	$224,546,270

Department	Q1 Actuals	(Rolling) Annual Budget				Annual
		Quarter 1	Quarter 2	Quarter 3	Quarter 4	Total
General inpatient	$16,512,150	$17,337,758	$18,204,645	$19,114,878	$20,070,622	$74,727,903
Intensive care inpatient	$18,391,554	$19,311,132	$20,276,688	$21,290,523	$22,355,049	$83,233,392
Emergency department	$17,831,953	$18,723,551	$19,659,728	$20,642,715	$21,674,850	$80,700,844
	$52,735,657	$55,372,441	$58,141,061	$61,048,116	$64,100,521	$238,662,139

Using Exhibit 11.2 as an example, the original annual budget shown at the top, reflects an estimated first quarter amount for three departments. The remaining three quarters of the budgeted year increase by 5% each quarter with an estimated total of $224,546,270 for the entire year. At the end of the first quarter, the organization's actual performance is different from the initial budget, so the actual figures are entered into the first quarter, with a rolling four-quarter budget being based on the actual figures instead of an estimate.

The **service-line budgeting** approach is a unique type of analysis that captures data based on the actual service line and workflow of the care provided. This approach captures revenues and expenses generated for a healthcare service across all departments that contribute to the delivery of that care. The service line analyzed is usually tied to a larger organizational initiative, with data capture to include all resources, supplies, and outcomes related to the service line. An example of this could start with a healthcare organization's initiative to decrease length of stay for routine (lower acuity) orthopedic surgical procedures or to possibly increase efficient use of skilled nursing hours. In this situation, the organization would track incurred nursing hours and labor expenses across the various departments to analyze trends and determine an accurate budget allocation (see Exhibit 11.3). This service-line view reflects the entire range of nursing services, allowing the organization to determine what the future needs would be to meet the goal of the estimated patient volume. Similar to the service-line approach is **program budgeting**, which addresses the revenue and expense estimates of an entire program and its associated initiatives. All service lines are considered in this type of budgeting and analysis to ensure the capture of all related inputs and outcomes. Program budgeting allows an organization's leadership to rank or score programs according to strategic importance, patient needs and outcomes, financial impact, or overall value. As we see in Exhibit 11.3, the nursing hours from the service-line budget are further detailed by initiative in the ambulatory center program budget. The two sample budgets show how the nursing hours budgeted for the ambulatory center are allocated to its various initiatives and projects. This example includes only the nursing labor expense portion, but the standard service-line and program budgets would likely include other required items such as revenue and income sources (patient services revenue and other operating revenue like cafeteria or gift shop); other labor expenses (other clinicians or contracted agency labor, housekeeping services, etc.); and materials, medical supplies, and other routine expenditures (space leasing, utilities, marketing, etc.).

EXHIBIT 11.3. Service-Line Budget and Program Budget

Nursing Unit	Previous Labor Hours (3yr Avg)	Previous Labor Expense (3yr Avg)	Budgeted Labor Hours	Budgeted Labor Expense
Medical units	80,000	$5,200,000	84,000	$5,460,000
Surgical units	75,500	$5,662,500	79,275	$5,945,625
Ambulatory center	62,350	$4,052,750	65,468	$4,255,388
Emergency department	91,495	$8,234,550	96,070	$8,646,278
	309,345	$23,149,800	324,813	$24,307,291

Ambulatory Center Initiatives	Previous Labor Hours (3yr Avg)	Previous Labor Expense (3yr Avg)	Budgeted Labor Hours	Budgeted Labor Expense
Ambulatory surgery	24,940	$1,621,100	26,187	$1,702,155
Dialysis center	12,470	$810,550	13,094	$851,078
Mobile diabetes clinic	6,235	$405,275	6,547	$425,539
Urgent care	18,705	$1,215,825	19,640	$1,276,616
	62,350	$4,052,750	65,468	$4,255,388

Zero-based budgeting is a budgeting approach that requires current justification for all budgeted items. This approach does not rely on prior performance, but instead requires the "ground-up" calculation for all expenses and revenues starting from zero. Workload calculations such as those explored in Chapter 8 often come into play with this approach, which can be overwhelming to do for all items or processes in a large healthcare organization. Each department, project, or function in the zero-based budgeting process would have to estimate the number of full-time equivalents, hours, pay rates, workload volumes, and so forth, as original calculations for budget inclusion. For this reason, zero-based budgeting is usually done in smaller organizations or new organizations (or service lines) with no prior performance history.

Budget Drafts, Reviews, and Adjustments

As stated in the previous section, each department is identified as a cost center or revenue center, which ultimately determines the types of budgets they will produce. The budgets are prepared in draft form, as further review and adjustments are still to be made. Revenue budgets project income for the upcoming FY and are based on volume estimates as well as anticipated payer agreements. Increases or decreases to patient volume and payer reimbursement contracts directly impact the projected revenue for a department and organization. These updates must be included in the drafted revenue budget before final review and approval occurs. Similarly, expense budgets are based on volume estimates but do not include revenue of any kind. Instead, expense budgets use the anticipated volume to estimate associated labor expense as well as supply expense (if the department is patient-driven) or the costs incurred by the department for performing administrative functions for the organization (human resources, finance, housekeeping, etc.). The draft operating budget includes the revenue draft and the expense draft, and reflects the remaining profit. This is done at the department level and then consolidated with all other departments to create the organization-level or total draft budget. Senior leadership reviews the draft operating budget and makes recommendations on adjustments. The adjustments could be broader changes that are applied across the organization, or they could be specific changes to a department's submission. An example of a broad adjustment is a required reduction in spending. If leadership has knowledge of a pending reimbursement or regulation change that may impact revenue, they may suggest an overall reduction in expenses if an increase in revenue isn't possible to absorb the change. Department-specific adjustments could be an adjustment to increase volume and associated revenue, or to minimize agency-provided staffing expenses. The review and adjustment phase happens in several iterations and management and senior leadership discuss the department's priorities, capacity, capabilities, and budgetary needs. When the inclusions of the budget have been decided, the final version of the budget is implemented with the start of the new FY.

Final Operating Budget and Implementation

Once approved, implementation of the final operating budget requires the entry of the budgeted figures and parameters into the accounting and finance information systems. All resources are then allocated as planned to enable departments to meet their budgeted targets. Resources include funding for the hiring of additional personnel, funding for material items, and space allocation or expansions as agreed upon in the operating budget. The budgeted revenues, expenses, and anticipated profit become the benchmarks for the FY's performance, with each department reviewing their actual performance monthly. For continuing processes that were already implemented and are included in prior operations, the budget implementation is somewhat seamless, with the only major change being the revised volume or financial targets. For newly budgeted items, the implementation may have begun several months ago, in preparation for the beginning of the new FY.

Budget Considerations and Challenges

A well-planned budgeting process is not without concerns or challenges, either during budget creation or implementation. There will always be situations over which we have no control, and those unprecedented situations will often impact the healthcare organization's financial situation. An example of this is the coronavirus pandemic, which impacted nations around the world. With surging rates of illness and expensive treatment options, healthcare organizations could not budget for the number of admissions, or the resources needed to care for those infected with the virus. The need for healthcare was immediate and ultimately required increased staffing (permanent employees as well as agency staffing), supplies, and technology. Effective medications were still being created and tested, and equipment such as ventilators were in short supply. Federal relief was distributed to help healthcare facilities maintain high levels of emergency care, which had essentially utilized the funding originally budgeted for routine care and operations. Virtual technologies became a mainstay during the pandemic, and although this treatment approach was successful in minimizing nonemergent visits to healthcare facilities, reimbursement is still inconsistent. Most insurers reimbursed providers at a rate of 100% for virtual office visits during the pandemic, as providers kept in-person visits reserved for COVID patients. Now, in the coronavirus endemic phase, some payers are attempting to pay for telemedicine sparingly, as necessary only for patients with mobility or access to care issues. Reimbursement for telemedicine remains widely debated, particularly with regard to mental health benefits and provider availability.

Increased demand requires not only additional human resources but additional material resources as well. Supply chain (covered in Chapter 15) delays can mean limiting the availability of healthcare services or paying drastically inflated prices to secure the items needed for care. Most healthcare organizations adjust their pricing annually to account for changes in pricing or labor rates, based on known factors or influences. Sudden shortages in supplies and increased pricing may not be foreseen and will therefore be unaccounted for in the current budget, causing cost overruns and other budgeting challenges. Mergers and acquisitions (referred to as M&As, covered in Appendix A) may also cause issues with budgeting, although these processes are planned and usually have detailed schedules for implementation. The challenge lies in the combination of multiple entities, whose financial processes may not perfectly align. Combining the historical data and budget information from different systems can be daunting if doing so while maintaining current operations. Payment model changes and healthcare financial legislation can directly impact the budgeting process if the changes are to be implemented during the current FY. If the financial changes were not communicated prior to the beginning of the FY and have not been incorporated into the budget, healthcare organizations would be required to absorb any cost increases, reimbursement shortfalls, or process changes without proper preparation.

CHAPTER SUMMARY

The operating budget is an important facet of organizational management in both the short term and long term. Participating in the annual budget preparation process helps leadership to communicate the purpose of the organization, its priorities, and key initiatives, as well as the path the organization will take to achieve them. At the department level, budget information helps to identify the core processes that are in place to create the desired output, whether the output is actually providing patient care (healthcare visits) or manufacturing a healthcare good (supplies, equipment, etc.). It helps employees to see the scope of work beyond their individual contribution to the process. It also helps everyone involved to see how revenues and expenses are generated, as well as how their department fits into the larger organization. The budgeting process is meticulously scheduled, with milestones and deliverables along the timeline, designed to be prepared, reviewed, and approved in advance of the FY start. Once implemented, performance can be measured using the budgeted volumes and dollars as standards, with additional variance analysis calculated at specific points throughout the year. Performance measurement, performance management, and variance analysis are covered in Chapter 13.

KEY TERMS FOR REVIEW

activity-based budgeting	fixed budgeting	revenue center
bottom-up budgeting	flexible budgeting	rolling budgeting
budget	incremental budgeting	service-line budgeting
budgeting approach	operating budget	statistics budget
budgeting process	profit estimations	top-down budgeting
cost center	program budgeting	zero-based budgeting
expense budget	revenue budget	

DISCUSSION QUESTIONS

1. Define the revenue budget and the expense budget. How do these relate to the operating budget?
2. Outline the steps in the budgeting process. Is there one step that drives everything else in the process? Explain your answer.
3. What are the key differences between the top-down and bottom-up budgeting information streams?
4. Discuss the concepts of revenue center and cost center. Can a department be considered both?
5. List and define the common approaches to budgeting. Does one approach appear to be better than the others?
6. Identify the differences between fixed budgeting and flexible budgeting. Will the results from these two approaches be the same?
7. Discuss at least three considerations or challenges that may impact the budgeting process in the healthcare sector.

PRACTICE PROBLEMS

Answers to this chapter's Practice Problems are available via Springer Publishing Connect™ by following the instructions on the opening page of this book and accessing Answers to Practice Problems on the Table of Contents.

1. If an organization has its operating budget as shown in Exhibit 11.4, with Quarter 2 through Quarter 4 increasing by 3% each (based on Quarter 1), construct a rolling budget, recalculating the four quarters based on the actual performance of inpatient services ($15,981,575), outpatient services ($18,943,649), and emergency department ($18,153,598).
2. Using the rolling budget annual total calculated for Problem 1 (based on Exhibit 11.4; excludes the actuals), construct an incremental budget using 7% as the inflation factor.

3. Using the data provided in Exhibit 11.4, calculate the contribution to the quarterly totals and the annual total made by each of the three departments.

EXHIBIT 11.4. Operating Budget (for Rolling Budget Calculation)

Department	Annual Budget				Annual
	Quarter 1	Quarter 2	Quarter 3	Quarter 4	Total
Inpatient services	$15,375,891	$15,837,168	$16,312,283	$16,801,651	$64,326,993
Outpatient services	$19,425,850	$20,008,626	$20,608,884	$21,227,151	$81,270,511
Emergency department	$17,295,650	$17,814,520	$18,348,955	$18,899,424	$72,358,549
	$52,097,391	$53,660,314	$55,270,122	$56,928,226	$217,956,053

4. The data provided in Exhibit 11.5 represents the statistics (volume) budget for the upcoming FY. Using this data, calculate the revenue budget for the department if expected revenue per case is $2,475.00 (all case types).

5. The data provided in Exhibit 11.5 represents the statistics (volume) budget for the upcoming FY. Using this data, calculate the expense budget for the department if expected expense per case is $1,969.00 (all case types).

6. Use the results from the revenue budget (Problem 4; based on Exhibit 11.5) and the expense budget (Problem 5; based on Exhibit 11.5) to construct a profit (net income) budget.

7. Using the annual total results from the profit budget (Problem 6; Exhibit 11.5), calculate the percentage contribution to the total profit, made by each of the three departments.

EXHIBIT 11.5. Statistical Budget Data

Surgical Services

Statistical Budget Data

Surgery Description	July	August	September	October	November	December	January	February	March	April	May	June	Annual Total
						Monthly Budgeted Volume						
Cardiac surgery	120	122	125	127	124	120	116	113	118	124	131	137	1,477
Neurological surgery	105	107	109	111	108	105	102	99	104	109	114	120	1,293
Orthopaedic surgery	225	230	234	239	232	225	218	211	222	233	245	257	2,771
Vascular surgery	160	163	166	170	165	160	155	150	158	166	174	183	1,970
Total surgeries	**610**	**622**	**634**	**647**	**629**	**610**	**591**	**573**	**602**	**632**	**664**	**697**	**7,511**

CHAPTER 11 CASE: UNDERSTANDING THE BUDGETING PROCESS

Budget preparation for Pantheon Health System is about to begin, and as the budget director you are responsible for the preliminary calculations at the organizational level. You have received draft budgets from several departments, and you must now create the final budgets using various budgeting approaches. Senior leadership has outlined the required assumptions and changes and will review the different budgets to determine the ideal path forward for the organization. (The assumptions will help you make changes to the draft figures as you construct the various budgets.) You have created the following draft statistics budget (Exhibit 11.6), as well as revenues, expenses, and profit budgets (Exhibit 11.7) to use as the basis for all assumptions. The drafts have been created with the revenue, expense, and profit budgets calculated using the statistics and per case rates. Revenue per case and expense per case used in these initial calculations are shown in Table 11.2. These case rates are used as a conversion factor, to translate case volumes (statistics) into budget dollars.

1. In the current draft budget, which service line currently contributes the most to total profit?

2. Flexible budget: Adjust the statistics budget to include an additional 5% monthly. Note the impacts on the revenue, expense, and profit budgets.

3. Incremental budget: The previous year's actuals resulted in an overall increase of 5% when compared to the budgeted annual figures. Increase the statistics annual totals by 5% for each department (this can be spread across the months for even distribution).

4. Reconstruct the provided budgets into quarterly formats with an annual total.

5. Rolling budget: Construct a rolling budget based on Quarter 1 statistics actuals of medical inpatient—1,450 cases; surgical inpatient—1,800 cases; ambulatory services—4,600 cases; urgent care services—12,100 cases.

6. With the changes implemented for the rolling budget, what is the resulting increase or decrease in profit?

7. If the revenue per case increased by 5% for inpatient services only, what would be the resulting change to revenue and profit? Assume no changes in original draft statistics figures.

8. If leadership set a goal of 3% reduction in expense per case for outpatient services only, what would be the resulting change to expense and profit? Assume no changes in original draft statistics figures.

9. Service-line budget: Leadership has decided to make changes to the surgical inpatient service line for the upcoming FY. For this service only: (a) increase the statistics volume by 10% for Quarter 2 and Quarter 4; (b) renegotiate contracts to increase revenue from the original $2,625 per case to a new rate of $2,700 per case; and (c) decrease expense per case from the original $2,050 per case to $1,900 per case. What is the impact to the service line's final revenue, expenses, and profit?

10. If leadership has set the goal of a final annual profit margin increase of 25% across all services, how might this be accomplished?

EXHIBIT 11.6. Pantheon Health System Statistics Budget

Service Description		July	August	September	October	November	December	January	February	March	April	May	June	Annual Total
	Monthly Budgeted Volume													
Medical inpatient		450	459	468	478	463	449	436	423	444	466	489	514	5,539
Surgical inpatient		600	612	624	637	618	599	581	564	592	621	653	685	7,386
Ambulatory services (outpt)		1,500	1,530	1,561	1,592	1,544	1,498	1,453	1,409	1,480	1,554	1,631	1,713	18,465
Urgent care services (outpt)		3,850	3,927	4,006	4,086	3,963	3,844	3,729	3,617	3,798	3,988	4,187	4,396	47,391
Total volume estimate		**6,400**	**6,528**	**6,659**	**6,793**	**6,588**	**6,390**	**6,199**	**6,013**	**6,314**	**6,629**	**6,960**	**7,308**	**78,781**

EXHIBIT 11.7. Pantheon Health System Revenues, Expenses, and Profit Budgets

Monthly Budgeted Revenue

Service Description	July	August	September	October	November	December	January	February	March	April	May	June	Annual Total
Medical inpatient	$1,113,750	$1,136,025	$1,158,746	$1,181,920	$1,146,463	$1,112,069	$1,078,707	$1,046,346	$1,098,663	$1,153,596	$1,211,276	$1,271,840	13,709,401
Surgical inpatient	$1,575,000	$1,606,500	$1,638,630	$1,671,403	$1,621,261	$1,572,623	$1,525,444	$1,479,681	$1,553,665	$1,631,348	$1,712,915	$1,798,561	19,387,030
Ambulatory services (outpt)	$412,500	$420,750	$429,165	$437,748	$424,616	$411,877	$399,521	$387,535	$406,912	$427,258	$448,621	$471,052	5,077,555
Urgent care services (outpt)	$481,250	$490,875	$500,693	$510,706	$495,385	$480,524	$466,108	$452,125	$474,731	$498,467	$523,391	$549,560	5,923,815
Total revenues	$3,582,500	$3,654,150	$3,727,234	$3,801,777	$3,687,725	$3,577,093	$3,469,780	$3,365,687	$3,533,971	$3,710,669	$3,896,203	$4,091,013	44,097,802

Monthly Budgeted Expenses

Service Description	July	August	September	October	November	December	January	February	March	April	May	June	Annual Total
Medical inpatient	$886,050	$903,771	$921,846	$940,283	$912,075	$884,713	$858,171	$832,426	$874,047	$917,750	$963,637	$1,011,819	10,906,588
Surgical inpatient	$1,230,000	$1,254,600	$1,279,692	$1,305,286	$1,266,127	$1,228,143	$1,191,299	$1,155,560	$1,213,338	$1,274,005	$1,337,705	$1,404,591	15,140,346
Ambulatory services (outpt)	$165,000	$168,300	$171,666	$175,099	$169,846	$164,751	$159,808	$155,014	$162,765	$170,903	$179,448	$188,421	2,031,021
Urgent care services (outpt)	$288,750	$294,525	$300,416	$306,424	$297,231	$288,314	$279,665	$271,275	$284,839	$299,080	$314,034	$329,736	3,554,289
Total expenses	$2,569,800	$2,621,196	$2,673,620	$2,727,092	$2,645,279	$2,565,921	$2,488,943	$2,414,275	$2,534,989	$2,661,738	$2,794,824	$2,934,567	$31,632,244

Monthly Budgeted Profit

Service Description	July	August	September	October	November	December	January	February	March	April	May	June	Annual Total
Medical inpatient	$227,700	$232,254	$236,899	$241,637	$234,388	$227,356	$220,536	$213,920	$224,616	$235,846	$247,639	$260,021	$2,802,812
Surgical inpatient	$345,000	$351,900	$358,938	$366,117	$355,133	$344,479	$334,145	$324,121	$340,327	$357,343	$375,210	$393,971	$4,246,684
Ambulatory services (outpt)	$247,500	$252,450	$257,499	$262,649	$254,770	$247,126	$239,713	$232,521	$244,147	$256,355	$269,172	$282,631	$3,046,533
Urgent care services (outpt)	$192,500	$196,350	$200,277	$204,283	$198,154	$192,209	$186,443	$180,850	$189,892	$199,387	$209,356	$219,824	$2,369,525
Total profit	$1,012,700	$1,032,954	$1,053,613	$1,074,686	$1,042,445	$1,011,170	$980,837	$951,412	$998,982	$1,048,931	$1,101,377	$1,156,447	$12,465,554

Table 11.2

PER CASE RATES

Service Description	Revenue Per Case	Expense Per Case
Medical inpatient	$2,475	$1,969
Surgical inpatient	$2,625	$2,050
Ambulatory services (outpt)	$275	$110
Urgent care services (outpt)	$125	$75

HEALTHCARE FINANCE COURSE PROJECT: CONSOLIDATION FOR PHASE II

The second phase of the course project is the consolidation phase. For consolidation, students will combine the zero-based SurgiFlex calculations from Phase I with the rest of the healthcare organization as presented in Phase II. The phase includes the following worksheets/calculations:

- Worksheet #7: Consolidated Operating/Utilization Data (Case Volumes)
- Worksheet #8: Consolidated Salary and Wage Calculations
- Worksheet #9: Consolidated Revenue Calculations
- Worksheet #10: Consolidated Nonsalary Expense Calculations
- Worksheet #11: Master Supply List

Review the "Course Project: Phase II" section of Chapter 16. All other worksheets in the second phase are to be created by the student, using the data provided for the first month of each sheet. All worksheets are to be connected (for consolidation) to the SurgiFlex utilization data (Worksheet #1), as well as other relevant worksheet calculations in Phase I. Be sure to review the Microsoft Excel® Reference Guide located in the Appendices as needed.

CHAPTER 12

The Capital Budget, Investments, and Financing Decisions

OBJECTIVES

1. Understand the differences between the capital budget and the operating budget.
2. Define and illustrate the time value of money (TVM) concepts.
3. Describe the overall capital project analysis process.
4. Perform the various calculations for a capital project financial assessment.

INTRODUCTION

There are many facets to managing a healthcare organization's financial performance, which includes routine revenues and expenses, as well as the larger items that impact the ability to provide healthcare services. These high-dollar or capital items affect several departments or functional areas within the organization, often requiring interdisciplinary analysis of both the current state without the project and future state with the project. In general, the organization and the population served must benefit from the purchase or implementation of the capital project, but due to funding restraints, the decision must be made as to what projects will be funded. This chapter explores the concept of capital budgeting and discusses the process by which items are proposed, defended, and ultimately funded. We will examine calculations relative to assessing the current and **future values** (FVs) of capital projects, as well as the potential impacts on the bottom line.

THE CAPITAL BUDGET

The **capital budget** is the planned funding of new, nonoperating expenditures and investments. These are not included in the operating budget and are supported by separate sources of funding. Capital budgeting is an important part of the healthcare organization's budgeting and financial control process, capturing and analyzing major expenses and purchases. Like the operating budget, the capital budget is prepared annually and is routinely reviewed for performance. The dollar threshold for what qualifies as capital varies by organization; however, in most cases, large expenses such as buildings, land, vehicles, equipment, organization-wide systems, or other high-dollar items are considered capital. The life span of these items must be greater than

1 year and the justification for the item must be presented. The data included in the proposal must also include any historical data and potential benefits that support the funding and implementation of the project. Departments seeking capital funding will often outline internal resources and available alternatives in the proposal to give decision makers a clear picture of what would be required for implementation. All of this information is collected and analyzed by leadership (or others responsible for funding decisions) to determine which capital projects will ultimately receive funding. The capital budgeting process has a review and implementation timeline independent of the operating budget, and includes the stages reflected in Figure 12.1.

Figure 12.1

The capital budgeting process

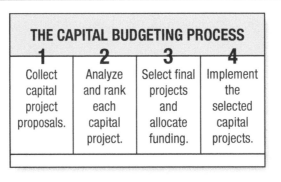

Capital project proposals can be submitted by any department within the healthcare organization that has a need for large project funding. Proposal preparation involves all departments or functions that would benefit from or utilize the newly implemented items. When capturing costs and benefits, the proposals must include all processes impacted by the new project—project implementation timeline, human and material resources, space and location requirements, ongoing upkeep, and maintenance. When all of the information has been compiled and submitted for consideration, the proposals are analyzed and ranked by the decision makers. Capital project analysis, as covered in the remaining sections of this chapter, is a detailed process that examines the shorter- and longer-term impacts of the project, while considering both financial and nonfinancial criteria. Initial investment amount, cashflows, and revenues are assessed for the financial analysis, while stakeholders' needs and benefits are reviewed for the nonfinancial criteria. Projects with the highest ranking or those that are the most feasible are selected and approved for funding and implementation. The proposal inclusions provide benchmarks and metrics for project performance measurement, with routine review and analysis taking place just as with the items included in the operating budget. Performance measurement and management, as well as variance analysis, are covered in Chapter 13.

CAPITAL PROJECT ANALYSIS

Capital project analysis is the evaluation process that examines the feasibility and profitability of long-term projects. Every project submitted for capital budget approval is reviewed to ensure the soundness of the investment decision. Many healthcare organizations, especially those that may be not-for-profit, do not have endless resources for capital projects, and must therefore be selective of the project's funding. **Capital rationing** is the concept of having more capital projects than available capital funding, which results in an evaluation and selection process. Project evaluation can include several types of financial analyses and other metrics, with each designed to indicate a different facet of potential risk and performance. **Risks** are potentially negative impacts to the organization, affecting those involved in the capital project or the larger organization. Ideally, risks are mitigated and avoided once identified, with plans put in place for those risks that are unavoidable.

Capital Project Time Frame Assessment

At the onset of the analysis, the decision makers determine the project type, the project time frame, and the project scope as listed in Table 12.1, which may ultimately help determine the order in which projects are reviewed and approved.

Table 12.1

CAPITAL PROJECT TIME FRAME AND SCOPE

Project Type	Project Time Frame	Project Scope
Replacement	Immediate to short term	Required replacement of existing infrastructure or equipment; outdated technology or inoperable equipment
	Short term to medium term	The infrastructure or equipment is functional but is nearing the end of the product life cycle or the next generation is available
Expansion	Short term to medium term	Expansion of current services as required by legislation, licensure, or medical regulations
	Medium term to long term	Expansion of current services to increase market share or competitiveness
Health and environmental	Immediate to short term	Required mediation of a health concern for stakeholders (patients, employees, etc.) or functionality of equipment (such as product recalls)
	Short term to medium term	Upgrades to existing processes, systems, and equipment because the next generation is available

Although exact parameters may vary by organization, capital project time frames are typically defined as:

- immediate to short term: 0 years to 2 years
- short term to medium term: 2 years to 5 years
- medium term to long term: 5 years to 10 years

For replacement projects, the organization must have a clear knowledge of when the replacement must take place. If the infrastructure, system, or equipment must be operational for patient care or other daily operating functions, then the replacement must be funded in the immediate to short-term time frame. An example of this may be inoperable imaging or laboratory equipment. These are essential for patient care and must be available at all times. Important key items such as these will usually receive a higher project ranking and higher likelihood of funding. Replacement projects that are still operational but aging would be funded in the short-term to medium-term time frame. Items of this project type are not hindering daily operations but may be showing signs of aging or requiring increased maintenance costs. Major systems, like Enterprise Resource Planning (ERP) software systems that connect all facets of the organization, or heating, ventilation, and cooling (HVAC) systems for all of the organization's buildings, are examples of projects that show signs of aging, with replacement of these large and expensive initiatives phased in over the medium term.

For expansion projects, the time frames are a bit more flexible depending on the reason for the requested expansion. Required expansions would be projects mandated by medical or federal legislation. An example of this would be the changes implemented by the Patient Protection and Affordable Care Act (PPACA), which impacted several key processes in the healthcare sector. When the PPACA legislation was passed in 2010, one of the requirements for states electing to expand Medicaid services was to create an online "marketplace" or exchange, where potential beneficiaries could enroll in the various plans. This change required information technology (IT) teams and payers working together to design new integrative, easily accessed platforms for Medicaid services. Examples of clinical treatment changes implemented by the PPACA would be the free annual wellness visits for Medicare patients and women's wellness cancer screenings. With this change, clinicians had to expand their visit capacity to accommodate the increased volume, and payers had to adjust their systems to absorb the entire cost for the visits. Implementation deadlines were given, so organizations were able to plan the required changes in the short-term to medium-term time frame. Optional expansions are capital projects that can be implemented at any time, due to the noncritical nature of the project. If increased market share and competitiveness are the underlying reasons for the expansion, the projects can be developed and implemented over the medium-term to long-term time frame. These projects often impact routine operations at multiple levels, as well as the organization's overall financial position, and will ideally be present for the entire life of the organization.

Health and environmental projects are assessed and ranked in accordance with the severity of issue or scope of impact. For projects that directly impact the safety of patient or employees, a higher project ranking and likelihood of funding would be assigned. An example of this would be issues with a hospital's water supply or air filtration system. This poses an immediate health concern for everyone and would need priority attention in the immediate to short-term time frame. Health and environmental system upgrades due to aging of equipment or the availability of next generation systems may not require immediate attention if they are still functioning properly. However, due to the importance of these systems in the healthcare sector, they would still be addressed in the short-term to medium-term time frame. After the initial project timeline assessment, the capital projects' financial assessment begins, which provides decision makers with investment projections such as cashflows and long-term profitability.

Financial and Economic Analysis of Capital Projects

The financial assessment of each project serves to further organize the list of prospective capital projects by examining the cashflows and profitability of each. In this portion of project analysis, each capital project proposal submitted for consideration must include:

- an estimation of cash inflows and outflows,
- a risk assessment,

 an estimated cost of capital, and

 a complete financial assessment.

To assess these items, several factors are considered such as initial cost incurred, cash outflows, and cash inflows, as well as items outside of the organization's control like interest rates and inflation. **Cashflow** is the movement of cash as specifically related to the implementation and ongoing activities of a project. Cash **outflows** represent money leaving the organization, and cash **inflows** represent money coming into the organization. An example of a cash outflow would be the initial purchase price of equipment for a project or a down payment for an office space lease agreement. An example of a cash inflow would be a large grant or donation used to fund a project or routine revenues received during the life span of a project. Ideally, a project's cash inflows are greater than its cash outflows, meaning the return is greater than the investment. When assessing cashflows, an important question answered by the estimate is the length of time it will take to recover the amount of the initial investment. This **payback period** is typically represented in years and is calculated using the initial cash outflows and the estimated cash inflows (see Box 12.1).

BOX 12.1

Payback Period Formula

Payback Period = Investment Costs ÷ Annual Cashflow

To illustrate the payback calculation, consider the following scenario: A hospital intends to build a new, fully automated parking garage, offering parking options for patients, visitors, and the guests of the partners renting space on site. The parking garage will have a life span of approximately 20 years, and leadership would like to see if it's worth the initial investment. Construction costs will total $200,000 and annual revenues are estimated to be $50,000 per year. We calculate the payback period as: $200,000 ÷ $50,000 = 4 years. In this example, the hospital will recover its initial investment in 4 years. After the payback period, there are 16 years left in the life span of the garage with $50,000 of annual revenue, which means $800,000 of income for this project. Although this example includes only an initial investment, projects may have additional costs incurred such as repairs, maintenance, or other annual fees. These cash outflows would all be included in the investment costs used as the numerator in the payback period calculation, which would increase the number of years for payback.

Project cashflows are also used for the overall financial valuation of capital projects across its expected life span. Cashflows and the value of money are impacted by interest rates throughout the economy, and project cashflows are no different. The **time value of money** (TVM) concept states that money today is more valuable than the same amount of money in the future. TVM calculations capture all estimated cashflows for the life of the capital project, as influenced by interest. These calculations help answer the question of whether or not the capital project is worth the investment. TVM looks at the FV of current cashflows as well as the **present value** (PV) of anticipated cashflows occurring later in the project's life span. FV cashflow analysis is called compounding, as it compounds the cashflows over time. Our formula for FV can be represented as:

$FV = PV \times (1 + r)^n$, where:

PV = present value, initial investment, or cashflow;

r = interest rate; and

n = number of periods, time frame for the investment; exponential power.

These elements are all needed to perform the FV calculation (and the PV calculation). To illustrate the FV calculation, let's examine a basic example using the information given in Exhibit 12.1.

EXHIBIT 12.1. Future Value Calculation

Calculate the FV of $48,500 invested at a rate of 9% for 12 years.

$$FV = PV \times (1+r)^n$$

$$FV = \$48,500 \times (1 + .09)^{12}$$

$$FV = \$48,500 \times (1.09)^{12}$$

$$FV = \$48,500 \times 2.8127$$

$$FV = \$136,415.95$$

When calculating the FV, the interest rate is represented in decimal form for ease of calculation. This example states that the $48,500 will be worth approximately $136,416 (rounded) in 12 years. (It should also be noted that a common error is multiplying (1 + interest rate) by 12 instead of raising it to the 12th power). The PV cashflow analysis is referred to as discounting and estimates what a future amount would be worth today. The interest rate is referred to as the discount rate, and the formula for the PV calculation is the reciprocal of the FV formula. Using the same key elements, the PV formula can be represented as: $PV = FV \div (1+r)^n$. To illustrate, we can use the same information from the previous example, with the PV amount as the FV amount, in Exhibit 12.2.

EXHIBIT 12.2. Present Value Calculation

$$PV = FV \div (1+r)^n$$

$$PV = \$48,500 \div (1.09)^{12}$$

$$PV = \$48,500 \div 2.8127$$

$$PV = \$17,243.22$$

In this example, the FV dollar amount is "discounted" or reduced annually in response to the discount rate and is less than the initial future dollar amount. The future amount of $48,500 is discounted or reduced at a rate of 9% per year for 12 years, with the number of years used as the exponential power in the calculation. The final PV amount is $17,243 (rounded). With a series of cashflows, the PV is calculated for each one using the same method. The **net present value** (NPV) is the summation of the PVs of a series of cashflows, providing the overall value for the financial portion of the capital project. To illustrate how NPV is calculated, consider the cashflow information presented in Exhibit 12.3.

EXHIBIT 12.3. Net Present Value Calculation

A capital project has the following estimated cashflows and a project life span of 5 years. An initial funding grant was given to begin the initiative, which is reflected at Year 0 (startup). Using a 7% discount rate, calculate the NPV.

Years	FV (Cashflows)		Years	FV (Cashflows)	PV		Years	FV (Cashflows)	PV
0	$10,000		0	$10,000	$10,000		0	$10,000	$10,000
1	$1,100		1	$1,100			1	$1,100	$1,028
2	$1,500		2	$1,500			2	$1,500	$1,310
3	$2,300		3	$2,300			3	$2,300	$1,877
4	$2,100		4	$2,100			4	$2,100	$1,602
5	$3,000		5	$3,000			5	$3,000	$2,139
									$17,956

FV, future value; PV, present value.

When analyzing cashflows, Year 0 represents the start of the project. A positive number in Year 0 is a cash inflow, and could be the result of a donation, seed funding, grants, and so forth. A negative number in Year 0 is a cash outflow and could be the result of an initial purchase or outlay of cash to begin the project. In Exhibit 12.3, the initial $10,000 is grant funding and is therefore shown as a positive number. Using the PV formula for the initial Year 0 cashflow and the 7% discount rate: $PV = 10,000 \div (1.07)^0$. Remembering the fundamental mathematics power of zero rule, any number raised to the power of zero is 1 (because $n = 0$ for the startup year). So, the resulting PV for the first cashflow is: $PV = \$10,000 \div 1$ or $10,000. Performing similar calculations for the remaining cashflows produces the PVs shown in the third box of Exhibit 12.3, and the resulting NPV of $17,956. A final factor that may impact cashflows and the NPV of a project is salvage value. **Salvage value** is the sales price of the items purchased for the capital project, after the useful life with the organization. A simple example of salvage value would be the resale of office computer equipment at the conclusion of a corporate training initiative. The company purchased the computers for $25,000. The training sessions are estimated to generate 3 years of cashflows: $2,500, $3,000, and $3,500. At the end of the training sessions, the company plans to sell the computers to a neighborhood education center for $5,000. The receipt of the sales price is a cash inflow, and will be added to the final year's cashflow, making year 3 total $8,500. This not only increases the cashflows, but the NPV and profitability of the overall project.

The valuation of cashflows also supports calculations to determine the overall profitability of the capital project. The **profitability index** (PI), one such calculation used to gauge the value of a project, uses the NPV in its calculation. The PI is calculated by dividing the NPV by the investment costs. In a ratio such as this, the greater the investment cost, the lower the PI. Let's have a look at a PI example in Exhibit 12.4.

EXHIBIT 12.4. Profitability Index Calculation

A small hematology laboratory is planning to buy three new centrifuge machines to replace the outdated equipment they currently have. With the purchase of the new machines, they can process testing requests much faster as they prepare to address an increased volume of requests (and associated revenues). The initial outlay of cash for purchase is $5,000, the discount rate for the project is 5%, and the life span for the equipment is 7 years. Calculate the NPV and PI if the estimated cashflows for the centrifuge capital project are as shown in the table that follows.

Years	FV (Cashflows)	PV		Years	FV (Cashflows)	PV
0	$(5,000)	$(5,000)		0	$(5,000)	$(5,000)
1	$2,000	$1,905		1	$2,000	$1,905
2	$2,200			2	$2,200	$1,995
3	$2,500			3	$2,500	$2,160
4	$3,100			4	$3,100	$2,550
5	$4,000			5	$4,000	$3,134
6	$3,750			6	$3,750	$2,798
7	$2,150			7	$2,150	$1,528
						$11,070

PI = $11,070/$5,000
PI = 2.21

FV, future value; NPV, net present value; PI, profitability index; PV, present value.

As previously defined, NPV is the summation of PVs for all of the project's cashflows. The purchase price of $5,000 is a cash outflow and is therefore shown as a negative number for the Year 0 startup. The power of zero rule results in a Year 0 PV of −$5,000. The Year 1 PV formula with all inputs is: $PV = \$2,000 \div (1.05)^1$, PV (Year 1) = $1,905 (rounded). The remaining PVs are calculated using the same methodology, for an NPV of $11,070. The PI is then calculated by dividing the NPV by the initial investment amount, PI = NPV ÷ Initial Investment, PI = $11,070 / $5,000 = 2.21. When interpreting the PI, the ideal PI should be 1.0 or greater. At PI = 1.0, the project NPV and initial investment are equal, meaning the project will breakeven by producing cashflows in the exact amount of the investment. If the PI is greater than 1.0, the project cashflows will recover the initial investment as well as additional positive cashflows or income.

Additional financial assessments used to determine a capital project's value are the **internal rate of return** (IRR) and the **return on investment** (ROI). The IRR measures the capital project's annual growth and profitability, while the ROI measures the capital project's total life span growth and profitability. The IRR calculates the discount rate that makes the project NPV equal 0. This calculation is best performed using designated calculator functions or Microsoft Excel® to pinpoint the discount rate, as hand calculations would require the trial of multiple rates to narrow down the IRR. Using the cashflows from the previous example (Exhibit 12.4), we can use Excel's IRR function to determine what discount rate would make the NPV for the cashflows equal to zero, getting the results shown in Exhibit 12.5.

The IRR function in Excel gives an IRR of 46.29% to make the NPV for this project's cashflows equal 0. The power of zero rule applies to Year 0, so we can review the Year 1 calculation using the IRR. The Year PV calculation becomes: $PV = \$2,000 \div (1 + .4629)^1 = \$1,367$ (rounded). The same calculation can be performed for the remaining cashflows, resulting in a zero NPV. Performing the calculation by hand would require a series of "guesses" to get closer to the IRR. The ROI for

EXHIBIT 12.5. IRR Calculation (Using the Excel Function)

Years	FV (Cashflows)	PV
0	$(5,000)	$(5,000)
1	$2,000	$1,367
2	$2,200	
3	$2,500	
4	$3,100	
5	$4,000	
6	$3,750	
7	$2,150	

Years	FV (Cashflows)	PV
0	$(5,000)	$(5,000)
1	$2,000	$1,367
2	$2,200	$1,027
3	$2,500	$799
4	$3,100	$677
5	$4,000	$597
6	$3,750	$383
7	$2,150	$150
		$0

FV, future value; IRR, internal rate of return; PV, present value.

a project is calculated using the formula: ROI = (Net Profit ÷ Project Investment) × 100. Using the cashflows presented in Exhibit 12.4, we can illustrate the ROI calculation shown in Exhibit 12.6.

EXHIBIT 12.6. Return on Investment Calculation

Years	FV (Cashflows)	PV
0	$(5,000)	$(5,000)
1	$2,000	$1,905
2	$2,200	$1,995
3	$2,500	$2,160
4	$3,100	$2,550
5	$4,000	$3,134
6	$3,750	$2,798
7	$2,150	$1,528
		$11,070

$$ROI = (Net\ Profit \div Project\ Investment) \times 100$$
$$ROI = (\$16,070 \div \$5,000) \times 100$$
$$ROI = 321.41\%$$

FV, future value; PV, present value; ROI, return on investment.

Net profit in the calculation is the sum of the cash inflows for project years 1 through 7, totaling $16,070. The net profit is then divided by the investment amount of $5,000 for a result of 3.214. The 3.214 is multiplied by 100 for an ROI of 321.4%. This project is definitely lucrative, as it yields greater than a 300% return.

After the various ratios and returns are estimated, the projects may be further assessed for sensitivity. **Sensitivity analysis** examines the changes in project value and NPV as the inputs for the project change. Examples of changes would include interest rate changes, initial investment amount, cashflow amounts, or anticipated life span of the project. Testing the changes would be as simple as updating the original values in the PV, FV, or NPV formulas which would then result in changes to the IRR and ROI. Volatile changes in IRR and ROI translate to a capital project with unpredictable outcomes, which may deter decision makers.

After all proposals have been analyzed and ranked, the final proposals are chosen and approved for capital funding. The approved projects, even after the analysis and ranking process, must meet the financial and nonfinancial requirements for capital funding allocation. Projects must (a) meet the needs of the organization operationally and strategically, (b) be financially feasible in both the short term (including initial investment) and long term (returns and cash inflows), and (c) be desirable and acceptable by the stakeholders impacted by the project (patients, clinicians, employees, donors/investors, etc.). Decision makers must then determine how the projects will be funded.

CAPITAL PROJECT FINANCING DECISIONS

The approved capital projects must be funded in some way, and for many organizations, there are multiple ways of doing this. Organizations may choose to use equity or funds it already has access to, debt or funds it borrows, or a combination of the two options. The financing approach used may be determined by the return on equity (ROE), the return on debt, the overall return to stakeholders (in a for-profit situation), or the costs of each. The **cost of equity** is defined as the rate of return or ROI required by owners/shareholders to finance the capital investments. The **cost of debt** is the interest rate applied by external lenders to the borrowed funds. The **corporate cost of capital** (CCC) is the weighted combination of the cost of equity and the cost of debt, producing the organization's capital structure. The **capital structure** is the organization's mix of equity and debt financing, with the ideal capital structure being the scenario with the lowest aggregate risks and costs. The formula used for the calculation of CCC is shown in Box 12.2.

BOX 12.2

Corporate Cost of Capital Formula

$$\text{CCC} = [(\text{Percentage of Equity}) \times (\text{Cost of Equity})] + [(\text{Percentage of Debt}) \times ([\text{Cost of Debt}] \times [1 - T])]$$

In the CCC calculation, the percentage of equity and the percentage of debt are the amounts the capital projects are to be financed by that particular method. For example, if the equity percentage is 100%, it means that no funding will be borrowed for financing (debt percentage = 0). If the equity percentage is 50%, then the debt percentage will be 50%. The sum of the equity percentage and the debt percentage must equal 100%. To further examine the relationship between these formula elements, we can begin by illustrating a CCC example (Exhibit 12.7).

As detailed in Exhibit 12.7, Community Hospital must earn a minimum of 6.14% aggregate return to meet the requirements of the shareholders as well as the external lenders. If Community Hospital was exploring multiple equity and debt combinations, the combination with the lowest CCC represents the lowest aggregate risk and would be the best possible combination.

Assessing the financing decision is important to determine the project's potential impacts on the organization's overall financial position. ROE and return to investors (in for-profit healthcare

---

EXHIBIT 12.7. Corporate Cost of Capital Calculation

Community Hospital has added an additional patient wing and is exploring financing options for all of the equipment needed for the new patient rooms. The hospital plans to fund the equipment using 60% equity and 40% debt, and currently has a tax rate of 3%. The required ROI is 7% and the interest rate for an equipment loan is 5%. In this scenario, what is the CCC?

$$\text{CCC} = [(\text{Percentage of Equity}) \times (\text{Cost of Equity})] + [(\text{Percentage of Debt})$$
$$\times ([\text{Cost of Debt}] \times [1 - \text{T}])]$$

$$\text{CCC} = [(.60) \times (7\%)] + [(.40) \times ([5\%] \times [1 - .03])]$$

$$\text{CCC} = [(.60) \times (7\%)] + [(.40) \times (4.85\%)]$$

$$\text{CCC} = 4.2\% + 1.94\%$$

$$\text{CCC} = 6.14\%$$

---

organizations) may both be impacted by the new capital structure. To assess the impact, a side-by-side comparison of the financing options is calculated, as well as the associated ratios for ROE and return to investors. The financial statements containing the required figures for analysis are the balance sheet and the statement of operations (income statement). The assessment process is detailed in the example shown in Exhibit 12.8.

EXHIBIT 12.8. Financing Decision Comparison

American Cancer Research Center (ACRC) is an established research and treatment facility located in the Blue Ridge Mountains. ACRC is considering an expansion opportunity but must first fully analyze the organization's financial health before moving forward with the expansion. The organization currently utilizes an all-equity approach to financing. Earnings before interest and taxes (EBIT) is $13,000,000 and the organization holds $17,000,000 in assets. As a newly hired financial analyst, it is now your responsibility to perform the necessary calculations and provide a final report to the executive team. Prepare ACRC's financial statements, comparing its current all-equity financing approach to a possible 65% debt financing approach. Assume an interest rate of 9% and a tax rate of 33% for your calculations.

For the comparison, we must (a) create ACRC's balance sheet, (b) create ACRC's statement of operations, and (c) calculate return to investors and ROE.

The balance sheet for ACRC shows the assets, debt, and equity for the current all-equity financing as well as the proposed partial debt financing. Because debt is defined as an amount owed, there will be no debt figure in the equity column, since this is funding already owned/in-house.

- The debt figure for the 65% financing option is calculated by multiplying the asset amount by the proposed debt percentage: $17,000,000 × .65 = $11,050,000.

- Total is the net equity, calculated by subtracting the debt amount from the asset amount in each column, resulting in equity = $17,000,000 and debt = $17,000,000 − $11,050,000 = $5,950,000.

(continued)

EXHIBIT 12.8. Financing Decision Comparison (*continued*)

Balance Sheet		
	Equity Financing (100%)	Debt Financing (65%)
Assets	$17,000,000	$17,000,000
Debt	$ -	$11,050,000
Total equity	$17,000,000	$5,950,000

Statement of Operations		
	Equity Financing (100%)	Debt Financing (65%)
EBIT	$13,000,000	$13,000,000
Interest (9%)	$ -	$994,500
Taxable Income	$13,000,000	$12,005,500
Taxes (33%)	$4,290,000	$3,961,815
Net Incomev	$8,710,000	$8,043,685

The statement of operations or income statement always begins with income. In this scenario, ACRC's income is noted as EBIT in the amount of $13,000,000. Deducted from earnings are interest expense and taxes. Interest expense is applied to the amount owed/borrowed; therefore, there is no interest expense applied to the equity column (it's not a debt).

  Interest expense for the debt column is calculated using the amount borrowed, then subtracted from earnings: Interest Expense = $11,050,000 × .09 = $994,500; $13,000,000 − $994,500 = $12,005,500.

  Taxable income is the amount of income remaining after interest expense has been subtracted, $13,000,000 for the equity financing option and $12,005,500 for the debt financing option. Taxes are then applied to both columns, using a tax rate of 33%, producing net income: Equity = $13,000,000 − $4,290,000 (Taxable Income × Tax Rate) = $8,710,000; Debt = $12,005,500 − $3,961,815 = $8,043,685.

The ROE and return to investors are calculated using figures contained in the financial statements. ROE = Net Income ÷ Total Assets and Return to Investors = Net Income + Interest Expense. We can calculate this for both financing options:

  ROE (equity financing column) = $8,710,000 ÷ $17,000,000 = .5124 or 51.24%; ROE (debt financing column) = $8,043,685 ÷ $5,950,000 = 1.3519 or 135.19%.

  Return to Investors (equity) = $8,710,000 + $0 = $8,710,000; Return to Investors (debt) = $8,043,685 + $994,500 = $9,038,185.

The comparison of the financing options shown in Exhibit 12.8 is very important to the final capital project decision-making process. Although both options in Exhibit 12.8 are profitable, the debt financing option offers the highest ROE and return to investors. This happens due to the impact of the interest expense on the earnings, which reduces the taxable income (and amount of taxes paid) for the investment. These subtle financial impacts could be the deciding factor in capital project approval or capital project denial.

CHAPTER SUMMARY

Although the capital budgeting process is separate from the operating budgeting process, it remains equally important. Decisions made regarding capital investments often impact multiple units or divisions and the financial position of the entire healthcare organization. Securing funding for large projects makes it possible for some organizations to remain competitive in the healthcare sector, while providing the highest quality care with the most recent technologies. Such high-dollar projects require meticulous planning and thorough analysis of possible results with the intent of preparing the organization for all predictable outcomes. Internal or external funding also makes a difference and should tie directly into the organization's short-term and longer-term financial goals.

KEY TERMS FOR REVIEW

capital budget	cost of equity	present value
capital project analysis	future value	profitability index
capital rationing	inflows	return on investment
capital structure	internal rate of return	risk
cashflow	net present value	salvage value
corporate cost of capital	outflows	sensitivity analysis
cost of debt	payback period	time value of money

DISCUSSION QUESTIONS

1. Define "capital budget" and explain how it differs from a healthcare organization's operating budget.

2. How does the concept of capital rationing influence the selection and funding of capital projects?

3. What are cash inflows and outflows? How do they impact an organization's financial bottom line?

4. Discuss how a capital project's payback period is calculated. Does the time frame matter if the initial investment is recovered during the project's life span? Explain your answer.

5. Define TVM and its connection to FV and PV calculations.

6. What is the PI? What would be an ideal PI?

7. When considering a capital project's return, what are the two main ratios discussed in the chapter for project analysis? Is one ratio better or more reliable than the other?

8. List the elements included in the capital structure.

9. What is the formula/calculation for CCC? When interpreting the results of a CCC comparison, which would be the ideal CCC?

10. What is the purpose of a sensitivity analysis?

PRACTICE PROBLEMS

Answers to this chapter's Practice Problems are available via Springer Publishing Connect™ by following the instructions on the opening page of this book and accessing Answers to Practice Problems on the Table of Contents.

1. What is the compounded FV of the cashflows in Exhibit 12.9? Assume a 5-year timeline and a rate of 12%.

EXHIBIT 12.9. Cashflows for FV Calculation

Year	Cashflow
0	$3,500
1	$2,100
2	$1,200
3	$1,750
4	$2,000
5	$1,500

FV, future value.

---

2. Calculate the FV of $35,775 invested at a rate of 8% for 11 years.

3. Calculate the PV of $1,500, to be received in 3 years, at a rate of 7%.

4. A hospital invests $250,000 into the purchase of new infusion therapy machines. The new machines have a life expectancy of 5 years, and have the estimated cashflows in Exhibit 12.10.

EXHIBIT 12.10. Cashflows for Payback Period Calculation

Year	Cashflow
0	$(250,000)
1	$90,000
2	$97,000
3	$105,000
4	$110,000
5	$115,000

5. University Finance Corporation is examining several options for its capital structure (shown in Exhibit 12.11) to determine which is optimal. Calculate (a) the CCC for each of the following structures, then (b) identify which is the best/ideal structure.

EXHIBIT 12.11. University Finance Corporation Capital Structure Comparison

	Percent Debt	Cost of Debt	Cost of Equity	Tax Rate
A	30%	9%	12%	0%
B	58%	13%	24%	9.5%
C	75%	8%	18%	8.1%
D	27%	11%	13%	7.7%

CHAPTER 12 CASE: MOUNTAIN MEDICAL'S CAPITAL PROJECT ANALYSIS

Mountain Medical, a not-for-profit community hospital, is considering the proposed purchase of a new ERP software system. The price of the ERP system is $750,000, and it has a life expectancy of 10 years. The system will be sold at the end of the life span, with salvage value of $175,000 to be paid over the final 3 years. While this new system will have no impact on the number of employees connected to the system on any given day, it is expected to save the organization $3,000 per year in operating costs (due to automation, which requires fewer full-time equivalents [FTEs]). On average, the implementation instructors train 30 people per day for 300 days per year. ERP training materials cost approximately $25 per person. Grant funding provides reimbursement of $125 for each person registered for ERP training. Year one expenses for Mountain Medical include instructor labor ($105,000), building operations (rent and utilities of $30,000 and $20,000, respectively), and overhead of $5,000. Costs increase by 7% annually. Revenues increase by 9% annually. The cost of capital is 11%.

1. Calculate the net cashflows for this capital project.

2. How does the $3,000 annual savings in operating costs impact the cashflows?

3. Calculate the NPV for this project, utilizing the cashflows identified in Question 1.

4. The salvage value as stated in the case is $175,000. How does the salvage value impact the cashflows and the NPV?

5. If Mountain Medical decides to use partial debt financing for the purchase of the equipment, what would be the effects on the balance sheet, statement of operations, and ROE if the following holds true:

    The organization is considering financing 50% of the purchase.

    Assets will be $750,000, the price of the ERP.

    Operating income for Mountain Medical is $7,000,000.

    The organization's tax rate is 20%.

HEALTHCARE FINANCE COURSE PROJECT: FINANCIAL STATEMENT AND FINANCING DECISIONS FOR PHASE III

The third phase of the course project is the creation of the financial statements and financing decisions. For this final phase, students will combine the consolidated financials from Phase II to create a balance sheet, statement of operations, statement of cashflows, and proforma for their healthcare organization. The phase includes the following worksheets/calculations:

- Worksheet #12: Balance Sheet
- Worksheet #13: Statement of Operations
- Worksheet #14: Statement of Cashflows
- Worksheet #15: Proforma Statement
- Worksheet #16: Financing Options Comparison
- Worksheet #17: Performance Measurement and Ratio Analysis
- Worksheet #18: Dashboards (Graphs and Visual Elements)

Review the "Course Project: Phase III" section of Chapter 16. All other worksheets in the third phase are to be created by the student, using the data calculated in the previous consolidation phase. All worksheets are to be connected to both Phases I and II where applicable. Be sure to review the Microsoft Excel® Reference Guide located in the Appendices as needed.

CHAPTER 13

Financial Performance and Evaluation

OBJECTIVES

1. Understand and define the major indicators of financial health.
2. Outline the importance of variance analysis for performance measurement.
3. Calculate the various financial ratios used to determine financial position.
4. Identify the steps/stages of a formative evaluation.

INTRODUCTION

The financial health of an organization can provide insight into an organization's management practices and operational efficiency, as well as its leadership decision-making. All functions within the healthcare organization contribute to its financial health in some way, with some having a direct connection while others may be more indirect. To properly assess financial performance, we must ensure accurate and complete capture of operating data and financial data, as well as the proper context within which to interpret this information. Chapter 6 of the textbook introduces the concepts of performance measurement and key performance indicators (KPIs). In this chapter, we take a closer look at the indicators of financial health, and at how metrics such as KPIs contribute to the organization's overall assessment of performance. We will explore the financial performance trends relative to the financial statements and discuss the types of evaluations most useful for evidence-based organizational management.

INDICATORS OF FINANCIAL HEALTH

There are numerous indicators of financial health, and most organizations will choose to monitor indicators that tie directly into their mission and core values. There are, however, metrics that benefit every healthcare organization, no matter its focus or mission. These somewhat universal measurement categories are patient demand, healthcare services and production, resource allocation, and cost effectiveness. These categories contain several types of indicators that may be used to assess an organization's financial health, and in many cases are used collectively to reflect how the organization is run. For patient demand, an organization must have the capabilities to meet current demand, as well as to properly plan for anticipated or future demand. This could be inpatient services, outpatient services, telemedicine, pharmacy, or any combination of the services offered. Being responsive to patient needs is definitely a key factor in establishing community relationships and encouraging return business. Healthcare services and production may be specific to the organization, or what it is they offer. These are the products and services created to meet the demand of patients and consumers. Healthcare services would include patient visits, imaging services, laboratory work and testing, or even medical transportation. The production side includes personal use products, durable medical equipment or machines, and capital purchases. Resource allocation includes the efficient utilization of human resources, financial resources, and material resources. Clinicians and other healthcare sector professionals make the provision of services and the creation of products possible. As with any other resource, available professionals for our sector are not an endless supply. We must utilize our professionals effectively and efficiently, in the context of their specialization and available time. Financial resources also require prudent allocation, as the healthcare sector continues to address the issue of rising costs. As we continue to strive to provide the highest quality healthcare at the lowest possible cost, we must remain diligent in maximizing current resources and minimizing unnecessary spending. Material resources are extremely important for the provision of care, as healthcare professionals rely on materials for various treatments. Being dependent on the smooth operation of the supply chain, material resources must be monitored for utilization rates and reorder points to ensure that materials are available when needed by providers and the patients they serve.

To monitor, maintain, and improve the indicators of financial health, and ultimately the operations of the healthcare organization, requires the development and implementation of measurable, quantifiable metrics that can be documented over time. The metrics, or measured data, will be different for each area and are specific to function, product, or purpose. Ideally, the data will be captured over a specified length of time and reveal any anomalies, patterns, trends, or seasonality that occur. There are several methods that are routinely used to analyze performance and the associated data, but this chapter will focus on the following approaches: variance analysis, ratio analysis, and formative evaluations. Each of these methods of analysis approaches the organization's performance from a different angle; however, the methods may work together to improve the overall decision-making and financial health.

VARIANCE ANALYSIS

Every organization creates an annual budget as a guide or benchmark for routine operations and financial performance. In healthcare, as with other sectors, things may not always go according to plan when there are so many variables involved. Changes in patient visit volume, changes in reimbursement and legislation, or societal events may all contribute to unplanned variances from the budget. **Variance analysis** is the comparison of actual figures to the planned or budgeted estimates. Variance from what was budgeted is expected in some cases, but large variances could signal an emerging event that may impact future operations, or possibly missed information during the budgeting process. Variance analysis is performed for statistics or volume data, revenues, expenses, and profit to identify any areas that may need management attention or adjustments to the budget estimation methodology. Variances can be favorable or unfavorable, with different interpretations based on the category (as shown in Table 13.1).

In some cases, going above or below the budgeted estimate is a positive thing for an organization, while in other situations, the variance may be a cause for concern. For budgeted

Table 13.1

VARIANCE ANALYSIS BY CATEGORY

Category	Calculation	Interpretation
Statistics/Volume data	Actual–budget	Favorable: more volume than budgeted; unfavorable: lower volume than budgeted
Revenues	Actual–budget	Favorable: more revenue than budgeted; unfavorable: less revenue than budgeted (still should be equal to or more than breakeven)
Expenses (costs)	Budget–actual	Favorable: fewer expenses than budgeted (spending less is good); unfavorable: greater expenses than budgeted (spending more is not good)
Profit (net income)	Actual–budget	Favorable: higher profit than budgeted; unfavorable: less profit than budgeted

statistics or patient volume, a higher-than-budgeted number signifies growth and potentially increased revenue. Of course, there may be associated expenses, but if sound staffing and reimbursement structures are in place, the organization will usually fare well. A shortfall in volume, or decreased patient volume numbers, could mean an unforeseen shift in demand, and may also result in missed revenue targets. Revenue variances, like statistical variance, are favorable if they are more than the budgeted figure. Ideally, the additional revenue will be the result of increased patient activity, and not a sign of missed estimation during the operating budget preparation process. Less revenue could be the result of decreased patient activity or a change in the payer reimbursement structure. The key is ensuring that actual revenues recognized are still enough to cover all expenses, even if they are less than the budgeted target. If the revenues do not at least hit the breakeven point, there are much larger financial issues to address. Expenses is the one category where exceeding the budgeted estimation is always unfavorable, denoted by the flip in calculation to budgeted figure minus the actual figure. Spending more, without being associated with increased patient volumes and increased revenues, means a potential internal controls issue for expenses. Spending less is favorable because it translates to effective internal cost controls and monitoring of spending. Profit variances are directly connected to revenue and expense variances, as revenues minus expenses equal profit. Profit will be favorable if revenue exceeds expenses. Increased expenses, without the associated increase in patient volumes and increase in revenue, may result in diminished profit, or a potential loss position for the organization. To illustrate the variances for the categories, we can review the budgeted and actual items in Exhibit 13.1 and Exhibit 13.2.

EXHIBIT 13.1. Favorable Variance Analysis Calculations

	Actual	Budget	Variance ($)	Variance (%)	Interpretation
Revenues	$5,500,000	$5,250,000	$250,000	4.76%	Favorable
Expenses	$2,500,000	$3,000,000	$500,000	16.67%	Favorable
Profit (net income)	$3,000,000	$2,250,000	$750,000	33.33%	Favorable

In the scenario shown in Exhibit 13.1, the variances for revenue, expenses, and profit are favorable. The revenues category is $250,000 more than the budgeted estimate ($5,500,000 – $5,250,000), which means more revenue was earned. This is a favorable result because the revenue target (cash inflow) was exceeded. The expenses category is $500,000 less than the budgeted estimate ($3,000,000 – $2,500,000), which means that spending was reduced. This is a favorable result because the cash outflow was less than planned. The resulting profit is $750,000 ($3,000,000 – $2,250,000), which is the same as the sum of the revenues and expenses variances ($250,000 + $500,000). Increased revenues and reduced expenses have increased the estimated profit amount—an overall favorable result.

EXHIBIT 13.2. Unfavorable Variance Analysis Calculations

	Actual	Budget	Variance ($)	Variance (%)	Interpretation
Revenues	$5,150,000	$5,250,000	$(100,000)	−1.90%	Unfavorable
Expenses	$3,250,000	$3,000,000	$(250,000)	−8.33%	Unfavorable
Profit (net income)	$1,900,000	$2,250,000	$(350,000)	−15.56%	Unfavorable

---

Exhibit 13.2 shows examples of unfavorable results for revenues, expenses, and profit. Revenues in this scenario are $100,000 less than the budgeted amount. This is unfavorable because it is a cash inflow shortfall, resulting in fewer revenue dollars to cover expenses. The expenses category is unfavorable in this instance because actual spending was in excess of the budgeted estimate by $250,000. The resulting profit is unfavorable, with the actual figure being $350,000 less than the budgeting profit amount. This example reflects a scenario where there wasn't enough actual revenue to cover the actual expenses, with the result being a loss position for this budgeted period. The favorable and unfavorable results can vary, with categories being favorable or unfavorable in any given scenario. The data provided by variance analysis supports several organizational functions including internal planning and control, effective performance measurement and monitoring, benchmarking and projections, program/project management, and decision-making. Together, these functions identify problem areas as well as areas for improvement, assisting leadership with facilitating organizational growth, economic and financial stability, and a culture of effectiveness and efficiency.

RATIO ANALYSIS

The concept of ratio analysis was introduced in Chapter 6, but now we will examine the actual calculation of the more common ratios using figures from the financial statements and discuss how they translate the financial health of an organization. **Ratio analysis** assesses the organization's overall financial position, using the operating and financial information found in the prepared financial statements. Particularly, they are used to analyze asset management, debt management, liquidity, and profitability in comparison to competition or national standards and best practices.

Asset Management

Asset management and the financial ratios that support it assess the healthcare organization's utilization and growth of items with value. Assets include cash, owned inventory, research patents, machines and equipment, buildings and facilities, or other items held by the organization. There are many ratios used for asset management, with the items chosen at the organization's discretion. The examples we'll cover for asset management in our discussion will be:

- total asset turnover
- change in net assets
- inventory turnover

Total asset turnover is a ratio used to determine how well the organization uses its assets to generate revenue or income. Ideally, the more assets owned by the healthcare organization, the greater or stronger the stream of income will be. This of course will be dependent on the size of the organization as well as the variety of services and payers offered, but theoretically the ownership of assets should result in favorable cash inflows. To calculate total asset turnover, we use figures from the statement of operations and the balance sheet, resulting in the formula shown in Box 13.1.

BOX 13.1

Total Asset Turnover

Total Asset Turnover = Total Revenues ÷ Total Assets

To illustrate the total asset turnover ratio calculation, we use the figures presented in the financial statements in Exhibit 13.3.

EXHIBIT 13.3. Sample Financial Statements

Statement of Operations

	2022	2021
Revenues		
Inpatient revenue	$2,563,873	$2,294,666
Outpatient revenue	$1,709,249	$1,529,778
Other operating revenue	$299,119	$267,712
Total revenues	**$4,572,241**	**$4,092,156**
Expenses		
Wages and fringe benefits	$1,508,840	$1,403,221
Purchased/Contracted services	$1,131,630	$1,052,416
Supplies and other expenses	$497,917	$463,063
Interest expense	$32,048	$29,805
Depreciation and amortization	$213,656	$198,700
Total expenses	**$3,384,091**	**$3,147,205**

(continued)

EXHIBIT 13.3. Sample Financial Statements (*continued*)

Operating income (loss)	$1,188,150	$944,951
Nonoperating revenues and expenses		
Contributions (unrestricted)	$3,757	$4,020
Marketing expense (brochures and publications)	$(67)	$(65)
Investment income	$53,047	$50,395
Total nonoperating expenses	**$56,737**	**$54,350**
Excess of revenues over (under) expenses	**$1,131,413**	**$890,601**

Balance sheet

	2022	2021
Assets		
Current assets		
Cash and cash equivalents	$756,542	$703,267
Accounts receivable (patients)	$100,000	$100,000
Inventory and supplies	$235,000	$210,000
Prepaid expenses	$75,000	$68,000
Short-term investments	$145,369	$186,322
Total current assets	**$1,311,911**	**$1,267,589**
Investments (long-term)	$4,837,510	$4,729,581
Property and equipment	$2,377,859	$2,238,951
Limited-use assets	$3,689,512	$3,357,628
Fundraising/Charity	$590,000	$341,500
Total assets	**$12,806,792**	**$11,935,249**
Liabilities		
Current liabilities		
Accounts payable	$237,381	$215,950
Accrued expenses	$485,660	$480,000
Lease liabilities	$325,000	$300,000
Lines of credit	$125,000	$150,000
Total current liabilities	**$1,173,041**	**$1,145,950**
Insurance and pension liability	$275,000	$250,000
Long-term debt	$540,000	$585,490
Salvage receipts	$1,500,000	$1,500,000
Total liabilities	**$3,488,041**	**$3,481,440**
Net assets	**$9,318,751**	**$8,453,809**

As we review the financial statements, we see that the total revenues figure for the most current year (2022) is $4,572,241 and the total assets figure for the current year is $12,806,792, which makes the calculation:

$$\text{Total Asset Turnover} = \text{Total Revenues} \div \text{Total Assets}$$

$$= \$4,572,241 \div \$12,806,792$$

$$= .3570$$

The resulting .3570 or 35.70% means that for every dollar in asset value, the company generates 35 cents in revenue. A better ratio would be an equivalent return of one dollar of revenue for each dollar in asset value, but a positive total asset turnover ratio indicates that the organization still is making some efficient uses of the assets owned. **Change in net assets** is the percentage change of net assets from the previous fiscal year to the current fiscal year. To calculate this using the balance sheet data in Exhibit 13.3, we see that net assets for 2021 were $8,453,809 and net assets for 2022 were $9,318,751. The increase in net assets is $864,942 or 10.23% from 2021. **Inventory turnover ratio** measures the time between inventory purchase and inventory sales. The "turnover" determines how many times the organization has sold and repurchased its supplies. This calculation is primarily used by those responsible for inventory and supply chain management, but is a useful metric for large organizations with high rates of supply utilization.

Inventory turnover ratio is calculated by dividing the cost of goods sold by the average inventory. If an organization has annual cost of goods sold for 2022 as $750,000, and average inventory of $235,000 as shown in Box 13.2, the inventory turnover ratio becomes:

BOX 13.2

Inventory Turnover Ratio

Inventory Turnover Ratio = Cost of Goods Sold ÷ Average Inventory

$$= \$750,000 \div \$235,000$$

$$= 3.19$$

The resulting inventory turnover ratio of 3.19 indicates that the organization sells and restocks its entire inventory three times per year. A low or high value for inventory turnover is dependent upon the types of products used as well as the volume of sales. Items with shorter life spans or expiration dates, like medications and pharmaceuticals, will have to be replenished often, while those items that are more shelf stable, like bandages and some medical supplies, will have to be replaced less frequently.

Debt Management

Debt management ratios analyze the healthcare organization's use of debt in financing its operations and initiatives. Proper debt management supports an organization's credit rating, equity improvement strategy, and borrowing practices, providing insight on areas that may need adjustment. It helps with capital investment decisions as well as capital project financing. Debt management can also be used to determine adequate revenue amounts, to ensure that an organization is generating enough revenue to cover its debt obligations. The debt management ratios discussed in this section will be:

- debt ratio
- debt service coverage
- long-term debt to capitalization

The **debt ratio** measures if an organization has enough assets to cover its liabilities, and is calculated using the formula shown in Box 13.3.

BOX 13.3

Debt Ratio

Debt Ratio = Total Liabilities ÷ Total Assets

Using the data provided in the balance sheet from Exhibit 13.3, the debt ratio can be calculated using the total liabilities and total assets:

Debt Ratio = Total Liabilities ÷ Total Assets

= $3,488,041 ÷ $12,806,792

= .2724

In this scenario, the debt ratio is .2724, which means that the healthcare organization has almost three times more assets than liabilities. If the amount of liabilities is .2724 or 27.24%, the amount of assets is .7276 or 72.76%. **Debt service coverage ratio** measures an organization's cashflow in relation to its debt. The greater the cashflow, the more liabilities covered. Debt service coverage is calculated by using the formula shown in Box 13.4.

BOX 13.4

Debt Service Coverage Ratio

Debt Service Coverage Ratio = (Net Income + Depreciation + Amortization + Interest) ÷ Current Debt

Again, we can use the statement of operations and the balance sheet provided in Exhibit 13.3 to illustrate our calculation.

$$\text{Debt Service Coverage Ratio} = (\text{Net Income} + \text{Depreciation} + \text{Amortization} + \text{Interest})$$
$$\div \text{ Current Debt}$$

$$= (\$1{,}131{,}413 + \$213{,}656 + \$32{,}048) \div \$1{,}173{,}041$$

$$= \$1{,}377{,}117 \div \$1{,}173{,}041$$

$$= 1.1740$$

The debt service coverage ratio result of 1.1740 translates to the organization being able to meet over 100% of its current obligations. This measure uses current liabilities instead of all long-term items, because long term is calculated using a capitalization analysis. **Long-term debt to capitalization** assesses the organization's capital structure and its long-term financing. The calculation includes long-term debt and unrestricted assets (shown in Box 13.5).

BOX 13.5

Long-Term Debt to Capitalization Ratio

$$\text{Long-Term Debt to Capitalization} = \text{Long-Term Debt} \div (\text{Long-Term Debt} + \text{Unrestricted Net Assets})$$

$$= \$2{,}315{,}000 \div (\$2{,}315{,}000 + \$5{,}629{,}239)$$

$$= \$2{,}315{,}000 \div \$7{,}944{,}239$$

$$= .2914$$

For this calculation, the long-term debt amount is taken from the lower portion of the balance sheet in Exhibit 13.3 (insurance and pension liabilities + long-term debt + salvage receipts). The unrestricted asset figure uses the total net assets number ($9,318,751) and subtracts the limited use asset number ($3,689,512) for a result of $5,629,239. Typically, a long-term debt to capitalization ratio less than 1.0 is seen as favorable, because this means that an organization has not financed most of its long-term initiatives and still has borrowing power. If the ratio result is greater than 1.0, the organization is seen as higher risk, since most of its initiatives have been financed instead of adequately using its equity.

Liquidity

Liquidity is the ability to quickly convert assets to cash. Cash is essential for any organization and its ability to meet its short-term obligations. Cash and liquidity are needed for routine functions such as employee payroll, supply vendor payments, rentals and consignments, and other liabilities owed during the shorter term. The ratios most commonly used to calculate liquidity are:

- current ratio
- quick ratio
- days cash on hand

The **current ratio** and **quick ratio** both measure liquidity, using slightly different elements from the balance sheet. The current ratio is calculated by dividing current assets by current liabilities, while the quick ratio is calculated by dividing the liquid assets only by the current liabilities. Using the balance sheet from Exhibit 13.3, we can calculate the liquidity ratio as:

$$\text{Current Ratio} = \text{Current Assets} \div \text{Current Liabilities}$$

$$= \$1,311,911 \div \$1,173,041$$

$$= 1.1184$$

The current ratio result, which is greater than 1, means that the organization can cover 100% of its short-term obligations. For the quick ratio, the liquid assets will include all current assets except the inventory, for the calculation:

$$\text{Quick Ratio} = \text{Liquid Assets} \div \text{Current Liabilities}$$

$$= (\$1,311,911 - \$235,000) \div \$1,173,041$$

$$= \$1,076,911 \div \$1,173,041$$

$$= .9181$$

The quick ratio comes close to covering all of the short-term liabilities, but misses the mark a bit. The company is still able to use all its assets as included in the current ratio but may want to consider an increase to its cash reserves or possibly an increase to patient services revenue to have better quick ratio results. This does not automatically mean issues or concerns with cashflow, but it is an important indicator used by investors. **Days cash on hand** (DCOH) is an estimation of how long an organization could continue to operate by using only its cash. The formula for this calculation is shown in Box 13.6, and can be illustrated using the balance sheet in Exhibit 13.3.

BOX 13.6

Days Cash on Hand

Days Cash on Hand = Cash (including Cash Equivalents) + Short-Term Investments $\div$ [(Operating Expenses – Depreciation)/365 days]

$$\text{DCOH} = (\$756,542 + \$145,369) \div [(\$3,384,091 - \$213,656) / 365 \text{ days}]$$

$$= (\$901,911) \div (\$3,170,435 / 365 \text{ days})$$

$$= \$901,911 \div 8,686.12 \text{ days}$$

$$= 103.83 \text{ days}$$

In this situation, the organization would potentially be able to operate for 103.83 days, or a little over 3 months, before running out of cash. This is a relatively good cash position, because it allows the organization some time to possibly increase revenue and make other impactful financial changes.

Profitability

Profitability ratios analyze an organization's net income, with the ideal scenario being that of revenues exceeding expenses. The key ratios used for profitability analysis are:

- operating margin
- profit margin
- return on assets (ROA)

With the exception of the ROA, which uses the asset figures from the balance sheet, all the profitability ratios use data found on the statement of operations or income statement. Formulas for these ratios are provided in Box 13.7, with shown results calculated using data from the statement of operations in Exhibit 13.3.

BOX 13.7

Profitability Ratios Formulas

Operating Margin = Operating Income ÷ Operating Revenues

Profit Margin = Net Income ÷ Revenue

Return on Assets = Net Income ÷ Total Assets

Operating Margin = Operating Income ÷ Operating Revenues

$\qquad$ = \$1,188,150 ÷ \$4,572,241

$\qquad$ = .2598 or 25.98%

Profit Margin = Net Income ÷ Revenue

$\qquad$ = \$1,131,413 ÷ \$4,572,241

$\qquad$ = .2475 or 24.75%

Return on Assets = Net Income ÷ Total Assets

$\qquad$ = \$1,131,413 ÷ \$12,806,792

$\qquad$ = .0883 or 8.83%

Operating margin measures the operational efficiency of the organization. Generally, an operating margin of 10% to 15% is considered efficient, with much lower operating margins indicating potential issues with expenses. Operating income is the difference between revenues and expenses, so low figures in this portion of the calculation point to higher expenses. As long as revenues exceed expenses, the operating margin will be positive, but may be lower than desired if expenses are uncontrolled.

Profit margin also relies on the revenue for its calculation, but it uses net income instead of operating income. Net income includes nonoperating revenues and expenses, such as investment income, contributions, and marketing expense, as shown on the sample statement of operations in Exhibit 13.3. In this scenario, the healthcare organization has a profit margin of 24.75%, which means that it has fared well. It is not uncommon for smaller organizations or nonprofit organizations to have much lower profit margins.

Return on assets (ROA) measures how efficiently an organization uses its assets to generate revenue. On average, healthcare organizations such as hospitals have an ROA of about 5%. This healthcare organization has an ROA of 8.83%, which means it is potentially performing better than the sector or its competition.

The **DuPont analysis** is another profitability measure that combines multiple ratios to assess profitability and return on equity (ROE). This detailed look at the various ratios shows how the elements are connected and can ultimately improve an organization's financial performance. The DuPont calculation determines profitability or ROE using three ratios: total profit margin, total asset turnover, and equity multiplier. The ratios are calculated using various financial statement elements and can be represented by the equation shown in Box 13.8.

BOX 13.8

The DuPont Analysis Equation

ROE = Total Profit Margin × Total Asset Turnover × Equity Multiplier

ROE = (Net Income ÷ Total Revenue) × (Total Revenue ÷ Total Assets)
    × (Total Assets ÷ Total Equity)

Using the ratios that we have already calculated for total profit margin and total asset turnover, we can fill in a few of the variables in our equation. We use the financial statements from Exhibit 13.3 for the remaining numbers:

$$\text{ROE} = (\text{Net Income} \div \text{Total Revenue}) \times (\text{Total Revenue} \div \text{Total Assets})$$
$$\times (\text{Total Assets} \div \text{Total Equity})$$

$$\$1{,}131{,}413 \div \$9{,}318{,}751 = (\$1{,}131{,}413 \div \$4{,}572{,}241) \times (\$4{,}572{,}241 \div \$12{,}806{,}792)$$
$$\times (\$12{,}806{,}792 \div \$9{,}318{,}751)$$

$$.1214 = .2475 \times .3570 \times 1.3743$$

$$.1214 = .1214$$

$$12.14\%$$

As with any mathematical equation, the left and right sides of the equation must balance. In this DuPont analysis, both sides of the equation total .1214 or 12.14%. Translating the results, the company generates a 12.14% ROE, while effectively managing revenue targets (profit margin), assets (total asset turnover), and debt financing (relatively low equity multiplier).

All of the ratios discussed in this chapter are just select items from a much larger list of available financial and operating ratios. The purpose of ratios and ratio analysis is to provide foundational data for leadership's assessment of their organization's effectiveness and efficiency, and the overall financial resources available to achieve its mission. The data for the ratios is readily available in the routinely prepared financial statements, which makes the results traceable over time. As ratio results are trended, they provide a much larger picture of performance, as organizations strive to remain competitive in local markets and the healthcare sector as a whole.

FORMATIVE EVALUATIONS

The purpose of a **formative evaluation** is to assess the effectiveness and efficiency of the department, program, or initiative of the healthcare organization or the healthcare delivery system within the context of the established processes, procedures, guidelines, and standards. Formative evaluation is a systematic analysis, which includes review of all goals, objectives, and activities that contribute to the anticipated outcomes. Both quantitative and qualitative data are used in the evaluation process to help identify areas needing revision, improvement, or change. Some of the focal points of the analysis include accountability and oversight, program and process improvement, resource allocation, and project or initiative selection—all of which contribute to overall organizational improvement and the effectiveness of the financial management function. Formative evaluation is grounded in the concept of program theory and the activity-flow process. **Program theory** is the modeling process of how a project, initiative, or department workflow begins and ends. The models used in program theory are referred to as **logic models**, which are visual representations of inputs, activities, and outcomes that operationalize an organization's goals and objectives. Program theory and logic models answer the questions: (a) What do we need? (b) How do we get there? (c) What are the results? As the formative evaluation begins, evaluators must have a clear picture of the intended process and outcomes, to use as a benchmark for performance and possible change. The logic model provides a summary of the intended process, as well as identification of major stakeholders. Outcomes of the evaluation will provide clear guidance for leadership, as they determine what should be updated or changed to improve the overall operation of the healthcare organization. Items reviewed during the evaluation should be monitored routinely in efforts to constantly improve such a valuable resource. A sample logic model is shown in Figure 13.1.

Program Evaluation Steps

Program evaluation connects available resources, activities, and outcomes associated with an organizational goal or plan (such as the strategic plan). There are several approaches to program evaluation implementation, but all approaches will include the following steps/stages.

Step 1: Data Collection—Ideally, there are existing measurement metrics or data being collected by the organization. What data to request or utilize will be specific to the program or organization being analyzed and may come from a variety of sources. Different stakeholders may have access to and use different types of data, which should be included if relevant or excluded if not.

Step 2: Data Analysis—The analysis of data collected should include historical data for all relevant areas. Historical data analysis will uncover trends and patterns that may help explain any challenges with the workflow process or desired outcomes. Included in the data analysis is the validity of the data and the determination if it is in fact the correct data to be collected for the specific process or outcome.

Step 3: Summarize Findings and Report Generation—At the conclusion of the evaluation, the results and findings must be summarized in preparation for communication with leadership. The summary should not only include the data used in the evaluation, but the strengths

Figure 13.1

Sample logic model

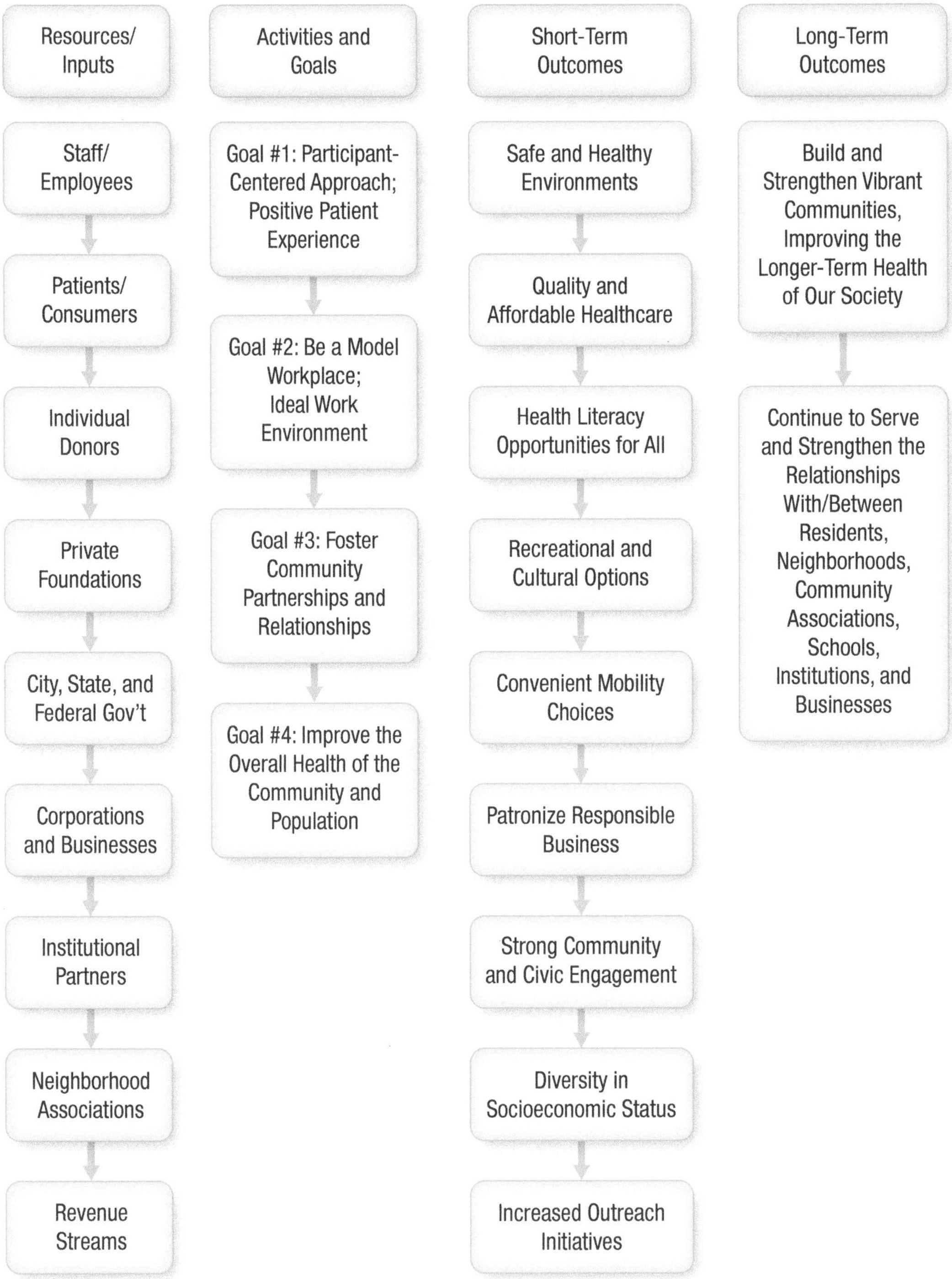

Resources/ Inputs	Activities and Goals	Short-Term Outcomes	Long-Term Outcomes
Staff/ Employees	Goal #1: Participant-Centered Approach; Positive Patient Experience	Safe and Healthy Environments	Build and Strengthen Vibrant Communities, Improving the Longer-Term Health of Our Society
Patients/ Consumers		Quality and Affordable Healthcare	
Individual Donors	Goal #2: Be a Model Workplace; Ideal Work Environment	Health Literacy Opportunities for All	Continue to Serve and Strengthen the Relationships With/Between Residents, Neighborhoods, Community Associations, Schools, Institutions, and Businesses
Private Foundations	Goal #3: Foster Community Partnerships and Relationships	Recreational and Cultural Options	
City, State, and Federal Gov't		Convenient Mobility Choices	
Corporations and Businesses	Goal #4: Improve the Overall Health of the Community and Population	Patronize Responsible Business	
Institutional Partners		Strong Community and Civic Engagement	
Neighborhood Associations		Diversity in Socioeconomic Status	
Revenue Streams		Increased Outreach Initiatives	

and weaknesses of the processes currently in place. Recommendations for moving forward should be a major part of the final report to assist with decision-making and evidence-based change.

Step 4: Report Dissemination—The final report is distributed to the designated stakeholders, as authorized by the organization's leadership. The report may consist of one document or several documents that contain data and findings specific to each stakeholder, area, or function. Communication of the findings should be in layman's terms, as appropriate for the organization and the stakeholders seeking to utilize the information.

In general, the formative evaluation should provide some foundational support for internal governance of the healthcare organization to include routine operations and longer-term planning. This impacts not only how they do business, but the financial health of the organization. Changes to operations and other areas in the healthcare organization may directly impact the information used in key finance department functions such as financial planning and decision-making, resource allocation and capital budgeting, cashflow management, and revenue recognition. The evaluation results should answer the following questions:

- What is the need for the program?
- Is the program relevant?
- Was the structure/logic of the program appropriate?
- Was the program implemented as intended?
- Was the program technically efficient?
- Was the program responsible for the outcomes that actually occurred?
- Did the program achieve its intended objectives?
- Was the program cost effective?
- Was the program cost beneficial?
- Was the program adequate?

The formative evaluation is utilization-focused for most healthcare organizations and must be completed within the contexts of industry constraints and regulations. For example, measurement metrics such as staffing and patient experience must be examined in the context of mandated staff–patient ratios, and not solely based on patient volume and salary expense. The evaluation should in some ways be interactive to ensure the buy-in of stakeholders for analysis and the implementation of subsequent changes. Upon the completion or close of the evaluation, the focus shifts from analysis and interpretation to performance measurement and management, with the ultimate goal being continuous improvement.

CHAPTER SUMMARY

The financial performance of an organization must be monitored and managed to ensure that the healthcare organization is viable and can continue providing important healthcare services to the population. Patient care truly comes first, but that cannot continue to happen for the longer term unless the organization is financially sound. The determination of financial health by variance analysis, ratio analysis, or formative evaluation is crucial for informed decision-making and establishment of benchmarks. The evaluations measure both financial and nonfinancial processes, with the purpose of measuring patient and consumer demand, healthcare service or material item production efficiency, efficient allocation of human and material resources, financial costs, and effectiveness and efficiency. A well-run, well-managed organization will routinely review its processes for identification of areas for improvement, as well as additional ways to achieve its mission.

KEY TERMS FOR REVIEW

asset management	formative evaluation	profitability ratios
change in net assets	inventory turnover ratio	program theory
current ratio	liquidity	quick ratio
days cash on hand	logic model	ratio analysis
debt management	long-term debt to	return on assets
debt ratio	capitalization	total asset turnover
debt service coverage ratio	operating margin	variance analysis
DuPont analysis	profit margin	

DISCUSSION QUESTIONS

1. Explain how the financial health of an organization impacts routine and longer-term operations.
2. Define "variance analysis" and discuss its purpose.
3. What is ratio analysis?
4. How does ratio analysis relate to a healthcare organization's financial statements?
5. Discuss the concept of asset management and the ratios used to support this concept.
6. What is debt management and what ratios are typically used to analyze it?
7. Define the term "liquidity." What are the benefits of "good" liquidity?
8. What information do profitability ratios provide?
9. Explain the formative evaluation process/steps.
10. What is program theory, and how does it relate to formative evaluation?

PRACTICE PROBLEMS

Answers to this chapter's Practice Problems are available via Springer Publishing Connect™ by following the instructions on the opening page of this book and accessing Answers to Practice Problems on the Table of Contents.

1. Perform a basic variance analysis on the line items shown in Exhibit 13.4. Are the variances for these items favorable or unfavorable? Explain your answer.

EXHIBIT 13.4. Variance Analysis Data (Practice Problem 1)

	Actual	Budget
Revenues	$6,492,580	$6,385,998
Expenses	$3,289,671	$3,119,550
Profit (net income)	$3,202,909	$3,266,448

---

2. Perform the revenue, cost, and profit variance analyses for both the simple and flexible budgets provided in Exhibit 13.5. Show the results in dollars and percentages.

EXHIBIT 13.5. Variance Analysis Data (Simple and Flex Budgets)

	Simple Budget	Flexible Budget	Actual
Patient visits	5,500	5,650	5,725
Patient revenue	$2,595,800	$2,595,800	$2,630,800
Salary expense	$785,590	$785,590	$790,000
Supply expense	$250,500	$250,500	$250,000
Profit	$1,559,710	$1,559,710	$1,590,800

For Practice Problems 3 to 7, use the statement of operations and balance sheet for Highland Hospital, shown in Exhibit 13.6.

EXHIBIT 13.6. Highland Hospital Statement of Operations and Balance Sheet

Highland Hospital
Statement of Operations
Year Ending June 30, 2022
(in thousands)

Revenue:	
Original publications	$27,500
Duplicate prints	$5,000
Citations/Royalties	$2,500
Total revenue	$35,000
Expenses:	
Salaries	$10,000

(continued)

EXHIBIT 13.6. Highland Hospital Statement of Operations and Balance Sheet (*continued*)

Printing materials	$3,000
Uncollectables	$100
Machine maintenance	$1,500
Depreciation	$150
Total expenses	$14,750
Net income	$20,250
Net assets (beginning yr.)	$700
Net assets/equity (end yr.)	$20,950

Highland Hospital
Balance Sheet
Year Ending June 30, 2022
(in thousands).

Assets:	
Cash and cash equivalents	$10,000
Printed copies (extras)	$9,000
Supplies	$400
Total current assets	$19,400
Net property and equipment	$7,750
Total assets	$27,150
Liabilities and net assets:	
Accounts payable	$2,000
Accrued expenses	$800
Current debt portion	$150
Total current liabilities	$2,950
Long-term debt	$3,000
Total liabilities	$5,950
Net assets/equity (end yr.)	$21,200
Total liabilities and net assets	$27,150

3. Referencing the Highland Hospital financial statements, calculate total asset turnover.

4. Calculate the operating margin and profit margin for Highland Hospital.

5. What is the ROE for Highland Hospital?

6. Perform a DuPont profitability analysis for Highland Hospital. Is the organization profitable according to the DuPont results?

7. Discuss the overall financial position and financial health of Highland Hospital.

CHAPTER 13 CASE: COMMUNITY HEALTH (OR NONPROFIT) PROGRAM EVALUATION

For this case, you must choose a community health program or nonprofit program on which to perform basic formative program evaluation. Choose a program that you are familiar with, or one that is well-known, with publicly available data. For your write-up of the formative evaluation, the following items must be included:

- community or population needs being satisfied
- available program resources (human, financial, and material)
- list of activities performed
- short-term outcomes
- long-term outcomes
- logic model (refer to Figure 13.1)
- literature review
- executive summary

To complete this assignment, you will have to perform a brief literature search to locate benchmarking data as demonstrated by competition or industry. This will help you make assumptions and offer improvements and suggestions for an organization with limited information. The information may be limited, but most organizations, particularly public ones, will have at least their mission, vision, and values statements online, as well as information on basic financial performance. In your final write-up (executive summary), be sure to answer the evaluation questions as noted in the "Program Evaluation Steps" section of this chapter.

HEALTHCARE FINANCE COURSE PROJECT: FINANCIAL STATEMENT ANALYSIS FOR PHASE III

The third phase of the course project is the creation of the financial statements and financing decisions. For this final phase, students will combine the consolidated financials from Phase II to create a balance sheet, statement of operations, statement of cashflows, and proforma for their healthcare organization. This chapter (Chapter 13) contains formulas and information needed for the creation of Worksheet #17: Performance Measurement and Ratio Analysis. This worksheet is to be drafted after the financial statements have been created to measure the financial performance of the organization and to assist with the decision-making needed for the proforma.

Review the "Course Project: Phase III" section of Chapter 16. All other worksheets in the third phase are to be created by the student using the data calculated in the previous consolidation phase. All worksheets are to be connected to both Phases I and II where applicable. Be sure to review the Microsoft Excel® Reference Guide located in the Appendices as needed.

Resource Management

Human Resources and Labor Management

1. Identify key employment legislation.
2. Discuss the core human resources (HR) functions and the department's role in the organization's strategic planning.
3. Define strategic human resources management (SHRM) and its potential impacts in healthcare.
4. Identify HR challenges that may be unique to healthcare.

INTRODUCTION

The human resources (HR) function in many organizations is responsible for the management of all personnel-related activities. Depending on the size and complexity of the company, this may in fact involve a large number of interrelated processes to keep things running smoothly. The HR department is often the entry point for new employees, as well as a key resource for existing employees with questions about benefits, salary, workplace communications, and the like. Being the organizer of such information is no easy feat, and for a large healthcare organization, the needs of the departments and employees require a great deal of coordination. Over time, the HR function has evolved from a primarily administrative focus to a planning focus, designed to help move the organization forward. In this chapter, we'll examine the key functions of HR and discuss how these functions satisfy the needs of the typical healthcare organization.

HUMAN RESOURCES AND EMPLOYMENT LEGISLATION

Regulations guiding the process of employment as well as the conditions of the workplace have been around for quite some time. Challenges with employee safety, hiring and pay equity, and fairness in ability and opportunity have been key drivers in drafting the legislation that now guides the HR function and the workplace. There have been many laws implemented over the years as guidance to workplace policies and procedures, most of which are still applicable today. For example, the **Civil Rights Act of 1964** was implemented to prohibit discrimination on the basis of race, color, sex, religion, or national origin for public accommodations and federally funded programs (U.S. Department of Labor, n.d.-a). The Act was expanded to include the prohibition of discrimination for voting and hiring practices. The **Occupational Safety and Health Act** (1970) was enacted to reinforce safe working conditions and workplace health standards. This Act holds employers accountable for knowingly exposing employees to hazardous conditions. The **Fair Labor Standards Act** (1938) introduced the minimum wage and overtime pay criteria. A series of amendments to the Act, and the implementation of the **Equal Pay Act** (1963), further expanded the law to eliminate pay disparities based on an employee's sex. The **Rehabilitation Act** (1973) was implemented to prohibit discrimination in the workplace against persons with disabilities. The Act was the foundational legislation to what we now know as the **Americans With Disabilities Act** (1990, 2008), which required accommodations in the workplace as well as public spaces (U.S. Department of Justice Civil Rights Division, 2020). The **Family and Medical Leave Act** (FMLA; 1993) requires employers to guarantee employment and unpaid leave to employees in the event of family medical concerns (U.S. Department of Labor, n.d.-b). The Act guarantees 12 weeks of unpaid leave per year. Other legislation such as the Veterans' Preference Act, Seasonal Worker Protection Act, and the Mine Safety and Health Act provide additional protections in the workplace designed to protect the well-being of employees.

STRATEGIC HUMAN RESOURCES MANAGEMENT

The routine activities of an organization, as well as the decision-making and longer-term planning, are designed to support the organization's goals and mission. There must be a strategy in place to achieve the mission, which should involve the effective and efficient utilization of resources, human and material. The concept of **strategic human resources management** (SHRM) is the application of the organization's strategic plan to the HR functions (Society for Human Resources Management, n.d.). The SHRM methodology supports business strategies by ensuring that the healthcare workforce meets the needs of the organization by receiving proper training, development, and compensation. The activities of SHRM include responsibility of the processes and practices for:

- recruitment and selection,
- training and development,
- performance and retention, and
- compensation and benefits.

HR professionals guide the flow of these processes, but rely heavily on the input and cooperation of the leadership team. The directors, managers, and supervisors throughout the organization provide firsthand information on the requirements for the positions available within their departments, as well as insight on existing employees' performance. SHRM is a partnership between HR professionals and leadership to ensure the right people are in place for the best organizational outcomes. In the healthcare sector, this means the hiring of clinicians, healthcare administration, and management personnel with the education, skills, and credentials required by their respective professions. A detailed look at each of the SHRM processes will further explain the need for this partnership.

Recruitment and Selection

The recruitment and selection process begins with a review of the available position and the related requirements. This **job analysis** is the first step in the recruitment and selection process, providing the foundational information for the role of the prospective employee. An in-depth job analysis identifies the tasks and activities that will be routinely performed, as well as any other responsibilities for the position. Ideally, identification of these items will consider the current and future needs of the department. For example, a department expanding its scope of services may add tasks to the job analysis that will help the department move toward its future state. Outcomes from the job analysis are summarized and included in the official job description used to advertise the available position. The **job description** is the written narrative that explains the details of the position and is shared with those inside and outside of the organization. Company background information, application deadlines, job location, and other basic information may be included in the job description, as HR professionals plan to attract the most qualified candidates. The decision must then be made on whether to fill the position by hiring an internal candidate, or by hiring an external candidate. Professional HR organizations have identified advantages as well as disadvantages for both internal and external candidates, with the most common elements noted in Table 14.1.

Table 14.1

RECRUITMENT ADVANTAGES AND DISADVANTAGES

Recruitment Type	Advantages	Disadvantages
Internal candidate	Lower cost to the organization	More training and development may be required
	Fill the position faster	Creates more positions to back-fill
	Existing knowledge of the organization	Existing knowledge limited by current position
	Positively impact employee morale	Negatively impact employee morale if not chosen
	Opportunities for advancement	Position entitlement
External candidate	No additional training needed (prior experience)	Not developing current employees
	Brings new ideas and expertise to the organization	May have difficulties with the company culture
	Opportunities to build new professional relationships	May have difficult relationships with candidates not chosen
		May lead to additional turnover (and vacant positions)
		Higher pay than some current employees

While every organization is different, there are common advantages and disadvantages to both internal and external recruiting. Cost to the organization, employee satisfaction and morale, skills and training, and compensation all influence the final decision on making an internal or an external hire. Final **selection**, or the process of choosing the ideal candidate, should be done according to skills, abilities, and experience of the candidate, as well as organizational fit.

Training and Development

Training and development of new and existing employees happens on multiple levels within the organization. **Role-specific training** prepares employees for the daily tasks and duties that they are required to perform. Examples of role-specific training are financial software training for a new accountant, or time-out patient safety training for a new surgical technician. **Organizational training,** which is typically required for all employees, provides information on company policies and industry regulations. New employee orientation, company ethics policy, **Health Insurance Portability and Accountability Act** (HIPAA) compliance, and Health and Human Services (HHS) guidelines are examples of required trainings for all employees. Training benefits the employee and the organization by improving productivity, engagement, professional relationships, and, potentially, mission achievement.

The challenge for many organizations is finding the most engaging method for delivery of the training. Some choose multiple modalities for training delivery to accommodate the different learning styles and interests of their employees. **In-person training** is the most traditional approach, with the instructor and employees present in the same workspace. For policy or information sessions, training may take place in a conference room or other basic training space. For procedural or hands-on sessions, training takes place in the actual work environment, like a medical unit or laboratory. The advantage of in-person training is the interaction and communication among colleagues, as well as immediate feedback from the instructor. **Virtual synchronous training** and **videoconferencing** are instructor-led learning sessions that take place at a designated time online. With these modalities, there is immediate feedback from the instructor, but the interaction with colleagues may not be as comfortable as the in-person session. **Asynchronous training** and **e-learning training** sessions rely on internet-based modules and presentations to deliver the information. There is no immediate instructor communication or collaboration with colleagues in these two training delivery methods, since employees take the training at a time convenient to them. In the healthcare sector, the need for training is a concerted effort as healthcare workers provide care in a myriad of settings and environments, with varying shifts (because many organizations have 24-hour operations), in multiple locations.

Performance and Retention

Employee performance and associated performance targets are largely dependent on the role of the employee. While there are some standard expectations such as time and attendance, job-specific performance targets drive the performance appraisal and management processes. A **performance appraisal** is the routine assessment of an employee's performance and progress compared to established goals and targets. Goal setting for performance measurement should include **SMART goals** (specific, measurable, attainable, relevant, and time-bound) and be designed to highlight strengths as well as opportunities for improvement (see Figure 14.1). The SHRM approach to performance moves away from the annual appraisal as the only source of feedback in favor of ongoing mentorship and improvement. This promotes employee growth and fosters a culture of engagement throughout the organization. Performance targets should be measurable and must be applicable to all employees in a specific role. Assessments must not be personal or subjective and should be consistent in measurement.

Ideally, the establishment of expectations and the performance appraisal process is a collaborative effort between the employee and reviewer (HR or management) to ensure that the outcomes are meaningful and beneficial. Performance appraisal outcomes should include clear direction on next steps, required deliverables, and at least a tentative timeline for future discussions and coaching. Coaching, guidance, and mentorship can be formal or informal, and may come from different levels or types of leadership. Line managers may provide guidance on best production practices, or the best time of day to complete a task with minimal interruptions. Mid-level or senior leadership may provide mentorship on professionalism or communication

Figure 14.1

SMART goals for performance

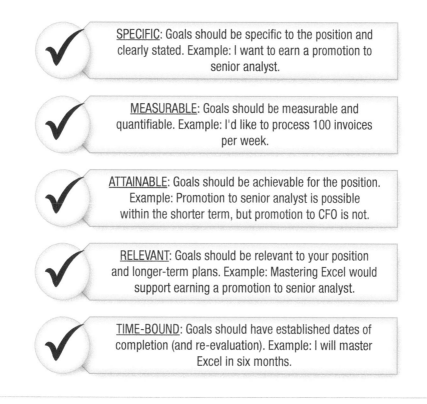

SPECIFIC: Goals should be specific to the position and clearly stated. Example: I want to earn a promotion to senior analyst.

MEASURABLE: Goals should be measurable and quantifiable. Example: I'd like to process 100 invoices per week.

ATTAINABLE: Goals should be achievable for the position. Example: Promotion to senior analyst is possible within the shorter term, but promotion to CFO is not.

RELEVANT: Goals should be relevant to your position and longer-term plans. Example: Mastering Excel would support earning a promotion to senior analyst.

TIME-BOUND: Goals should have established dates of completion (and re-evaluation). Example: I will master Excel in six months.

---

skills needed for the next promotion. Additional training may also be included in the outcomes if skill reinforcement, additional certification, or education is needed for goal achievement. Positive performance outcomes and effective, meaningful communication between the employee and management have a direct impact on employee retention.

Employee retention can be defined as an organization's ability and efforts to keep its employees, minimizing turnover. In healthcare, turnover may directly impact the ability to care for patients, particularly in the clinical and practitioner ranks. SHRM practices begin with identifying the underlying causes of employee turnover and developing strategies to mitigate the issues. SHRM promotes addressing the needs of employees holistically, instead of anecdotally. Common causes for employee turnover include burnout, no work–life balance, low or uncompetitive compensation, toxic company culture, feeling unappreciated, ineffective management, or limited opportunities for growth and advancement. While it is impractical to believe that an employer can meet all of the needs for every employee, there are some basic strategies that organizations can implement to help with employee retention. For example, a company can increase employee engagement efforts, improving the overall culture of the organization. Employee opinion and feedback are important not only for their sense of belonging, but for the knowledge retention and growth of the company. Flexible scheduling and routine analyses of workload and assignment distribution have been used by some organizations to address concerns of burnout and work–life balance. Scheduling changes and flexibility may provide support for the employee beyond the physical workplace. Issues with company culture should be addressed swiftly and decisively. Many organizations have implemented codes of conduct or ethics policies to address issues within company culture, intending to prevent the negative or uncomfortable behaviors from occurring in the first place. Salary surveys and industry position best practices can help ensure competitive pay and clearly defined career paths.

Compensation and Benefits

Compensation is the monetary value of a job or position paid to an employee for job performance. The amount of compensation is determined internally by the organization's budgeted amount and externally by the industry's standard compensation for the role. Adjustments in compensation may also be the result of an employee's qualifications, rank within the job category (e.g., junior manager vs. senior manager), and previous experience. Organizations determine a job's value by performing a **job evaluation**, which gathers all of the relevant data from internal and external sources. Job evaluation methods include:

- job classifications, which consist of pay grades with assigned salary ranges;
- quartile systems, which assign compensation in comparison to market salaries;
- point systems, which award different points for education, skills, and so forth; and
- industry pricing, which assigns compensation based on average industry pay.

Based upon the size and type of organization, as well as the scope of work for the position, variable compensation may be used to incentivize employees. **Variable compensation** is the awarding of pay (or other items of value) for increased performance or to promote fairness. Variable compensation includes items such as bonuses, commissions, or stock shares awarded to individual employees or teams that have contributed to the company's targets. Pay for shift-differential or location-specific pay are additional examples of variable compensation awarded to employees who, for example, may choose the least popular schedule or an undesirable commute.

Benefits, commonly referred to as fringe benefits, are nonsalary items offered to company employees in addition to their base pay. As with the job evaluation for salary determination, the "benefits package" is also assigned a dollar value and, to prospective employees, is often considered as important as the position's salary. Health insurance (including dental, vision, and disability), Social Security payments, unemployment benefits, company leave (vacation, sick, and medical), and retirement plans are examples of benefits employers typically offer as supplemental compensation. Available health plans, coverage options, and premium pricing vary by organization, with final costs based on employee selections. In most cases, new employees will have the opportunity to select benefits coverage at the onset of employment. After the initial year of benefits coverage, existing employees may update or change coverage during the company's **open enrollment period**. This is the annual time frame during which employees can change health plans or other benefits coverage for the next calendar year. Changes outside of the open enrollment period are only granted in the instance of a major lifestyle change, which includes childbirth or adoption, marriage or divorce, death of a covered dependent, or loss of previous coverage.

HUMAN RESOURCES CHALLENGES IN HEALTHCARE

Every sector undoubtedly has its challenges, but there are a few issues that are more prevalent in healthcare. Recruitment, specifically for medical and clinical personnel, has proven to be a challenge for several reasons. Available talent is scarce, as medical schools and clinical training programs have limited slots, producing a limited number of graduates. The cost of medical education and certification is exorbitant, with new graduates opting for the highest paid employment opportunities. The highest paid jobs are rarely in the areas that need healthcare the most, resulting in limited providers and care delivery shortages for underserved and rural populations. To counteract this trend, some federal agencies offer financial incentives (such as loan repayment and signing bonuses) to make these areas more attractive to new graduates. In recent years, the traveling practitioner has become more common, as nurses and others in the industry embrace increased pay for traveling specialists. The pandemic caused an almost immediate shift in demand and HR availability, resulting in lucrative opportunities for those willing to travel to meet the needs of the industry. Work burnout contributed to the growing population of traveling clinicians, as they were able to choose when and where they worked. Larger healthcare systems are attempting to find ways to address the turnover caused by the traveling clinician by creating internal traveling offices or agencies. The organization would have its current staff travel to meet the needs of other organizations in its network, paying a premium or travel rate to the employee. This allows the employee to travel for higher wages and allows the organization to retain the employee (instead of losing them to turnover).

Rapidly changing technology has been a double-edged sword in healthcare, improving the delivery of care for the patient, but requiring additional employee training (and incurred costs). The latest and greatest technology attracts top talent and new consumers, but that technology comes at a cost. The purchase of new technology often requires a sizeable capital budget, and smaller competing organizations may not have the capital. This may also impact recruiting, as new employees prefer to work in healthcare organizations with the latest technology. Integration of the new equipment may require upgrades of other supporting systems, as well as hands-on training for employees on the new systems. This leads to unanticipated expenses that may not have been captured in the budgeting process. Another facet of technology change is the increase in wearable technology and telemedicine. Depending on the specialization of the medical professional, or even their generation, some professionals may not be as tech-savvy as newer graduates. With upgraded systems and tech, some veteran clinicians may be more resistant to change, or may require more training than their counterparts. Technology and innovation move medical practice forward, but increasing costs continue to be a challenge for insurers, patients, and others who rely on healthcare products and services.

CHAPTER SUMMARY

This chapter provides an overview of the HR function and its importance in the development of the organization. Healthcare organizations must hire the appropriate personnel for their clinical functions as well as their managerial functions, with varying levels of education, skill, and workplace knowledge required for each. The demands of healthcare create an intense, high-turnover environment that must be managed for the patient and consumer, as well as for the professionals providing the services. While benefits, and in some instances salary, remain competitive in comparison to other industries, the scope of work, particularly among clinicians and specialists, can be extraordinary, requiring the best tools and equipment in the trade. SHRM will continue to make positive impacts on the healthcare organizations as we strive to remain at the forefront of advancement and retain talented employees while we do.

KEY TERMS FOR REVIEW

Americans With Disabilities Act

asynchronous training

benefits

Civil Rights Act of 1964

compensation

e-learning training

employee retention

Equal Pay Act

Fair Labor Standards Act

Family and Medical Leave Act

Health Insurance Portability and Accountability Act (HIPAA)

in-person training

job analysis

job description

job evaluation

Occupational Safety and Health Act

open enrollment period

organizational training

performance appraisal

Rehabilitation Act

role-specific training

selection

SMART goals

strategic human resources management

variable compensation

videoconferencing

virtual synchronous training

DISCUSSION QUESTIONS

1. Define and discuss the role of SHRM.

2. List and describe five key employment laws.

3. When we discuss work/position redesign, we think of flexibility. List three ways in which a workplace can offer flexibility of schedule.

4. What is the difference between a job evaluation and a job description?

5. What does the acronym FMLA stand for and what is its purpose? What does it guarantee, and what does it not?

6. How do organizations solve the employee retention problem? Provide three examples of strategies and solutions.

7. Discuss at least three different training modalities. Which appears to be the most effective?

8. Define and provide examples of variable compensation.

CHAPTER 14 CASE: REVAMPING THE JOB DESCRIPTION

HR management, often referred to as human capital management, is critical to the success and sustainability of any healthcare organization or system. This case study is designed to give students the opportunity to explore the full range of employee selection and performance measurement activities typically performed by healthcare HR organizations, using a competency-based approach. This approach matches the competencies of the job candidates with the culture, strategy, mission, vision, and values of the organization.

You will complete the case study focusing on one of the following positions (assigned or chosen, at the discretion of the professor):

- healthcare financial analyst
- director of operations
- patient services coordinator
- health information specialist/manager
- administrative assistant (unit clerk)
- emergency room nurse (RN or nurse practitioner)
- surgical technician (any specialty)
- call center manager (insurance or pharmaceutical)
- office manager/practice manager (specifically healthcare)
- chief executive officer (CEO; specifically healthcare)
- supply chain manager
- skilled nursing facility (SNF) or long-term care facility (LTC) administrator

Part I: Job Analysis

1. Collect existing industry information about the assigned position. Locate at least three (3) job descriptions/position postings. Examine and note the similarities and differences.

2. List the tasks for the position (consolidated from all postings). This list may be lengthy, but you'll narrow things down in the next step.

3. Identify the critical tasks.

4. Identify the critical competencies needed to effectively perform the job.

5. Link the critical tasks to the critical competencies.

6. Choose the selection and quality rating factors.

Several templates from the Government's Office of Personnel Management (OPM) are included to help you navigate the job analysis project. This first part of the project is crucial to the successful completion of the other parts of the project, as it lays the foundation for a sound recruiting process and candidate search.

Part II: Job Design

The purpose of the job design is to maximize or enhance organizational efficiencies and employee satisfaction.

1. What tasks should be changed, eliminated, or modified to make the job better for the employee?

2. What tasks should be changed, eliminated, or modified to make the job better for the organization?

Changes/modifications could be based on healthcare industry trends, new or updated technology, or changes in demand or demographics of the patient/consumer population.

Part III: Job Description and Specifications

You may refer to the job descriptions gathered in Part I for layout and formatting guidelines, choosing what you believe to be the best of the three (or combination of them).

1. The job description is the overview of the position, describing the characteristics or basic information: official title, duties, and work site/location. These items should be clear and concise, providing an accurate picture of the position.

2. The job specifications detail the knowledge, skills, and abilities (KSAs) required for the specific job tasks. This includes personal qualities that would be considered for a cultural fit. This is where you sell the company and position! This should make candidates want to apply.

Part IV: Recruitment and Selection

For this part of the project, you'll have to make a few important decisions to get the right candidate:

1. Internal or external hire? For the purposes of this project we'll use external candidates, but real-world scenarios include internal candidates as well.

2. Planning—what's the timeline for the candidate search? Are there budget constraints? What other organizational entities need to be on board and included in the process (payroll, employee health, IT for systems access, etc.)?

3. Sourcing/advertising—what venues will we use to advertise this position (job search engines, professional associations, company website, etc.)?

4. Interviews/Offer—will the candidates interview with the HR representative or department contact? Will there be a second round of interviews? Panel interviews? What's the salary range to keep in mind for the initial offer and/or counteroffer?

5. Onboarding—what are the steps taken to bring the newly hired employee into the organization? What departments/activities need to be scheduled?

Part V: Performance Evaluation/Appraisal

For the final step of the project, develop a performance evaluation form/template for the newly hired candidate. The evaluation must:

1. Focus on the essential tasks and job functions, completely describing each task.

2. Include measures of both quality and quantity, where applicable.

3. Utilize at least a 5-point Likert scale with appropriate weighting (if all tasks aren't weighted equally).

4. Suggest items for professional and career development.

5. Provide space/opportunity for employee feedback.

REFERENCES

Americans With Disabilities Act Ammendments Act of 2008. 122 Stat. 3553 (2008). https://www.govinfo.gov/app/details/STATUTE-122/STATUTE-122-Pg3553

Americans With Disabilities Act of 1990, 42 U.S.C. § 12101 (1990). https://www.ada.gov/pubs/adastatute08.htm

Fair Labor Standards Act, Ch. 676, §1, 52 Stat. 1060 (1938). https://uscode.house.gov/view.xhtml?path=/prelim@title29/chapter8&edition=prelim

Society for Human Resources Management. (n.d.). *Practicing strategic human resources management*. Retrieved February 22, 2023, from https://www.shrm.org/resourcesandtools/tools-and-samples/toolkits/pages/practicingstrategichumanresources.aspx

U.S. Department of Justice Civil Rights Division. (2020, February 28). *Guide to disability rights laws*. https://www.ada.gov/resources/disability-rights-guide

U.S. Department of Labor. (n.d.-a). *Legal highlight: The Civil Rights Act of 1964*. https://www.dol.gov/agencies/oasam/civil-rights-center/statutes/civil-rights-act-of-1964#:~:text=The%20Civil%20Rights%20Act%20of%201964%20prohibits%20discrimination%20on%20the,hiring%2C%20promoting%2C%20and%20firing

U.S. Department of Labor. (n.d.-b). *Summary of the major laws of the Department of Labor*. https://www.dol.gov/general/aboutdol/majorlaws

Healthcare Supply Chain Management

1. Understand the basics of supply chain management (SCM).
2. Explore qualitative and quantitative historical data analysis.
3. Define the various inventory management techniques.
4. Detail associated inventory costs and the impacts on an organization's financials.

INTRODUCTION

The concept of **supply chain management** (SCM) is built on theories of economic efficiency and has been applied to industries worldwide. It has been particularly useful in high volume areas, where high demand meets the need for the constant managing of costs. Healthcare, being a very large and complex sector, requires a host of support teams and materials to keep things running smoothly, all while attempting to control costs. Coordinating these supporting efforts is challenging, with activities interconnected throughout the system. Providers are at the forefront of patient care and healthcare service provision, connected to others through the supplies, materials, and machines used for diagnosis and treatment support. The process of creating and supplying these items to the hospitals, physicians' offices, and other healthcare facilities must be well organized, reliable, timely, cost effective, and flexible. This is where the SCM best practices are applied. In this chapter, we'll explore the basics of SCM and discuss how these concepts have been implemented into healthcare operations. A high-level review of demand and inventory management is included as we connect the ideas of supply, control, and efficiency.

WHAT IS THE SUPPLY CHAIN?

The **supply chain** is the manufacturing and distribution process from raw materials to the final sale of goods and services. The supply chain includes all parties involved in meeting the customer's needs (customers can be both internal and/or external). For healthcare, this means producers of medical supplies, pharmaceuticals, and large-scale medical equipment, to sales and consumption by the consumer (usage in hospitals, retail pharmacies, home care, etc.). The goal of the supply chain, as with most other healthcare initiatives, is to provide the highest quality care or service, according to organizational specifications, at the least possible cost—the maximization of value. The collaborative efforts of all included in the healthcare supply chain (see Figure 15.1) play an important role in the creation of value.

Figure 15.1

The healthcare supply chain

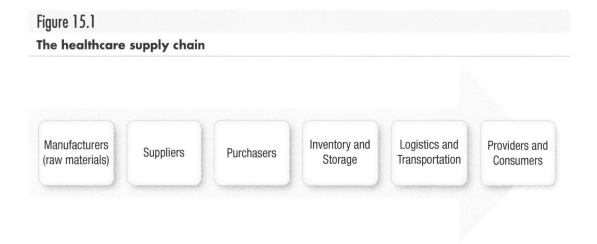

Manufacturers begin the supply chain with the processing of raw materials used in the creation of healthcare goods. All tangible supplies and equipment are comprised of base elements or some combination of base elements—plastics, metals, composites, and so forth, are all used to create the items used in the delivery or support of patient care. Suppliers buy the manufactured goods to meet the demand of consumers in the healthcare supply chain. Suppliers sell the items bought from manufacturers to members of multiple supply chains, especially those items that are universal and used by most in healthcare (bandages, gauze, etc.). Purchasers buy goods in bulk in most cases, then parcel the items out as ordered throughout the network. As with suppliers, purchasers can be members of multiple supply chains and networks, maximizing resources and purchasing power. Inventory and storage is the next link in the supply chain, as purchasers decide where and how to store their acquired items. This is highly dependent upon the needs and requirements of the last two pieces of the chain: logistics and consumers. Consumers with a high turnover of supplies will require orders and deliveries more frequently. The frequency will often determine the type of transportation used as well as the location of the storage facility. Providers and consumers who use the healthcare products in direct care may opt for storing a portion of the inventory in their own storage facilities for ease of access and reduced delivery or wait times. Managing this process takes a great deal of planning and coordination, as well as the decision on the types of inventory management methods that work best. **Supply chain length** is one of the key performance measures used to analyze the efficiency of a supply chain. Shorter supply chains are considered more efficient than longer supply chains. Shorter supply chains often have fewer "middle men" and have a more direct relationship with the consumer. They often have decreased delivery times and can get the end products delivered to the consumer faster. Supply chain length is measured in days, and is calculated using the three inputs shown in Box 15.1.

BOX 15.1

Supply Chain Length

$$\text{Length (in Days)} = \text{DRM1} + \text{DWIP2} + \text{DFG3}$$

1. DRM = Day of Raw Materials
   = Raw Materials Inventory × (365 / Cost of Raw Materials)

2. DWIP = Days of Work in Progress
   = Semi-Finished Goods × (365 / Cost of Production)

3. DFG = Days of Finished Goods
   = Finished Goods Inventory × (365 / Cost of Sales)

INVENTORY MANAGEMENT METHODS

Supply expense in healthcare is second only to labor and wage expenses incurred by healthcare organizations. **Inventory management** is the ordering, procurement, utilization, and recordkeeping of a healthcare organization's purchased goods. Those responsible for the inventory management portion of the healthcare system work to ensure: (a) responsiveness to consumer needs, (b) efficient ordering and delivery times, (c) workflow (and partnership) reliability, and (d) availability of the needed products. There are several methods utilized for inventory management, as shown in Table 15.1, with the chosen methods being specific to the organization and its functions.

Table 15.1

INVENTORY MANAGEMENT METHODS

Inventory Management Method	Method Description
Base stock	Inventory held onsite/in-house to meet the expected routine utilization. Example: bandages, alcohol, gloves
Safety stock	Amount of inventory kept above the base stock to avoid shortages. Example: extra items stored in case of delivery delays
Just-in-time	Inventory received when needed, not far in advance of scheduled usage. Example: implants delivered the morning of surgery
Stockless	Inventory items/supplies ordered and delivered at the time of use, stocked by the supplier. Example: items delivered directly to the departments or medical units
Consignment	Inventory items owned by the supplier, borrowed by the consumer. Example: borrowed surgical instruments for unanticipated emergency volume

Most healthcare organizations maintain some type of **base stock**, or routine supplies used for every patient or consumer interaction. Base stock in a physician's office would be examination gloves, bandages, cotton swabs, or any other medical supply used for just about every patient.

Examples of base stock in a pharmacy would be prescription bottles or syringes used for immunizations. **Safety stock** builds on base stock by keeping a few additional items to avoid running out. These items would be the high-volume supplies included in the base stock, kept at a level to last until the next scheduled order or delivery. The **just-in-time** inventory system delivers the needed supply as close to the time of utilization as possible. This method of inventory management is best used for planned, scheduled utilization, instead of high-volume or emergency items. A scheduled knee replacement could use the just-in-time method, but items needed for daily operation of the emergency department would not benefit from such a system. The **stockless** inventory system skips on-site storage completely and delivers the requested items directly to the medical unit or department. This is common with emergency departments that have extremely high volume and supply turnover, and simply can't wait for what may be a lengthy supply replenishment process. The **consignment** inventory method leaves ownership of the supply item with the supplier, while the consumer borrows it for use. This arrangement is seen quite frequently in situations where the borrowed item is expensive and only needed for a limited time. An example of this would be surgical instrument kits, which typically cost thousands of dollars each. A local disaster may require several emergent life-saving surgeries, and a facility may not have enough to satisfy this short-term need. They would borrow the surgical instruments on consignment, then return the items to the supplier upon completion of the surgeries. Although these methods can be implemented as stand-alone processes, they are often used in some combination to manage the different types of supplies used within the organization. Scheduled surgical services, for example, may use all of these methods at some point, while a typical lower acuity inpatient unit would rely more on the base stock and safety stock methods.

THE IMPORTANCE OF DEMAND

The purpose of the supply chain is to provide the healthcare goods needed (and wanted) by providers. For that to happen effectively, supply chain managers must have an idea of what the providers are requesting and what the healthcare sector needs: the demand. **Demand** (in economic terms) is the desire of a consumer to purchase a particular good or service. As applied to the healthcare SCM process, this means the goods or supplies that providers and other healthcare consumers want to buy. The challenge is determining exactly how much of each item to buy at a given price point. Some healthcare systems (with adequate resources) have secured specialized software systems to appropriately manage their supply chain functions. The systems are often integrated into the organization's Enterprise Resource Planning (ERP) systems, as well as the general ledger, to meticulously track each transaction relative to supply and inventory purchases. Analyzing demand and supply chain activities helps to answer the following important questions:

- How much of an item to order?
- When to place the order?
- Are there carrying costs associated with the inventory?
- How do we adjust for the variations in product life cycle?
- Do we need changes in delivery or transportation terms?

The quantity of an item ordered is dependent upon the organization's utilization and the type of inventory management method used. Base stock and safety stock both usually have a targeted supply amount to maintain, but just-in-time, stockless, and consignment methods may not have a targeted amount or routine order quantity. The timing of when to place the order is determined by an established reorder point. The **reorder point** is the designated level of the supplies that prompts an automatic order or restock. Reorder points are typically implemented with base stock and safety stock methods. **Carrying costs** are the costs incurred by an organization for storing and maintaining an inventory. Carrying costs and the organization's ability to absorb it directly influence the decision on what type of method to use. Organizations with owned storage space may incur fewer costs than those needed to rent space or those outsourcing the SCM function. The **product life cycle** is the time frame from initial purchase through the product's expiration date or required replacement. Items such as medicines, laboratory reagents, or medical solutions all have expiration dates, at which point they are no longer usable. Proper inventory management tracks the dates of such items to ensure they are used before they expire (before sold, resulting in lost revenue). Some items may not have a specific expiration date but may be replaced by the latest version, rendering the initial item without value. The answers to all of these questions point to possible changes in delivery or transportation terms, as the needs of the organization and the demands of the consumers change. To further explore the financial implications of SCM, we can examine some basic calculations that most healthcare organizations use in their inventory decision-making.

Forecasting Demand

As the foundational element of SCM, demand must be properly estimated at the beginning and at critical points throughout the process. The forecasting or prediction of demand involves the interpretation of both qualitative and quantitative data, and the calculation of several indicators for demand adjustments. *Qualitative* measures include the Delphi method and the market research method, both of which are used with quantitative methods. The **Delphi method** of forecasting demand uses industry experts to predict the parameters and outcomes for the organization's supply chain. This team of consultants relies on the best practices of SCM to suggest demand levels and associated inventory management methodologies. The **market research** approach to demand forecasting analyzes the organization's demand and inventory practices in the context of current industry competition. While both of these qualitative methods are useful, they are rarely used as stand-alone forecasting methods. A great deal of consideration must be given to the actual performance of the organization before the adoption of industry or competitor approaches. The *quantitative* demand forecasting methods rely on historical data for prediction of future supply chain performance. Several of these methods require complex statistical analyses that are best done using statistical software packages or programmed modules in the SCM software system, but some of the basic calculations can be done using Microsoft Excel® or a standard financial calculator.

Descriptive analytics or descriptive statistics is often the first step in quantitative demand forecasting. **Descriptive analytics** is a statistical summation of the historical data, highlighting the main characteristics or categories of the collected information. Descriptive analytics answer the basic questions of "How many do we have?" and "What types do we have?" without determining specifics to be applied to future data. An example of descriptive analytics routinely performed in the finance department would be the calculation of payer mix or the aging schedule. For supply chain data, descriptives would summarize the item count and size of a particular medical supply, or possibly summarize the item count of a supply from various vendors. To illustrate a supply chain related example, we can review the data presented in Table 15.2.

The data in Table 15.2 show a list of bandage orders for 1 month, containing vendor, item, and pricing information. There are several ways to summarize the data, which could be

Table 15.2

SUPPLY VENDOR DATA

Vendor	Order No.	Item Desc.	Quantity	Unit Price	Total Price
Coastal Supply	1	Small bandages	25	$12.99	$324.75
MedEx	2	Medium bandages	50	$16.25	$812.50
State Medical	3	Large bandages	50	$21.50	$1,075.00
State Medical	4	Small bandages	30	$13.95	$418.50
MedEx	5	Medium bandages	55	$16.25	$893.75
MedEx	6	Large bandages	65	$22.25	$1,446.25
Coastal Supply	7	Small bandages	28	$12.99	$363.72
Coastal Supply	8	Medium bandages	53	$15.99	$847.47
Coastal Supply	9	Large bandages	56	$19.99	$1,119.44
State Medical	10	Large bandages	55	$21.50	$1,182.50

represented as basic calculations or graphically (possibly for a dashboard or executive report). Descriptive analytics for this data highlight a few key summary points:

- Number of supply orders: 10

- Vendor summary statistics: Coastal Supply has 40% of the month's orders, MedEx has 30% of the month's orders, and State Medical has 30% of the month's orders.

- Item description statistics: Small bandages make up 30% of the bandage orders, medium bandages make up 30% of the bandage orders, and large bandages make up 40% of the bandage orders.

The data contain a total of 10 individual bandage orders from three different vendors. Coastal Supply has the most orders with four of 10 (or 40%), while MedEx and State Medical have three orders each. When reviewing the item description data, we can determine that most of the bandage orders were for large bandages, which comprise 40% of the orders (four of 10), with small bandages and medium bandages making up 30% each of the total orders. These basic calculations give a basic summary of the supply order data presented. Additional calculations can be performed on the price data, which can be shown numerically, like the vendor and item description data, or graphically, as shown in Figure 15.2.

In Figure 15.2, we see just two possible visual representations of total price by vendor. The first graph shows vendors as a percentage of the total price, which is $8,483.88. Coastal Supply contributes 31% (rounded) of the total price ($2,655.38 / $8,483.88 = .3129), MedEx contributes 37%, and State Medical contributes 32%. The second graph shows vendor contributions as dollar amounts instead of percentages, summarizing the dollar amounts for each vendor's orders. Coastal Supply orders total $2,655.38 (the sum of $324.75, $363.72, $847.47, and $1,119.44), MedEx totals $3,152.52, and State Medical totals $2,676.00. Data chosen for the calculations or the graphs are determined by those performing the analysis and the items/categories being analyzed.

Another type of descriptive measure used for quantitative analysis is central tendency. **Central tendency** is a method that describes individual data points in relation to an entire data set. The most common central tendency calculations are mean, median, and mode. The **mean** is the mathematical average of a set of data. The **median** is the number that sits in the middle of the

Figure 15.2

Total price by vendor

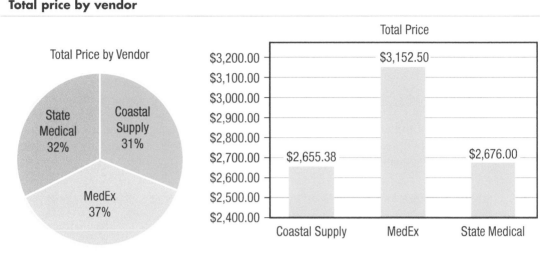

data set. The **mode** of a data set is the number or data point with the highest frequency. These concepts can be illustrated using the data shown in Table 15.3.

Table 15.3

CENTRAL TENDENCY DATA SET

Patient	Age	Patient	Age
1	25	21	22
2	31	22	25
3	28	23	30
4	35	24	37
5	22	25	41
6	38	26	33
7	41	27	29
8	40	28	27
9	22	29	34
10	26	30	35
11	27	31	23
12	34	32	23
13	24	33	28
14	33	34	39
15	35	35	21
16	39	36	25
17	32	37	22
18	30	38	31
19	21	39	27
20	23	40	32

The information in Table 15.3 shows the ages of 40 patients. To calculate the mean, or mathematical average of the patient ages, we add up all of the patients' ages and divide by the number of patients.

mean = Sum of All Ages ÷ Number of Patients

mean = 1,190 ÷ 40

mean = 29.75

The calculation of the mean uses the data in the existing sequence, while the determination of the median requires the reordering of the data (Table 15.4). When the list of ages is reordered, the ages range from 21 years to 41 years.

Table 15.4

CENTRAL TENDENCY DATA SET REORDERED

Patient	Age	Patient	Age
1	21	21	30
2	21	22	30
3	22	23	31
4	22	24	31
5	22	25	32
6	22	26	32
7	23	27	33
8	23	28	33
9	23	29	34
10	24	30	34
11	25	31	35
12	25	32	35
13	25	33	35
14	26	34	37
15	27	35	38
16	27	36	39
17	27	37	39
18	28	38	40
19	28	39	41
20	29	40	41

The median identifies the number in the middle of a data set, and since this list of patient ages represents an even number of patients (40 patients), there is no one age located in the middle of the list. In situations such as this, the median will be calculated by taking the average of the two middle numbers (29 and 30), for a median patient age of 29.5. Using this reordered data set, we can also identify the mode, which is the number with the highest frequency—in this case, the patient age that appears the most. Looking at the list of ages, we can see that the mode in the range of patient ages is 22 years. Together, these three measures of central tendency provide a concise summary of the patient age data set.

Time-Series Analysis and Moving Averages

There are many factors that can impact inventory ordering, utilization, and product pricing, with some resulting changes being more routine than others. Analysis of an organization's historical data is an important part of demand forecasting, which identifies trends, patterns, seasonality, and changes in actual performance. One of the most common approaches to historical data analysis is time-series analysis. **Time-series analysis** in supply chain and inventory management uses data from a previous time frame to estimate future demand. Time-series data include prior ordering, pricing, sales, and utilization data to determine what vendor and ordering activity a company should move forward with. If a small neighborhood clinic typically orders 25 boxes of flu tests per month at a price of $75 per box, the monthly price would be $1,875. When reviewing the clinic's historical data, the supply analyst notices fluctuations in the data. To illustrate a very basic example of this, we use the summary data shown in Table 15.5.

Table 15.5

MONTHLY SALES DATA

Month	Number of Orders	Total Price
January	27	$2,329
February	31	$2,674
March	25	$1,875
April	25	$1,875
May	25	$1,875
June	25	$1,875
July	25	$1,875
August	25	$1,875
September	25	$1,875
October	25	$1,875
November	27	$2,329
December	30	$2,588

In this example, we can see that March through October reflects 25 orders per month, with the price for each month of $1,875. The months of November through February, however, show an increase in the number of orders as well as the monthly prices. These variations represent seasonality as the clinic experiences flu season, with increased boxes ordered as well as a 15% increase in vendor cost per box. During flu season, vendors charged $86.25 per box instead of the $75 charges during non-flu months. Identifying the seasonality in the data will inform the demand forecast for next year, which should include some type of adjustment for the anticipation of flu season. Analysis of historical data can also be done by calculating the **moving average** of the data, creating subsets of smaller time frames and identifying trends in the data. Using the original sales data from Table 15.5, Figure 15.3 illustrates how the moving average is calculated.

Figure 15.3

Moving average calculation

Month	Number of Orders	Moving	Average
January	27		
February	31		
March	25	27.67	(Jan - Mar)
April	25	27.00	(Feb - Apr)
May	25	25.00	(Mar - May)
June	25	25.00	(Apr - Jun)
July	25	25.00	(May - Jul)
August	25	25.00	(Jun - Aug)
September	25	25.00	(Jul - Sep)
October	25	25.00	(Aug - Oct)
November	27	25.67	(Sep - Nov)
December	30	27.33	(Oct - Dec)

Using this data, we begin the moving average calculation with the first 3 months, calculating the average orders for January through March by summing the number of orders and then dividing by the number of months ($27 + 31 + 25 = 83$; $83 / 3 = 27.67$). We then "move" the 3-month average to include the next 3 months, which would be February through April. Following the same calculation, we calculate the new moving average as: $31 + 25 + 25 = 81$, $81 / 3 = 27.0$. Moving averages is just another way of capturing seasonality or fluctuations in historical data.

Today's inventory management systems have the ability to capture and analyze large amounts of data. These systems can be customized to include data specific to an organization or industry, and can be integrated into other operating or financial systems. Integration allows healthcare organizations to have SCM activities recorded accurately and in a timely fashion in the financial systems (general ledger and financial statements), based on appropriate inventory levels and ordering practices.

FINANCIAL IMPLICATIONS

The function of SCM may not fall solely on the finance department, but the financial impacts directly tie to the healthcare organization's financial performance. The costs incurred for the operation of the supply chain, as well as the prices paid for the actual supplies and goods, impact the bottom line, as do the stocking and storage of the purchased items. Costs incurred for storage of inventory are referred to as carrying costs. Carrying costs are calculated to reflect the cost of total inventory storage, but may also be calculated to show costs of specific items or items held at a specific location. As an example, let's review the scenario in Box 15.2.

In this scenario, the clinics are paying almost one quarter of the inventory's value in storage costs. The carrying costs are incurred by each clinic until the supplies are utilized or sold; therefore, to minimize costs and maintain (or increase) profits, the clinics and Regional Health System (RHS) would want to utilize/sell the products and supplies quickly. The amount of

BOX 15.2

Regional Health System Carrying Costs

Regional Health System (RHS) is a large system with five community clinics. RHS maintains a central warehouse, which stores all of the medical equipment and supplies for the system. To accurately show expense contributions for each of the clinics, RHS decides to charge each clinic for a portion of the incurred supply chain expense. To calculate the monthly carrying cost percentage for each clinic, RHS includes these items:

Warehouse space rental: $7,000
Warehouse labor: $20,000
Logistics/Transportation: $4,000
Cost of goods (sales price): $125,000
Carrying Cost (%) = (Costs Incurred ÷ Cost of Goods)
= ($31,000 ÷ $125,000)
= .248 or 24.8%

carrying costs influences inventory management method decisions, as healthcare organizations determine how they will store purchased items (stocked, just-in-time, stockless, or consignment).

CHAPTER SUMMARY

This chapter highlights only a few of the important factors in healthcare SCM. As healthcare delivery continues to expand its services, so must the availability of the supplies and products that support it. Research, development, and technological advancements improve the function of some products and often shorten the life span of others. The supply chain must be adaptive and efficient, while helping providers maintain the highest level of healthcare quality. As healthcare costs continue to increase, strategies such as volume pricing and streamlining of supply lists are more important than ever. Supply needs and inventory management methods vary by organization, but quality, cost savings, and improved operating efficiencies will continue to be among the common elements in healthcare delivery.

KEY TERMS FOR REVIEW

base stock	just-in-time	safety stock
carrying costs	market research	stockless
central tendency	mean	supply chain
consignment	median	supply chain length
Delphi method	mode	supply chain management
demand	moving average	time-series analysis
descriptive analytics	product life cycle	
inventory management	reorder point	

DISCUSSION QUESTIONS

1. Define SCM. How is it different from inventory management?
2. List and discuss the inventory management methods presented in the chapter.
3. What is descriptive analytics?
4. Identify the three main types of central tendency. How are they calculated?
5. How can carrying costs impact an organization's financial position?
6. When it comes to supply chain length, what length is best? Explain your answer.
7. Discuss how the product life cycle influences SCM activities.

PRACTICE PROBLEMS

Answers to this chapter's Practice Problems are available via Springer Publishing Connect™ by following the instructions on the opening page of this book and accessing Answers to Practice Problems on the Table of Contents.

1. A company would like to further hone its business model by forecasting demand for its other healthcare services. They plan to use the moving average approach, using three quarters for each of the moving average calculations. Complete the moving averages in Table 15.6.

Table 15.6

MOVING AVERAGES DATA

Time (Quarter)	Demand (Actual)	Moving Averages
1	222	
2	261	
3	263	
4	187	
5	346	
6	288	
7	298	
8	318	
9	494	
10	456	
11	420	
12	533	
13	494	
14	565	
15	586	
16	579	
17	577	
18	577	
19	577	
20	577	

2. Using the supply ordering information presented in Table 15.7, calculate the descriptive analytics for vendor, supply item, and price data (calculations only).

Table 15.7

DESCRIPTIVE ANALYTICS DATA

Vendor	Order No.	Item Desc.	Quantity	Unit Price	Total Price
East Medical Supply	1	5 mL syringes	100	$6.99	$699.00
West Medical Supply	2	10 mL syringes	150	$15.99	$2,398.50
East Medical Supply	3	20 mL syringes	200	$19.99	$3,998.00
East Medical Supply	4	20 mL syringes	150	$19.99	$2,998.50
West Medical Supply	5	5 mL syringes	100	$15.99	$1,599.00
Central Medical Supply	6	20 mL syringes	75	$22.99	$1,724.25
West Medical Supply	7	5 mL syringes	75	$7.99	$599.25
Central Medical Supply	8	10 mL syringes	50	$16.99	$849.50
Central Medical Supply	9	5 mL syringes	25	$8.99	$224.75
West Medical Supply	10	10 mL syringes	125	$15.99	$1,998.75
West Medical Supply	11	20 mL syringes	125	$20.99	$2,623.75
East Medical Supply	12	20 mL syringes	100	$19.99	$1,999.00
East Medical Supply	13	20 mL syringes	200	$19.99	$3,998.00
East Medical Supply	14	5 mL syringes	75	$6.99	$524.25
Central Medical Supply	15	5 mL syringes	150	$8.99	$1,348.50

3. Using the supply ordering information presented in Table 15.7, calculate the descriptive analytics for vendor, supply item, and price data (graphs only).

4. Calculate the central tendency measures for the patient wait times shown in Table 15.8.

Table 15.8

PATIENT WAIT TIMES DATA

Patient	Wait Time (Minutes)
1	15
2	10
3	15
4	12
5	10
6	10
7	7
8	17
9	15

(continued)

Table 15.8	
PATIENT WAIT TIMES DATA (_continued_)	
Patient	Wait Time (Minutes)
10	20
11	13
12	11
13	10
14	15
15	20

5. Refer to Table 15.5. Increase the monthly order volume to reflect a 3% increase in order volume and a 5% increase in price (for inflation). What are the new totals for the months? Calculate the updated 3-month moving averages.

CHAPTER 15 CASE: HISTORICAL DATA ANALYSIS (FOR SUPPLY CHAIN MANAGEMENT)

In 2021, the Centers for Medicare & Medicaid Services (CMS) expanded their imaging payment coverage for cancer patients. Family View is considering the implementation of PET scans for its growing cancer patient population, and to hopefully boost their revenue. It already offers MRI and CT scans, but this new service will require a list of equipment and storage facilities to accommodate the increased volume of patients. The financial analysis team must estimate the impacts of the new service line and determine its feasibility for the organization. Demand for next year's imaging services are provided in Table 15.9. Using the data presented in Table 15.9, estimate:

1. Total supply costs per month, if imaging supply costs are $155 per procedure.

2. Percentage contribution of the new PET scan services to total imaging services (monthly and total/annual calculations).

3. Additional warehouse/storage labor expense for new personnel:
   inventory manager @ $60.00 per hour (1 full-time equivalent [FTE])
   data analyst @ $50.00 per hour (1 FTE)
   inventory clerks @ $25.00 per hour (3 FTEs)

4. Carrying costs to include labor costs and the following expenses:
   additional warehouse space rental: $10,000
   transportation/delivery: $2,000
   cost of goods: $100,000

Table 15.9

FAMILY VIEW IMAGING DATA

	January	February	March	April	May	June	July	August	September	October	November	December	Total
CT	2,110	2,047	1,985	1,926	2,099	2,288	2,494	2,369	2,251	2,138	2,395	2,682	**26,784**
MRI	1,496	1,496	1,663	1,496	1,496	1,663	1,496	1,496	1,663	1,496	1,496	1,663	**18,620**
PET	3,970	3,851	3,735	3,623	3,949	4,305	4,692	4,458	4,235	4,023	4,506	5,047	**50,394**
Total	**7,576**	**7,394**	**7,383**	**7,045**	**7,544**	**8,256**	**8,682**	**8,323**	**8,149**	**7,657**	**8,397**	**9,392**	**95,798**

Course Project: SurgiFlex Robotic Surgery System

OBJECTIVES

1. Explain how costs of healthcare services are categorized.

2. Understand fundamental principles, concepts, generalizations, theories, and models of healthcare financial management.

3. Perform basic budgeting tasks for healthcare organizations.

4. Analyze and explain the content of financial statements and financial ratios for healthcare organizations.

5. Apply financial management concepts to a case study for problem diagnosis, problem-solving, and decision-making.

6. Demonstrate improved spreadsheet calculation skills.

COURSE PROJECT: AN INTRODUCTION

The SurgiFlex Robotic Surgery System was purchased by your hospital. It was an expensive capital purchase ($3.5 million) and hospital executives aren't totally convinced it was worth it. They have asked you to compile and present data for the first year of operation (fiscal year ending in June) to help them determine whether they'll keep the SurgiFlex Robotic Surgery System moving forward or liquidate it and eliminate the robotic surgery service line.

The financial analysis workbook you will create over the semester includes standard operating and financial data, as well as SurgiFlex-specific information. The data listed in this chapter is to be used for the various calculations throughout the financial analysis workbook and referenced in the business plan portion of the project. There will be several additional calculations that you must perform to complete the workbook. The SurgiFlex Financial Analysis project is comprised of three phases of work, with specific requirements and inclusions for each phase.

COURSE PROJECT: EXCEL WORKBOOK SETUP

Step 1: To begin the course project, you must create the Microsoft Excel® workbook that will contain all of the calculations for the course project. Select a name for your healthcare organization.

Suggested nomenclature for your workbook is to begin with your last name, followed by the name of your hospital/healthcare organization (Smith—Lakeside Research Hospital).

Step 2: To set up your workbook, you must create and label the following worksheets which cover the assignments for the duration of the project. The worksheet tabs hold a limited number of characters so the names of each will have to be abbreviated.

- Worksheet #1—SurgiFlex Operating Data (Surgical Case Volume)
- Worksheet #2—SurgiFlex Salary and Wage Calculations
- Worksheet #3—SurgiFlex Revenue Calculations
- Worksheet #4—SurgiFlex Nonsalary Expense Calculations
- Worksheet #5—SurgiFlex Breakeven Calculations
- Worksheet #6—SurgiFlex Supply Vendor Analysis Calculations
- Worksheet #7—Consolidated Operating/Utilization Data
- Worksheet #8—Consolidated Salary and Wage Calculations
- Worksheet #9—Consolidated Revenue Calculations
- Worksheet #10—Consolidated Nonsalary Expense Calculations
- Worksheet #11—Master Supply List
- Worksheet #12—Balance Sheet
- Worksheet #13—Statement of Operations
- Worksheet #14—Statement of Cashflows
- Worksheet #15—Proforma Statement
- Worksheet #16—Financing Options Comparison
- Worksheet #17—Performance Measurement and Ratio Analysis
- Worksheet #18—Dashboards (Graphs and Visual Elements)

Step 3: Create a worksheet heading/title block for each worksheet in your workbook. All financial worksheets must include: (a) the organization's name, (b) the worksheet's title, and (c) the fiscal year or financial period covered by it. (For additional examples, refer to the financial statement discussions in Chapter 6.)

COURSE PROJECT: PHASE I: SURGIFLEX ROBOTIC SURGERY SYSTEM CALCULATIONS

Now that you have set things up, you can start completing the worksheets (noted in the previous list) with the relevant calculations. Use the following information to draft your worksheets.

Worksheet #1: SurgiFlex Operating Data: To begin the calculations for Phase I of the course project, create this worksheet using the data and format shown in Exhibit 16A.1 (see Chapter 16 Appendix, Exhibit 16A.1). The operating data in the worksheet represents the surgical case volume for our SurgiFlex system. Patients and consumers, and in this instance surgical case volume, drive the healthcare organization and launch the healthcare finance functions. On this starting worksheet, column headings include: (a) the category, (b) the months of the fiscal year covered, and (c) the annual total for the fiscal year.

- **Categories:** The categories on each worksheet represent the various elements or variables used in the calculations for that sheet. Worksheet #1 includes categories reflecting the types of surgeries performed by the SurgiFlex System (single surgeries and double surgeries). Each variable is to be entered on a separate row, with monthly totals (each column), variable annual totals (each row), and grand totals required for each worksheet.

- **Fiscal year months:** The months for the fiscal year covered for the project and in the accompanying worksheets are for July 2021 through June 2022. The time frame can be adapted based on student or instructor preferences.

- **Annual total:** Each line item or variable contained within the worksheets should have an annual total summarizing the 12 months of activity. Each sheet should also have a grand total.

Worksheet #2: SurgiFlex Salary and Wage Calculations: For each SurgiFlex surgical case type (single surgeries and double surgeries), you must perform workload calculations to estimate the salary and wage expense for this surgical service. As with many healthcare procedures, care is provided by a team of clinical professionals, each with varying roles and wage rates. Although many are salaried, the course project uses hourly wage rates to convey the understanding of basic wage and benefits calculations. For each surgical case, the SurgiFlex clinical team includes the personnel noted in Table 16.1 at the noted hourly rates.

Table 16.1

SURGIFLEX SURGICAL TEAM FTES AND WAGES

Required FTEs	Clinician Title	Hourly Rate/Wage (Per FTE)
1.0	Surgeon/Specialist	$485.00
1.0	Anesthesiologist	$405.00
1.0	Registered nurse	$90.00
2.0	Surgical technicians	$65.00
Fringe benefits rate: 33%		

FTE, full-time equivalent.

For each single surgery, assume one clinical team and 3 hours per surgery. For double surgeries, assume two clinical teams and 4 hours per surgery. You must reference/link the volume data from Worksheet #1 into these calculations. The double surgery case volume does not need to be doubled for the calculations. The fringe benefits amount is to be applied as 33% of salaries. The fringe benefits amount can be applied per full-time equivalent (FTE) or for the entire team since the same rate is applicable to each person.

Worksheet #3: SurgiFlex Revenue Calculations: Every healthcare organization must estimate patient services revenue that will be based on the number of surgeries/cases performed. For SurgiFlex, the revenue estimates will be based on the operating data created in Worksheet #1.

There are three different payers to consider for the robotic surgical service, with reimbursement rates and case volume as noted in Table 16.2.

Table 16.2

SURGIFLEX REIMBURSEMENT PER CASE BY PAYER

Payer	Per Case Reimbursement	Cases Covered
Medicare	$3,500	30% of cases
Medicaid	$1,750	15% of cases
Commercial	$8,950	55% of cases

You must reference/link the volume data from Worksheet #1 into these calculations. You must also calculate the total reimbursement per case (by adding the per case rates) which will be used in the breakeven analysis.

Worksheet #4: SurgiFlex Nonsalary Expense Calculations: This worksheet contains supply costs per surgical case and a calculation for the allocation of the annual maintenance costs. The supply costs value for each SurgiFlex single surgery case is $3,500 and for each double surgery case is $4,000. You must reference/link the volume data from Worksheet #1 into these calculations. The annual maintenance cost agreement is $350,000, which must be allocated proportionately to the single and double surgery lines. For proper allocation based on the single and double contribution to total surgeries, review and apply the allocation methodology from Chapter 8.

Worksheet #5: SurgiFlex Breakeven Calculations: For this simplified breakeven calculation, you are answering the question: "How many single surgery and double surgery cases must we perform at a given price point to cover all related SurgiFlex expenses?" The expenses to consider in this calculation include the SurgiFlex salary and wage information and the SurgiFlex nonsalary expenses. The data from these two worksheets (Worksheet #2 and Worksheet #4) must be referenced/linked into these calculations. The price point for the calculations is the per case reimbursement total from Worksheet #3. The number of cases needed for breakeven must show single surgery cases needed, double surgery cases needed, and total cases needed.

Worksheet #6: SurgiFlex Supply Vendor Analysis Calculations: You must select a supply vendor for the SurgiFlex surgical service from the vendor proposals submitted. Refer to Exhibit 16A.2 (see Chapter 16 Appendix, Exhibit 16A.2) for the summary data from each vendor proposal. There are several metrics to consider, but you must determine which vendor will work best for this surgical service. There are three vendors bidding for the business, and this analysis represents the additional administrative costs associated with securing supplies. The top portion of the proposal data spreadsheet contains the summary data from each proposal. You must create Excel formulas in the bottom portion of the spreadsheet and choose the ideal vendor based on the selection criteria in the text that follows.

Calculations for Vendor Comparison:

1. Economic Ordering Quantity (EOQ) = [Square Root of (2 × Fixed Cost per Order × Annual Usage)] / (Carrying Cost × Purchase Price)

2. Total Carrying Costs = (Order Quantity / 2) × Carrying Costs × Purchase Price

3. Total Ordering Costs = (Annual Usage / Ordering Quantity) × Fixed Cost per Order

4. Total Inventory Costs = Total Carrying Costs + Total Ordering Costs

5. Reorder Point = (Annual Usage / Days per Year) × Delivery Time

The ideal vendor should be chosen based on the following selection criteria:

- largest safety stock (provides the ability to remain operational/productive during unforeseen emergencies),

- total carrying costs of less than $15,000,

- total ordering costs of less than $10,000,

- total inventory costs of less than $25,000, and

- highest reorder point (allows for longer periods of time between orders).

COURSE PROJECT: PHASE II

Now that you've set things up and have completed the SurgiFlex calculations in Phase I, you can start completing the consolidated worksheets with the relevant calculations and bring in the master supply list! The second phase starts with the supply list because it's also linked into the consolidated sheets (like the rest of the SurgiFlex Phase I calculations). Phase II is the "consolidated" phase of the project because it incorporates the SurgiFlex data into the organization-level data. Note that SurgiFlex figures from Phase I do not change with seasonality percentages. As with the Phase I calculations, there should be categories, monthly calculations, and totals on all worksheets, with the exception of the master supply list.

Worksheet #11: Master Supply List: The master supply list is the supply list for the entire healthcare organization and will be referenced/linked into Worksheet #10. For now, simply copy and paste the master supply list provided in Exhibit 16A.3 (see Chapter 16 Appendix, Exhibit 16A.3). Be sure to add a heading/title block and do a summation on total costs.

Worksheet #7: Consolidated Operating/Utilization Data: This worksheet combines the SurgiFlex operating data from Worksheet #1 with the rest of the healthcare organization's operating data (patient/procedure volumes). To create this worksheet, use the data and format shown in Exhibit 16A.4 (see Chapter 16 Appendix, Exhibit 16A.4). The data provided is for the first month of the fiscal year (July). After the first month of data has been completed, the remaining months must increase or decrease to reflect seasonality. The increases or decreases should be entered as formulas and should be based on the prior month (August changes based on July, September changes based on August, etc.). The seasonality changes are:

- Aug to Oct: ↓2%

- Nov to Jan: ↑7%

- Feb to Apr: ↓4%

- May to June: ↑11%

Worksheet #8: Consolidated Salary and Wage Calculations: This data represents the medical (non-SurgiFlex) salaries from the rest of the organization, given for month one (July). Remaining months of medical salaries must fluctuate with the same percentage changes used in Worksheet #7. Increased cases/volume often means increased labor hours in the clinical setting, so labor dollars must change as well. SurgiFlex salaries must be linked in from Worksheet #2.

- medical salaries: $2,495,500

- surgical salaries: $3,750,000

- fringe benefits: 33% of salaries

Worksheet #9: Consolidated Revenue Calculations: Revenue (non-SurgiFlex) is given for month one in Table 16.3. Remaining months must fluctuate with the same percentage changes used in Worksheet #7. SurgiFlex revenue must be referenced/linked in from Worksheet #3.

Table 16.3	
NON-SURGIFLEX REVENUE	
Category and Payer	**Revenue (July)**
Inpatient revenue—Medicare	$4,498,550
Inpatient revenue—Medicaid	$1,925,775
Inpatient revenue—commercial	$9,675,325
Outpatient revenue (all payers)	$5,595,225
Ancillary revenue (all payers)	$975,000

Worksheet #10: Consolidated Nonsalary Expense Calculations: Expenses noted in the list that follows are given for month one. Remaining months must fluctuate with the percentage changes used in Worksheet #7. SurgiFlex supplies must be linked in from Worksheet #4. In addition, the following items must be represented:

- facility maintenance: $735,000

- utilities: $80,000

- patient transportation: $165,000

- marketing: $100,000

- supplies total: linked total from the master supply list (Worksheet #11)

- vendor total inventory costs (chosen vendor linked from Worksheet #6)

COURSE PROJECT: PHASE III

Now that you've completed the SurgiFlex and consolidated calculations, you can begin the final phase of the workbook—the financial statements and performance measurement items. Remember, you've already done most of the work for these; now it's time to pull it all together. Be sure to reference the textbook for the formatting of these statements.

Worksheet #12: Balance Sheet: This financial statement details the hospital's assets and liabilities. Use the following data for this financial statement; see formatting examples in the textbook. Just use these categories; no other data is required at this time. (Data is summarized **annually** using formulas.)

- cash and cash equivalents: $10,875,000

- prepaid expenses: $65,000

land: $3,225,900

amortization: $40,000

accounts payable: $75,000

notes payable: $35,000

equipment (non-SurgiFlex): $5,000,000

Worksheet #13: Statement of Operations: Also called an income statement, this is a summary statement for the entire 12-month period. The data comes from the consolidated revenue and consolidated expenses worksheets (Worksheets #8–#10). For purposes of this project, the data must be summarized **quarterly** using Excel formulas (required).

Worksheet #14: Statement of Cashflows: This financial statement details the cash transactions of the hospitals (inflows and outflows). Use the following data for this financial statement; operations, investing, and financing subsections must be used. See formatting examples in the textbook. Just use these categories; no other data is required at this time. (Data is summarized **annually** using formulas.)

new equipment purchase (SurgiFlex): $3,500,000

salvage receipts (old equipment): $2,775,000

cash from patients (copays): $425,000

interest paid: $55,000

taxes paid: $.00

fundraising/charity donations and receipts: $980,000

bonds/securities purchase: $550,000

interest earned: $725,000

Worksheet #15: Proforma Statement: This financial statement is a forecast anticipating future financial performance. Link in the annual totals for each category from the statement of operations (Worksheet #13). For the financial projections, incorporate the following anticipated changes for the next 4 years:

inpatient revenue: ↑8% annually

outpatient revenue: ↑4% annually

SurgiFlex revenue: ↑4% annually

all salaries: ↑2% annually

all supplies: ↑1% annually

All other line items remain static.

Worksheet #16: Financing Options Comparison: This worksheet will contain a financing comparison for the SurgiFlex surgical service purchase of $3.5 million. For these calculations, compare a 100% equity financing approach with a 60% debt financing approach, using the purchase price as the asset value. For your calculations, use the following data:

earnings for interest and taxes (EBIT): $1,500,000

interest rate: 6%

tax rate: 30%

Include the return on equity (ROE) and return to investors (ROI) percentages on this worksheet. Reference Chapter 8 for an example of this capital structure calculation.

Worksheet #17: Performance Measurement and Ratio Analysis: Financial ratios are measures of an organization's performance and use figures that are already represented in the financial statements. Financial ratios should be calculated *after* you've created the financial statements. The formulas for these ratios are in Chapter 13 of the textbook. The following ratios must be represented in your workbook (assigned ratios are subject to change):

- total margin (profit margin)
- return on assets
- return on equity
- debt ratio
- total assets turnover

Worksheet #18: Dashboards (Graphs and Visual Elements): The dashboard/performance measurement graphs will be based on the data calculated on the various worksheets of your workbook. Your graphs can be any style: line, bar, combined, and so forth. Required dashboard items (separate graphs) are:

- statement of operations net income (all years)
- proforma net income (all years)
- consolidated revenue (showing each service line)
- consolidated expense (showing each service line)
- SurgiFlex revenue
- SurgiFlex expense
- SurgiFlex profit margin

Do NOT include the grand totals on your graphs; it will skew the visual representation of your data.

CHAPTER SUMMARY

This course project explores the various types of operating costs within a healthcare organization and details how these costs are captured in the organization's financial processes and reporting. It is designed to help students synthesize the key concepts learned throughout the healthcare finance course with the core functionality of Microsoft Excel. This software was chosen because it is often the "go to" or preferred software for data collection, budget dissemination, and routine financial analysis. Organizations that can be represented within this project span the entire health system (hospitals, physician practices, assisted living facilities, homecare agencies, etc.), and can be further developed to expose students to the interdisciplinary nature of healthcare (functions such as finance, marketing, and human resources are present and impact all types of healthcare organizations). All areas within the healthcare organization, whether direct to patient care or indirect services, participate in the financial process, even if only minimally. The course project is designed to showcase how the costs from these areas are incorporated.

ADDITIONAL COURSE PROJECT DISCUSSION QUESTIONS AND ASSIGNMENTS

1. Executive summary: The executive summary gives a high-level overview of your entire project, start to finish. Draft an executive summary for submission to your organization's leadership team.

2. Financial analysis summary: The financial analysis summary is a sound discussion of your Excel workbook. For this summary, discuss the overall financial picture of the hospital both with and without the implementation of the SurgiFlex system. Key items to include in the summary are (not limited to; add others as needed):

   - occupancy rate

   - average length of stay

   - operating margin: (Total Revenue – Total Expenses) / Total Revenue

   - average collection period, average daily sales

   - changes (increases and decreases) in volume

   - changes (increases and decreases) in revenue and expense

   - overall impact of the SurgiFlex system

3. What/who within the organization would be affected by the implementation of the SurgiFlex Robotic Surgery System? We have calculated data for the service-specific staffing, but other departments will surely be impacted.

4. Performance measurement and management: Perform a brief literature search to locate information on other robotic surgical systems. Compare them to the work you've done for SurgiFlex and suggest some changes or updates for the leadership team. Things to consider may include:

   - What routine reports and/or benchmarking is needed?

   - What corrective actions/activities are needed to keep things on task?

   - How would you market the service?

   - Should there have been a change in the financing option chosen?

   - What would make things better in the future? How could things be changed to make things run more smoothly?

   - What recommendations or changes would you make for human resources, capabilities, capacity, leadership, patient focus, and so forth?

Chapter 16: Appendix

EXHIBIT 16A.1 SurgiFlex Operating Data

Your Hospital Name
SurgiFlex Operating Data (Surgical Case Volume)
Fiscal Year Ending June 2022

Category	Jul-21	Aug-21	Sep-21	Oct-21	Nov-21	Dec-21	Jan-22	Feb-22	Mar-22	Apr-22	May-22	Jun-22	**Total**
SurgiFlex Single Surgery (SS) Cases	220	220	235	220	220	235	220	220	235	220	220	235	**2,700**
SurgiFlex Double Surgery (DS) Cases	110	110	130	110	110	130	110	110	130	110	110	130	**1,400**
SurgiFlex Total Surgical Cases	330	330	365	330	330	365	330	330	365	330	330	365	**4,100**
Inpatient Days Per Case	4.5	4.5	4.5	4.5	4.5	4.5	4.5	4.5	4.5	4.5	4.5	4.5	**4.5**
Total SurgiFlex Inpatient Days	1,485	1,485	1,643	1,485	1,485	1,643	1,485	1,485	1,643	1,485	1,485	1,643	18,450

These must be formulas!

These must be formulas!

EXHIBIT 16A.2. SurgiFlex Supply Vendor Proposal Data

Your Hospital Name
SurgiFlex Vendor Analysis
Fiscal Year Ending June 2022

	Vendor #1: Towson Healthcare	Vendor #2: Tiger Clinical Resources	Vendor #3: Golden Medical
Annual usage (supply bundles)	3,500	3,500	3,500
Purchase price (per supply bundle)	$3,925	$3,775	$3,850
% Carrying cost	25.0%	27.0%	28.0%
Delivery time (days)	5	1	3
Fixed cost per order	$78	$65	$72
Days per year	360	345	350
Safety stock quantity	7	4	5
Discount %	N/A	N/A	N/A
Discount quantity	N/A	N/A	N/A
Order quantity	30	30	30

	Vendor #1: Towson Healthcare	Vendor #2: Tiger Clinical Resources	Vendor #3: Golden Medical
EOQ			
Total carrying costs			
Total ordering costs			
Total inventory costs			
Reorder point (number of supply bundles)			

These must be formulas, as noted for Worksheet #6.

EOQ, economic ordering quantity.

EXHIBIT 16A.3. Master Supply List

Item Number	Category	Description	Quantity	Price Per Unit	Total Price
1	Syringe/Needle	Syringe with needle, sterile, 1 mL or less	50	$1.75	$87.50
2	Syringe/Needle	Syringe with needle, sterile 2 mL	50	$1.75	$87.50
3	Syringe/Needle	Syringe with needle, sterile 3 mL	50	$1.75	$87.50
4	Syringe/Needle	Syringe with needle, sterile 5 mL or greater	50	$1.75	$87.50
5	Syringe/Needle	Noncoring needle	50	$1.75	$87.50
6	Miscellaneous	Syringe, bulb type (infant nasal aspirators, ear and ulcer bulb syringes)	25	$0.99	$24.75
7	Syringe/Needle	Needle, sterile, any size, each	50	$1.75	$87.50

(continued)

EXHIBIT 16A.3. Master Supply List (*continued*)

Item Number	Category	Description	Quantity	Price Per Unit	Total Price
8	Infusion supply	Intravenous administration set (with or without infusion pump), hypodermoclysis administration set, connecting device, heparin lock caps	250	$5.75	$1,437.50
9	Diabetic supply	Infusion set for external insulin pump, nonneedle cannula type	30	$20.95	$628.50
10	Diabetic supply	Infusion set for external insulin pump, needle type	30	$20.95	$628.50
11	Diabetic supply	Syringe with needle for external insulin pump, sterile, 3 cc	30	$20.95	$628.50
12	Diabetic supply	Normal, low and high calibrator solution/chips	30	$20.95	$628.50
13	Infusion supply	Disposable drug delivery system, flow rate of 50 mL or greater per hour	30	$35.99	$1,079.70
14	Infusion supply	Disposable drug delivery system, flow rate of less than 50 mL per hour	30	$35.99	$1,079.70
15	Urologic supply	Insertion tray without drainage bag and without catheter (accessories only)	200	$14.99	$2,998.00
16	Urologic supply	Insertion tray without drainage bag with indwelling catheter, foley type, two-way latex with coating (teflon, silicone, silicone elastomer or hydrophilic, etc.)	200	$14.99	$2,998.00
17	Urologic supply	Insertion tray without drainage bag with indwelling catheter, foley type, two-way, all silicone	200	$14.99	$2,998.00
18	Urologic supply	Insertion tray without drainage bag with indwelling catheter, foley type, three-way, for continuous irrigation	200	$14.99	$2,998.00
19	Urologic supply	Insertion tray with drainage bag with indwelling catheter, foley type, two-way latex with coating (teflon, silicone, silicone elastomer or hydrophilic, etc.)	200	$14.99	$2,998.00

(continued)

EXHIBIT 16A.3. Master Supply List (*continued*)

Item Number	Category	Description	Quantity	Price Per Unit	Total Price
20	Urologic supply	Insertion tray with drainage bag with indwelling catheter, foley type, two-way, all silicone	200	$14.99	$2,998.00
21	Urologic supply	Insertion tray with drainage bag with indwelling catheter, foley type, three-way, for continuous irrigation	200	$14.99	$2,998.00
22	Urologic supply	Irrigation tray with bulb or piston syringe, any purpose	200	$14.99	$2,998.00
23	Urologic supply	Irrigation syringe, bulb or piston, each	200	$14.99	$2,998.00
24	Urologic supply	Male external catheter with integral collection chamber, any type, each	200	$14.99	$2,998.00
25	Urologic supply	Female external urinary collection device; meatal cup, each	200	$14.99	$2,998.00
26	Urologic supply	Female external urinary collection device; pouch, each	200	$14.99	$2,998.00
27	Ostomy supply	Ostomy faceplate, each	150	$1.50	$225.00
28	Ostomy supply	Skin barrier; solid "4 × 4" or equivalent, each	150	$1.75	$262.50
29	Ostomy supply	Ostomy clamp, any type, replacement only, each	150	$4.99	$748.50
30	Ostomy supply	Adhesive, liquid or equal, any type	20	$3.99	$79.80
31	Ostomy supply	Ostomy vent, any type, each	150	$1.75	$262.50
32	Ostomy supply	Ostomy belt, each	150	$1.75	$262.50
33	Ostomy supply	Ostomy filter, any type, each	150	$1.75	$262.50
34	Ostomy supply	Ostomy skin barrier, liquid (spray/brush etc)	150	$1.75	$262.50
35	Ostomy supply	Ostomy skin barrier, powder	150	$1.75	$262.50
36	Ostomy supply	Ostomy pouch, drainable with faceplate attached, plastic, each	150	$1.75	$262.50
37	Ostomy supply	Ostomy pouch, drainable with faceplate attached, rubber, each	150	$1.75	$262.50
38	Tracheostomy supply	Tracheostoma filter, any type, any size, each	100	$17.99	$1,799.00

(continued)

EXHIBIT 16A.3. Master Supply List (*continued*)

Item Number	Category	Description	Quantity	Price Per Unit	Total Price
39	Tracheostomy supply	Moisture exchanger, disposable, for use w/ invasive mechanical ventilation	100	$17.99	$1,799.00
40	Tracheostomy supply	Tracheal suction catheter, closed system, each	100	$17.99	$1,799.00
41	Tracheostomy supply	Tracheostomy, inner cannula	100	$17.99	$1,799.00
42	Tracheostomy supply	Tracheal suction catheter, any type other than closed system, each	100	$17.99	$1,799.00
43	Tracheostomy supply	Tracheostomy care kit for new tracheostomy	100	$17.99	$1,799.00
44	Tracheostomy supply	Tracheostomy cleaning brush, each	250	$17.99	$4,497.50
45	Tracheostomy supply	Oropharyngeal suction catheter, each	250	$17.99	$4,497.50
46	Wound care supply	Wound pouch, each	100	$1.00	$100.00
47	Wound care supply	Alginate or other fiber gelling dressing, wound cover, sterile, pad size 16 sq. in. or less, each dressing	100	$2.99	$299.00
48	Wound care supply	Alginate or other fiber gelling dressing, wound cover, sterile, pad size more than 16 sq. in. but less than or equal to 48 sq. in., each dressing	100	$2.99	$299.00
49	Wound care supply	Alginate or other fiber gelling dressing, wound filler, sterile	100	$2.99	$299.00
50	Wound care supply	Composite dressing, sterile, pad size 16 sq. in. or less, with any size adhesive border, each dressing	100	$2.99	$299.00
51	Wound care supply	Composite dressing, sterile, pad size more than 16 sq. in. but less than or equal to 48 sq. in., with any size adhesive border, each dressing	100	$2.99	$299.00
52	Wound care supply	Composite dressing, sterile, pad size more than 48 sq. in., with any size adhesive border, each dressing	100	$2.99	$299.00

(*continued*)

EXHIBIT 16A.3. Master Supply List (*continued*)

Item Number	Category	Description	Quantity	Price Per Unit	Total Price
53	Wound care supply	Contact layer, sterile, 16 sq. in. or less, each dressing	100	$2.99	$299.00
54	Wound care supply	Contact layer, sterile, more than 16 sq. in. but less than or equal to 48 sq. in., each dressing	100	$2.99	$299.00
55	Wound care supply	Contact layer, sterile, more than 48 sq. in., each dressing	100	$2.99	$299.00
56	Wound care supply	Foam dressing, wound cover, sterile, pad size 16 sq. in. or less, without adhesive border, each dressing	100	$2.99	$299.00
57	Wound care supply	Foam dressing, wound cover, sterile, pad size more than 16 sq. in. but less than or equal to 48 sq. in., without adhesive border, each dressing	100	$2.99	$299.00
58	Wound care supply	Foam dressing, wound cover, sterile, pad size more than 48 sq. in., without adhesive border, each dressing	100	$2.99	$299.00
59	Wound care supply	Foam dressing, wound cover, sterile, pad size 16 sq. in. or less, with any size adhesive border, each dressing	100	$2.99	$299.00
60	Wound care supply	Foam dressing, wound cover, sterile, pad size more than 16 sq. in. but less than or equal to 48 sq. in., with any size adhesive border, each dressing	100	$2.99	$299.00
61	Wound care supply	Foam dressing, wound cover, sterile, pad size more than 48 sq. in., with any size adhesive border, each dressing	100	$2.99	$299.00
62	Wound care supply	Foam dressing, wound filler, sterile, per gram	100	$2.99	$299.00
63	Wound care supply	Gauze, nonimpregnated, nonsterile, pad size 16 sq. in. or less, without adhesive border, each dressing	100	$2.99	$299.00

(*continued*)

EXHIBIT 16A.3. Master Supply List (*continued*)

Item Number	Category	Description	Quantity	Price Per Unit	Total Price
64	Wound care supply	Gauze, nonimpregnated, nonsterile, pad size more than 16 sq. in. but less than or equal to 48 sq. in., without adhesive border, each dressing	100	$2.99	$299.00
65	Wound care supply	Gauze, nonimpregnated, nonsterile, pad size more than 48 sq. in., without adhesive border, each dressing	100	$2.99	$299.00
66	Wound care supply	Gauze, nonimpregnated, sterile, pad size 16 sq. in. or less, with any size adhesive border, each dressing	100	$2.99	$299.00
67	Wound care supply	Gauze, nonimpregnated, sterile, pad size more than 16 sq. in. but less than or equal to 48 sq. in., with any size adhesive border, each dressing	100	$2.99	$299.00
68	Wound care supply	Gauze, nonimpregnated, sterile, pad size more than 48 sq. in., with any size adhesive border, each dressing	100	$2.99	$299.00
69	Wound care supply	Gauze, impregnated with other than water, normal saline, or hydrogel, sterile, pad size 16 sq. in. or less, without adhesive border, each dressing	100	$2.99	$299.00
70	Wound care supply	Gauze, impregnated with other than water, normal saline, or hydrogel, sterile, pad size more than 16 sq. in., but less than or equal to 48 sq. in., without adhesive border, each dressing	100	$2.99	$299.00
71	Wound care supply	Gauze, impregnated with other than water, normal saline, or hydrogel, sterile, pad size more than 48 sq. in., without adhesive border, each dressing	100	$2.99	$299.00

(*continued*)

EXHIBIT 16A.3. Master Supply List (*continued*)

Item Number	Category	Description	Quantity	Price Per Unit	Total Price
72	Wound care supply	Gauze, impregnated, water or normal saline, sterile, pad size 16 sq. in. or less, without adhesive border, each dressing	100	$2.99	$299.00
73	Wound care supply	Gauze, impregnated, water or normal saline, sterile, pad size more than 16 sq. in. but less than or equal to 48 sq. in., without adhesive border, each dressing	100	$2.99	$299.00
74	Wound care supply	Gauze, impregnated, water or normal saline, sterile, pad size more than 48 sq. in., without adhesive border, each dressing	100	$2.99	$299.00
75	Wound care supply	Gauze, impregnated, hydrogel, for direct wound contact, sterile, pad size 16 sq. in. or less, each dressing	100	$2.99	$299.00
76	Wound care supply	Gauze, impregnated, hydrogel, for direct wound contact, sterile, pad size greater than 16 sq. in., but less than or equal to 48 sq. in., each dressing	100	$2.99	$299.00
77	Wound care supply	Gauze, impregnated, hydrogel, for direct wound contact, sterile, pad size more than 48 sq. in., each dressing	100	$2.99	$299.00
78	Wound care supply	Hydrocolloid dressing, wound cover, sterile, pad size 16 sq. in. or less, without adhesive border, each dressing	100	$2.99	$299.00
79	Wound care supply	Hydrocolloid dressing, wound cover, sterile, pad size more than 16 sq. in. but less than or equal to 48 sq. in., without adhesive border, each dressing	100	$2.99	$299.00
80	Wound care supply	Hydrocolloid dressing, wound cover, sterile, pad size more than 48 sq. in., without adhesive border, each dressing	100	$2.99	$299.00

(continued)

EXHIBIT 16A.3. Master Supply List (*continued*)

Item Number	Category	Description	Quantity	Price Per Unit	Total Price
81	Wound care supply	Hydrocolloid dressing, wound cover, sterile, pad size 16 sq. in. or less, with any size adhesive border, each dressing	100	$2.99	$299.00
82	Wound care supply	Hydrocolloid dressing, wound cover, sterile, pad size more than 16 sq. in. but less than or equal to 48 sq. in., with any size adhesive border, each dressing	100	$2.99	$299.00
83	Wound care supply	Hydrocolloid dressing, wound cover, sterile, pad size more than 48 sq. in., with any size adhesive border, each dressing	100	$2.99	$299.00
84	Wound care supply	Hydrocolloid dressing, wound filler, paste, sterile	100	$2.99	$299.00
85	Wound care supply	Hydrocolloid dressing, wound filler, dry form, sterile, per gram	100	$2.99	$299.00
86	Wound care supply	Hydrogel dressing, wound cover, sterile, pad size 16 sq. in. or less, without adhesive border, each dressing	100	$2.99	$299.00
87	Wound care supply	Hydrogel dressing, wound cover, sterile, pad size more than 16 sq. in. but less than or equal to 48 sq. in., without adhesive border, each dressing	100	$2.99	$299.00
88	Wound care supply	Hydrogel dressing, wound cover, sterile, pad size more than 48 sq. in., without adhesive border, each dressing	100	$2.99	$299.00
89	Wound care supply	Hydrogel dressing, wound cover, sterile, pad size 16 sq. in. or less, with any size adhesive border, each dressing	100	$2.99	$299.00

(*continued*)

EXHIBIT 16A.3. Master Supply List (*continued*)

Item Number	Category	Description	Quantity	Price Per Unit	Total Price
90	Wound care supply	Hydrogel dressing, wound cover, sterile, pad size more than 16 sq. in. but less than or equal to 48 sq. in., with any size adhesive border, each dressing	100	$2.99	$299.00
91	Wound care supply	Hydrogel dressing, wound cover, sterile, pad size more than 48 sq. in., with any size adhesive border, each dressing	100	$2.99	$299.00
92	Wound care supply	Hydrogel dressing, wound filler, gel	100	$2.99	$299.00
93	Wound care supply	Specialty absorptive dressing, wound cover, sterile, pad size 16 sq. in. or less, without adhesive border, each dressing	100	$2.99	$299.00
94	Wound care supply	Specialty absorptive dressing, wound cover, sterile, pad size more than 16 sq. in. but less than or equal to 48 sq. in., without adhesive border, each dressing	100	$2.99	$299.00
95	Wound care supply	Specialty absorptive dressing, wound cover, sterile, pad size more than 48 sq. in., without adhesive border, each dressing	100	$2.99	$299.00
96	Wound care supply	Specialty absorptive dressing, wound cover, sterile, pad size 16 sq. in. or less, with any size adhesive border, each dressing	100	$2.99	$299.00
97	Wound care supply	Specialty absorptive dressing, wound cover, sterile, pad size more than 16 sq. in. but less than or equal to 48 sq. in., with any size adhesive border, each dressing	100	$2.99	$299.00
98	Wound care supply	Specialty absorptive dressing, wound cover, sterile, pad size more than 48 sq. in., with any size adhesive border, each dressing	100	$2.99	$299.00

(continued)

EXHIBIT 16A.3. Master Supply List (*continued*)

Item Number	Category	Description	Quantity	Price Per Unit	Total Price
99	Wound care supply	Transparent film, sterile, 16 sq. in. or less, each dressing	100	$2.99	$299.00
100	Wound care supply	Transparent film, sterile, more than 16 sq. in. but less than or equal to 48 sq. in., each dressing	100	$2.99	$299.00
101	Wound care supply	Transparent film, sterile, more than 48 sq. in., each dressing	100	$2.99	$299.00
102	Wound care supply	Wound filler, gel/paste, not otherwise specified	100	$2.99	$299.00
103	Wound care supply	Wound filler, dry form, per gram, not otherwise specified	100	$2.99	$299.00
104	Wound care supply	Gauze, impregnated, other than water, normal saline, or zinc paste, sterile, any width, per linear yard	100	$2.99	$299.00
105	Wound care supply	Gauze, nonimpregnated, sterile, pad size 16 sq. in. or less, without adhesive border, each dressing	100	$2.99	$299.00
106	Wound care supply	Gauze, nonimpregnated, sterile, pad size more than 16 sq. in. less than or equal to 48 sq. in., without adhesive border, each dressing	100	$2.99	$299.00
107	Wound care supply	Gauze, nonimpregnated, sterile, pad size more than 48 sq. in., without adhesive border, each dressing	100	$2.99	$299.00
108	Wound care supply	Packing strips, nonimpregnated, sterile, up to 2 inches in width, per linear yard	100	$2.99	$299.00
109	Wound care supply	Eye pad, sterile, each	100	$2.99	$299.00
110	Wound care supply	Eye pad, nonsterile, each	100	$2.99	$299.00
111	Wound care supply	Conforming bandage, nonelastic, knitted/woven, nonsterile, width less than 3 inches, per yard	100	$2.99	$299.00

(continued)

EXHIBIT 16A.3. Master Supply List (*continued*)

Item Number	Category	Description	Quantity	Price Per Unit	Total Price
112	Wound care supply	Conforming bandage, nonelastic, knitted/woven, nonsterile, width greater than or equal to 3 inches and less than 5 inches, per yard	100	$2.99	$299.00
113	Wound care supply	Conforming bandage, nonelastic, knitted/woven, nonsterile, width greater than or equal to 5 inches, per yard	100	$2.99	$299.00
114	Wound care supply	Conforming bandage, nonelastic, knitted/woven, sterile, width less than 3 inches, per yard	100	$2.99	$299.00
115	Wound care supply	Conforming bandage, nonelastic, knitted/woven, sterile, width greater than or equal to 3 inches and less than 5 inches, per yard	100	$2.99	$299.00
116	Wound care supply	Conforming bandage, nonelastic, knitted/woven, sterile, width greater than or equal to 5 inches, per yard	100	$2.99	$299.00
117	Wound care supply	Self-adherent bandage, elastic, nonknitted/nonwoven, width less than 3 inches, per yard	100	$2.99	$299.00
118	Wound care supply	Self-adherent bandage, elastic, nonknitted/nonwoven, width greater than or equal to 3 inches and less than 5 inches, per yard	100	$2.99	$299.00
119	Wound care supply	Self-adherent bandage, elastic, nonknitted/nonwoven, width greater than or equal to 5 inches, per yard	100	$2.99	$299.00
120	Wound care supply	Tubular dressing with or without elastic, any width, per linear yard	100	$2.99	$299.00
121	Respiratory supply	Tubing, used with suction pump, each	250	$5.99	$1,497.50
122	Respiratory supply	Administration set, with small volume nonfiltered pneumatic nebulizer, disposable	250	$5.99	$1,497.50

(*continued*)

EXHIBIT 16A.3. Master Supply List (*continued*)

Item Number	Category	Description	Quantity	Price Per Unit	Total Price
123	Respiratory supply	Small volume nonfiltered pneumatic nebulizer, disposable	250	$5.99	$1,497.50
124	Respiratory supply	Administration set, with small volume filtered pneumatic nebulizer	250	$5.99	$1,497.50
125	Respiratory supply	Large volume nebulizer, disposable, unfilled, used with aerosol compressor	250	$5.99	$1,497.50
126	Respiratory supply	Large volume nebulizer, disposable, prefilled, used with aerosol compressor	250	$5.99	$1,497.50
127	Respiratory supply	Corrugated tubing, disposable, used with large volume nebulizer, 100 feet	250	$5.99	$1,497.50
128	Respiratory supply	Water collection device, used with large volume nebulizer	250	$5.99	$1,497.50
129	Respiratory supply	Filter, disposable, used with aerosol compressor or ultrasonic generator	250	$5.99	$1,497.50
130	Respiratory supply	Dome and mouthpiece, used with small volume ultrasonic nebulizer	250	$5.99	$1,497.50
131	Tracheostomy supply	Tracheostoma valve, including diaphragm, each	350	$19.99	$6,996.50
132	Tracheostomy supply	Replacement diaphragm/ faceplate for tracheostoma valve, each	350	$14.99	$5,246.50
133	Tracheostomy supply	Filter holder or filter cap, reusable, for use in a tracheostoma heat and moisture exchange system, each	350	$14.99	$5,246.50
134	Tracheostomy supply	Filter for use in a tracheostoma heat and moisture exchange system, each	350	$14.99	$5,246.50
135	Tracheostomy supply	Housing, reusable without adhesive, for use in a heat and moisture exchange system and/or with a tracheostoma valve, each	350	$14.99	$5,246.50

(continued)

EXHIBIT 16A.3. Master Supply List (*continued*)

Item Number	Category	Description	Quantity	Price Per Unit	Total Price
136	Tracheostomy supply	Adhesive disc for use in a heat and moisture exchange system and/or with tracheostoma valve, any type each	350	$14.99	$5,246.50
137	Tracheostomy supply	Filter holder and integrated filter without adhesive, for use in a tracheostoma heat and moisture exchange system, each	350	$14.99	$5,246.50
138	Tracheostomy supply	Housing and integrated adhesive, for use in a tracheostoma heat and moisture exchange system and/or with a tracheostoma valve, each	350	$14.99	$5,246.50
139	Tracheostomy supply	Filter holder and integrated filter housing, and adhesive, for use as a tracheostoma heat and moisture exchange system, each	350	$14.99	$5,246.50
140	Tracheostomy supply	Tracheostomy/laryngectomy tube, noncuffed, polyvinylchloride (pvc), silicone or equal, each	350	$14.99	$5,246.50
141	Tracheostomy supply	Tracheostomy/ laryngectomy tube, cuffed, polyvinylchloride (pvc), silicone or equal, each	350	$14.99	$5,246.50
142	Tracheostomy supply	Tracheostomy/laryngectomy tube, stainless steel or equal (sterilizable and reusable), each	350	$14.99	$5,246.50
143	Tracheostomy supply	Tracheostomy shower protector, each	350	$4.99	$1,746.50
144	Tracheostomy supply	Tracheostoma stent/stud/ button, each	350	$4.99	$1,746.50
145	Tracheostomy supply	Tracheostomy mask, each	350	$4.99	$1,746.50
146	Tracheostomy supply	Tracheostomy tube collar/ holder, each	350	$4.99	$1,746.50
147	Infusion supply	Heparin flush solution, 10 units/mL	1,000	$7.99	$7,990.00
148	Infusion supply	Heparin flush solution, 100 units/mL	1,000	$7.99	$7,990.00

(continued)

EXHIBIT 16A.3. Master Supply List (*continued*)

Item Number	Category	Description	Quantity	Price Per Unit	Total Price
149	Infusion supply	Syringe, normal saline/0.9% sodium chloride flush	1,000	$7.99	$7,990.00
150	Orthopaedic implants	Surgical supply sets: ortho	50	$49.99	$2,499.50
151	Neurology implants	Surgical supply sets: neuro	50	$49.99	$2,499.50
152	Cardiology implants	Surgical supply sets: cardio	25	$69.99	$1,749.75
			Total	——>	**$205,192.70**

EXHIBIT 16A.4. Consolidated Operating Data

Your Hospital Name
SurgiFlex Consolidated Operating Data
Fiscal Year Ending June 2022

Category	Jul-21	Aug-21	Sep-21	Oct-21	Nov-21	Dec-21	Jan-22	Feb-22	Mar-22	Apr-22	May-22	Jun-22	Total
Medical Inpt Days	22,375												22,375
Surgical Inpt Days (non-SurgiFlex)	2,105												2,105
SurgiFlex Inpt Days (Cases)													–
Outpt Visits	3,865												3,865
Total Discharges	6,495												6,495
Inpt Ancillary	5,348												5,348
Outpt Ancillary	4,631												4,631
Total of Patient Activities	44,819												**44,819**
Licensed beds	985												
Avg Length of Stay (ALOS)	3.77												
Occupancy Rate	80.17%												

Notes:
1. Enter the July numbers for all except SurgiFlex.
2. Link in the July SurgiFlex Total Inpatient Days from Worksheet #1.
3. Total patient activities sums all items.
4. Licensed beds = 985 for all months (no changes).
5. ALOS = sum of all inpt days/total discharges.
6. Occupancy rate = sum of inpt days/days in that month, then divide by licensed beds.
Remember: formulas required.
Remember: title, categories, monthly columns and totals annual totals required.
Refer to the requirements documents for July numbers for other consolidated sheets; link in the SurgiFlex numbers.

APPENDICES

Wrapping Up: A Summary of the Healthcare Industry Today

HEALTHCARE INDUSTRY CHALLENGES: MOVING US FORWARD

Though it remains resilient and steadfast in its mission, the healthcare industry is not without its fair share of issues. Demand for healthcare services continues to increase, as does the availability of providers. The challenge for healthcare systems, then, is meeting the needs of many while maintaining effective and efficient operations—often working only with limited resources and funding. As evidenced by pandemic and endemic data, the healthcare system still has work to do on many fronts, one of the most important being addressing health disparities. The COVID-19 pandemic exposed many of our shortcomings regarding equity in healthcare, which impact communities of various size, location, income, and ethnicity.

While providing equal access to care and improving the overall health of our citizens remain the overarching goals of our healthcare system, the path to achieving these goals is not so straightforward. Our complex system needs to remain patient-centered, and any implementation strategies need to have equity and inclusivity at their core in order to effect any meaningful short-term or long-term changes. This will require the consistent commitment, cooperation, and collaboration of stakeholders at all levels, including patients, providers, nonprofits, and other entities. It is only when we work together across many different levels of power and organization that we can develop a more just, accessible, and equitable healthcare system. The national *Healthy People* initiative is focused on addressing the underlying influences of health disparity such as race, ethnicity, geography, and socioeconomic status, reinforcing the need for cultural awareness. Specific items such as education, income level, and family structure are significant in the determination of these influences, and ultimately affect the type and quality of care a patient has traditionally received. To address these disparities and improve our healthcare delivery system, we must continue to focus on the facets of healthcare that impact the overall health of our population.

Access to Care

The most important part of the systems improvement process is streamlining the patient's first interaction with the healthcare system, that is, improving the patient's ability to identify their initial need for care and their access to the necessary forms of care. There are several major factors that drive the success of this beginning stage including: (a) patient responsibility, (b) ability to pay and/or insurance coverage, and (c) healthcare service and facility availability. These items often act as the "springboard" by which the mechanisms of the healthcare delivery system are initiated, and they must be refined in order for overall system improvement to occur. During the pandemic, many did not seek care because they had no health insurance, or only had extremely limited coverage. In some instances, there was no healthcare even available in some neighborhoods. No access to care and no ability to pay presents an impossible situation for a patient in need. Relief funds as issued by the Department of Health and Human Services and other government health agencies addressed the financial needs of many by making COVID-19 testing and vaccinations free for patients, no matter their insurance status or ability to pay. For severe cases requiring inpatient hospitalization, healthcare expenses were exorbitant, especially for those uninsured or underinsured.

The patient (or responsible family members) must also be able to recognize when medical attention is needed, ideally prior to an emergent situation. Community health and wellness initiatives, preventive screenings, and specific cultural health education efforts all help people identify existing conditions and risks that may affect disparate populations differently. This may involve identifying and acknowledging linguistic, religious, or ethnic differences in order to gauge how health education and access to care can best be tailored to meet the needs of specific populations. It has been proven that many minority communities have a distrust of the healthcare system and will delay care or treatment as long as possible. Traditionally, the ability to pay has guided the decision-making of those seeking care, and for lower income families it wasn't always possible to afford the necessary care until the implementation of the Patient Protection and Affordable Care Act (PPACA) of 2010. This act provided healthcare coverage to those previously uninsured and underinsured, removing the ability to pay dilemma. Although many opposed this legislation, the Act's patient-centered focus has resulted in tremendous improvements in public health, due to both increased preventive screenings and improved access to treatment for existing conditions.

Finally, healthcare services must be widely available to patients in both number of locations and breadth of disciplines. Health needs for disparate communities are oftentimes different from the rest of the populations, with one main area of concern being the prevalence of conditions categorized as chronic diseases (hypertension, heart disease, diabetes, etc.). There must be adequate numbers of providers and ancillary medical services available to treat the growing numbers of patients with these conditions. The need for mental health services and related care has also come to the forefront of the healthcare industry, as the stigma around mental health has become less prevalent. Telehealth and telemedicine have helped resolve some access to care issues, providing valuable assistance for those needing basic medical consultations or those with limited transportation options. However, challenges with virtual access to care can arise if patients or households are without the reliable means to access the internet, further reinforcing the need for additional access considerations in order to promote the most equitable and accessible health system possible.

Quality of Care

The quality of a patient's healthcare must be evaluated and improved upon on both sides of the equation, taking into consideration both the patient and the healthcare professional's assessment of the quality of care. According to the American Hospital Association, hospitals should take the lead on this task, keeping the following focal points in mind: (a) time spent with patients, (b) quality-centered resources, (c) disclosure and transparency, (d) improved data collection, (e) facility governance, (f) public health initiatives, and (g) additional professional development opportunities. Improving these items will allow clinicians to accurately assess patient needs and provide the appropriate care, while retaining competent staff dedicated to the betterment of the system. The patients receiving care must also be satisfied with the quality of their experience, and should be comfortable with the safety of the environment and their treatment. Professionals must be aware of all patient concerns and possible predispositions, which entails a strong awareness of cultural differences and being well-versed in the treatment of disparate populations. Communication between the professional and the patient must be improved to identify and address health issues, which only comes with time spent during visits. Fostering an environment of mutual trust and respect is crucial in developing an effective care plan. Although largely relying on changes made for in-person interactions, improvements to quality of care may also involve the systems used to support those interactions, ultimately impacting the rising costs of healthcare.

Cost of Care

The rising cost of healthcare has been an area of concern for all stakeholders in the healthcare industry. With the exception of pandemic relief funding, paying for healthcare services has been, in some cases, impossible for many consumers. To date, the healthcare industry recognizes approximately $4.1 trillion in expenditures, with all major payers (private and government) contributing to a constantly changing revenue stream ($4.3 trillion if pandemic costs are included). With many factors impacting the costs of care, there are some major contributors to the financial picture we see today. Approximately 75% of the country's total healthcare expenditure goes to the diagnosis and ongoing treatment of chronic illnesses, and the lost productivity they create, affecting 133 million Americans. Most of the occurrences of chronic illness are, in fact, preventable. Community health education will drastically reduce the number of people stricken with these life-threatening illnesses, as changes in lifestyle choices are essential for the larger picture of health improvement. Early detection is also a vital tool in mitigating emergent treatment for those at risk due to lifestyle choices as well as genetic disposition. The challenge for the industry is securing or uncovering the resources needed for expanded community education and preventive screenings.

Advancements in technology have also been a major contributor to rising healthcare costs, although improved technologies do provide an overall benefit to the industry. Healthcare technologies help providers identify undetected or new illnesses, and often provide the necessary support for treatment. New technologies face the challenge of meeting the clinical needs of the providers while also being affordable and accessible enough for the patients and consumers, which requires steep research and development efforts. Upgrades to machinery and operating systems are often absorbed by providers and health systems without being directly billable or associated with revenue. As with any industry, remaining viable requires recovery of expenses in the most basic sense, even if a defined profit margin isn't part of the scenario. Donations and capital funding sources have been the mechanisms by which technology is secured, particularly in health systems struggling to maintain financial viability.

Barriers to Change

Every plan comes with its own set of challenges and obstacles, and the improvements to the healthcare delivery system are no exception. Experts at the Agency for Healthcare Research and Quality, a U.S. Department of Health and Human Services agency, states that healthcare utilization issues as well as healthcare costs are among the "mainstay" barriers to an improved health system. As the previously mentioned solutions to healthcare disparities are implemented, these mainstays will surely grow in size. Increased coverage and access, as provided by the PPACA of 2010, improved quality of care as well as preventive care and community education, and will rapidly infuse the current health system with new patients at all levels of care. How will we absorb this excess demand and still maintain high standards of care? Will the clinician–patient interaction suffer because of volume?

Improving the availability of healthcare workers is a central concern as we are moving toward a major shortage of physicians, nurses, and other direct care staff. Rising demand and increased need for patient care has not led to an increase in the number of professionals trained and employed in the field. Medical schools nationwide struggle to find instructors (because qualified instructors often choose higher-salary industry positions) and must therefore continue to limit the number of potential clinicians admitted to their programs. Patient safety and possibly the quality of care could be compromised if the shortage of clinical professionals continues unchecked. Healthcare visits may also be shortened to allow doctors to see more patients, but this would surely affect patient satisfaction and care. The combined efforts of facilities, small offices, nonprofits, and contractors will be needed to combat this problem of limited staffing, which introduces additional operating difficulties as well as costs.

Healthcare expenditures will continue to increase along with our various improvements, due to a myriad of both controllable and unanticipated costs. More patients mean more visits and more treatments, as well as more ancillary services such as testing and pharmaceuticals. The short-term effect will be greater bottom-line costs, but the long-term benefit will be a healthier society due to increased prevention and early detection efforts.

SYSTEMS DESIGN AND STRUCTURAL CHANGES: CHALLENGES FOR HEALTH ADMINISTRATORS

Future healthcare leaders must make hard decisions on how to accomplish success in all areas of operations. Access, quality, and costs are at the forefront of what every healthcare organization must consider. These decisions mean examining current operations and determining if a change is in fact necessary; in some cases, this prompts a systems merger decision. The overall goals of a merger are to maximize care delivery, reduce operating costs, and improve availability of services and providers. The thinking here is that the merged system benefits from fewer duplicated services, increased utilization by a potentially larger patient base, and consolidated administrative costs, which further reduce the overall operating costs of the newly formed organization. Merged systems are often created in the wake of a saturated or supersaturated market, which may directly impact smaller organizations' ability to provide healthcare goods and services.

Impacts (both short-term and long-term) to the organization and its employees are predicated on proper communication of situation—why is the merger necessary? Financial factors, health policies, and changing population needs all drive merger decisions. On the operations side of things, mergers are usually prompted by one or several of the following dilemmas: (a) declining inpatient volumes in multiple diagnoses or categories of care, (b) misaligned or insufficient capacity, (c) changing funding and reimbursement landscape, and (d) fragmented service delivery—duplicative services and excessive waste. On the larger, more strategic side of things, reasons for a merger would include increased market share or an attempt at market dominance and vertical/horizontal systems efficiencies. As the industry strives to remain consumer-oriented, increased competition and untraditional methods of healthcare delivery (such as e-medicine, telehealth, and other virtual methods) become key factors in system restructuring decisions, presenting ongoing challenges for leadership. Integrated systems have several benefits for all stakeholders involved. The first, and usually the foundation of the cost-savings element of a merger, is the decrease in administrative costs. This decrease is the direct result of the consolidation of (nonclinical) administrative and operations functions. Secondly, integrated systems tend to reduce the number of competing organizations, which serves to eliminate duplicative services in the service area. This theoretically leads to increased utilization and the accompanying revenues. A third benefit of integrated healthcare delivery systems is shared accountability and responsibility to the community being served. All members of the integrated system work toward a common mission, vision, and values, creating foundational efficiencies for the newly formed organization.

To prepare future healthcare administrators for these potential structural system-wide changes, the healthcare management and administration pedagogy must reflect this newly created integrated healthcare delivery system, providing the specialized skill sets needed for industry competencies. What are the pedagogical needs to accommodate these things? Merger success and sustainability requires the combined efforts of both clinical and nonclinical administrators throughout the organization. Leadership must possess several different types of competencies and be "boundary spanners" to make this new integrated, interprofessional collaborative network successful. These boundary spanners would not only have the knowledge needed for their respective areas but have a broader sense of how the services they provide impact the larger organization. This entails the understanding of operating procedures as well as financial ones. Effective, sustainable mergers and systems changes must form a new leadership structure, create integrated operations, and establish ongoing measurement metrics to gauge the success of the merger. This also requires the premerger discussion on employee satisfaction and retention. Patients aren't cared for without employees—so how do we keep our employees happy and committed? Lack of good work–life balance and work burnout became painfully evident during the pandemic, and the healthcare industry must do more to address these issues moving forward. Flexible work scheduling, virtual work options, and adequate staffing are just a few ways that organizations can improve work–life balance and ultimately employee satisfaction.

IMPACTS OF COVID-19: WHAT IS NEXT FOR THE U.S HEALTH SYSTEM?

The COVID-19 pandemic revealed several shortcomings of our healthcare system, some known and some relatively new. Our response was a clear indicator of how available resources are often taken for granted, and ultimately how unprepared we were for times of crisis and emergency response. The shift from primary care to emergent care with heavy respiratory support has shifted the financial focus from scheduled surgeries and elective procedures to higher-priced, just-in-time inventory management strategies. The unanticipated intensity and rapid spread of the pandemic has managed to disrupt even the strongest and largest providers, causing them to rethink the dynamics and overall structure of their health delivery systems. Some organizations have changed the scope of their operations, realigned services, and merged with other providers in efforts to meet the population's health needs while controlling operating expenditures.

So, what's next for U.S. health systems? Healthcare mergers and acquisitions are creating more integrated healthcare delivery systems, which can include just about all facets of care. These newly formed integrated delivery systems will be the new look of healthcare delivery postpandemic. Solid strategic planning and performance measurement are needed to make these new systems work effectively and efficiently. Meaningful performance measurement requires a gauge and a context, providing criteria for measurement as well as the scope in which to operate. These underlying or "root cause" purposes often assist the performance measurement effort by clarifying long-term outcomes and ongoing strategies, which are undoubtedly needed as organizations become more comprehensive and complex. All of the models, no matter the sector, include four key strategic initiatives or "perspectives" by which organizations should capture data and ultimately measure performance. The *financial* perspective focuses on metrics such as resource allocation and acquisitions, aiming to promote effective and efficient fiscal practices. The *customer* perspective focuses on customer satisfaction, public value, and the relationships of both internal and external interactions. The *internal business process* perspective captures the current picture of an organization's workflow and helps identify how these could possibly be improved. Lastly, the *learning and growth* perspective focuses on the development and motivation of employees, which truly determines the success of organizational change.

The future of healthcare financial management will depend on more than perfecting the existing processes and procedures. We will be required to challenge ourselves, to make continuous improvements in a complex industry. Changing regulatory environments and reimbursement structures will continue to impact the landscape, but we still must remain steadfast on our journey toward ideal effectiveness, efficiency, and evidence-based financial practices. In recent years we've worked diligently to improve access to care and foster quality patient experiences. While strides have been made to address increasing healthcare expenditures, we must continue with diligent research and analysis to find the most impactful and sustainable shorter-term and longer-term solutions to the problems we face today.

Microsoft Excel® Reference Guide

Note: This Microsoft Excel® Reference Guide serves as an introduction to the functions of Excel, as needed for this Healthcare Finance course. This is by no means an exhaustive guide to Excel functionality or utilization.

THE BASICS

Microsoft Excel® spreadsheets are designed for data organization, management, and analysis, with the ability to perform a host of calculations. Each data point is entered into a **cell**, which is the intersection of a **column** and **row**. Columns are the vertical locations in a spreadsheet and rows are the horizontal locations in the spreadsheet. The cell reference (data location) is then used as an element in various formulas, functions, and calculations. Cell references are always noted with the column first (alphabetical), followed by the row (numeric). In Figure A.1, the word "Sample" is located in cell A1 (Column A, Row 1).

Figure A.1

Spreadsheet layout in Excel

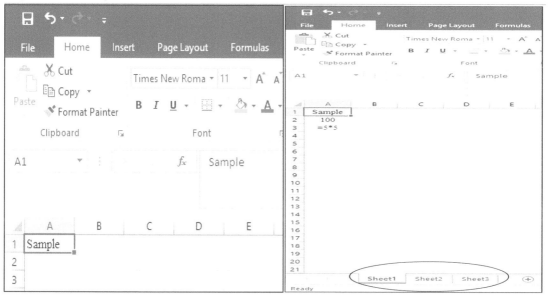

The **ribbon** or control panel at the top of the spreadsheet contains many of the same functions as other Microsoft applications (such as clipboard, font, and alignment). These will operate the same in Excel, and will be used to change the appearance and position of the data. Other options in the ribbon allow for customization of the spreadsheet, meeting the specific needs of the organizer. Columns and rows can be added or deleted, data within the cells can be formatted, and information and styles can be copied or pasted. When launched, Excel opens with at least one spreadsheet shown (standard is three spreadsheets). Multiple spreadsheets in one file is referred to as a **workbook**, with a workbook containing hundreds of worksheets dependent upon computer memory. Additional spreadsheets can be added by the user as needed, using the circled plus sign next to the worksheet names. Worksheets are often referred to as **tabs**, and are titled Sheet1, Sheet2, and Sheet3 when the application is initially launched. The tabs can be renamed/customized by double-clicking on the worksheet name, then entering a new worksheet name. Tab functions can also be accessed by right-clicking on the tab to show the tab/worksheet menu for renaming, color changes, moving, copying, hiding, or inserting additional worksheets.

THE DATA

Excel can store and manage different types of data, with each type acknowledged differently by the Excel application: those with numerical value and those without numerical value. **Labels** are words, phrases, or basic text entered into a cell, with no numerical value. Labels are therefore unable to be used in a calculation. **Constants** are numbers that are data entered/typed into a cell that has a numerical value. Constants can be represented as numbers, percentages, or decimals that can be used in calculations or other numbers-based operations. **Formulas** are the equations used to perform mathematical operations using the data entered into the cells. Since formulas are mathematical in nature, they rely on constants and other built-in functions of Excel, and cannot use labels. Figure A.2 shows examples of the Excel data types.

Figure A.2

Data types in Excel

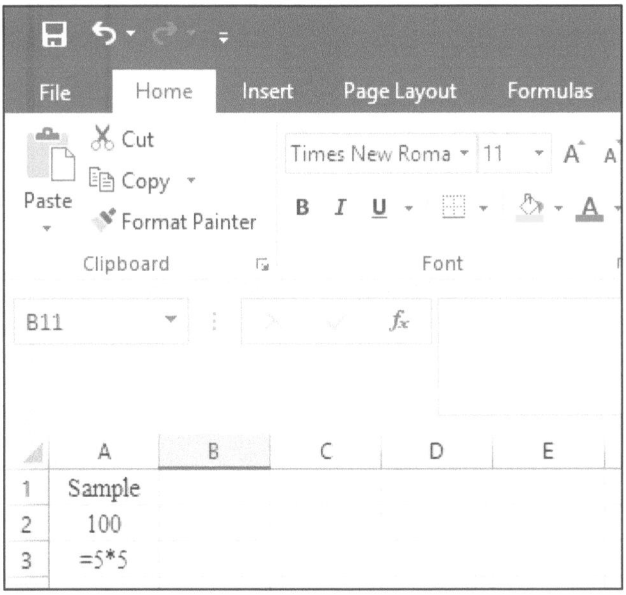

Here, the word "Sample" located in cell A1 is a label and cannot be used for calculations. As with other applications (like Microsoft Word®), labels and other text can be sorted as part of a list or formatted using the ribbon. The number "100" located in cell A2 is a constant. This number was typed into the cell as an actual number, which can be used for calculations. In cell A3, we have an example of a basic formula, multiplying 5 times 5. Formulas are entered into the cell, but only the results are returned. So, in the actual spreadsheet, the number returned in cell A3 will be 25. Typically, labels are left-justified in the cells, with constants and numerical values returned from formulas being right-justified in the cells. (The examples shown in Figure A.2 are centered for demonstration purposes.)

Data as entered into a spreadsheet can be any type of data you need to store, manage, or analyze. The data can be a list of names, a list of item descriptions, or a list of sales figures or salaries. Lists of labels and descriptions can be formatted and sorted alphabetically; numbers such as sales figures or salaries can be sorted from smallest to largest (or vice versa) or can be referenced/included in formulas, functions, and calculations.

In Figure A.3, we see the standard ribbon features for formatting and alignment as used in most applications. For formulas and functions, we will rely heavily on the Excel-specific features, which will customize our data for input and analysis. The "number" section of the ribbon is what we will use to format our numerical values as general numbers, dates, accounting or currency, or percentages. The cell in the spreadsheet will show the result or output of the calculation, so we rely on the **formula bar** to show the formulas or functions behind that calculation. Now that we've covered the basics, let's discuss the creation of basic Excel formulas.

Figure A.3

Data formatting and Excel features

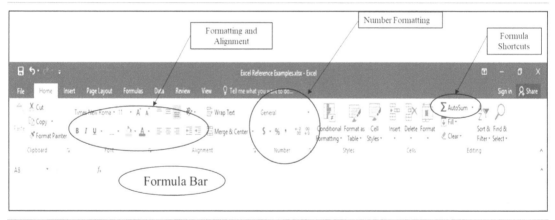

THE FORMULAS

Formulas and functions in this Excel guide are just some of the more common items to be used for this course. There are hundreds of other items beyond the scope of what we cover here, spanning from basic to extremely complex. To begin our discussion of basic formulas, remember that every formula begins with the equal sign (=). The equal sign prompts Excel for a calculation or function. In the Figure A.2 formula example, the equal sign precedes the numbers to be used in the calculation. Much of the symbolism used in Excel formulas is the same as the keys on a standard calculator. Mathematical operations will work the same way: sum/addition (+), subtraction (−), product/multiplication (*), and division (/). These symbols can be typed directly into a formula, with some accessible through the AutoSum option (∑) as shown in Figure A.3. Average, Count, MIN (minimum or smallest value), and MAX (maximum or largest value) are also available with the AutoSum option.

What You Want to Do	How to Do It	Comments
To enter a formula:	Always begin with "=". Enter the formula using numbers, cell references, mathematical operations, and functions.	When selecting a function, Excel will insert the "=" automatically. Place your formula where you want the results to appear.
To reference a cell:	Always begin with "=". Type the cell reference or click the cell you want to reference/include in your calculation.	When referencing a cell or data on a different spreadsheet, simply click the desired cell or data and Excel will add the reference.
To insert/delete a column or row:	Right-click where the column or row is to be inserted/deleted. From the drop-down menu, select insert/delete. Or select insert/delete from the ribbon "Cells" section.	Both methods of access accomplish the same task.
To use mathematical operations in formulas:	For sum/addition, type: + For subtraction, type: − For multiplication, type: * For division, type: / For greater/less than, type: > or <	The symbols used for the operations in Excel are the same as those used in basic math or on a calculator. For multiplication, "= product" is also used.
To use AutoSum functions (∑): Sum, Average, Count Numbers, Max, Min	Click the AutoSum ∑ in the "Editing" panel of the ribbon and select the desired function. Press enter for the results.	When you select a function, Excel highlights the data to be included in the calculation (usually adjacent rows/columns). If a different range of data is to be included, simply highlight the correct data. Place your function where you want the results to appear.
To create charts/ graphs:	Click on the "Insert" tab/page at the top of the ribbon. Highlight the data to be included in the chart/graph. Choose a specific layout or "Recommended Charts" to see possible results. Select the desired chart layout, then "ok."	Once selected, the chart can be customized with a title and color changes. The chart/graph can also be moved to other worksheets without being "detached" from the source data.

The items discussed in this Reference Guide should be adequate for the completion of the course project and basic data analyses. Additional functionality provides more in-depth data modeling by using other key Excel features.

- Using the "Formulas" tab, students may access the Function Library which provides Logic Functions, Corporate Finance Functions, Trigonometry Functions, and a host of other mathematical and statistical formulas.

- Using the "Data" tab will allow students to import large data sets from various databases and query platforms for analysis. These functions will also assist students with managing their data sets (identifying and deleting duplicates, data validation, data consolidation, and basic data forecasting).

Adding the Excel "Data Analysis Toolpak" to the "Data" tab brings more complex statistical analysis functionality. This is a free add-in for the program, which is used for data analysis processes such as regression analysis, descriptive statistics, exponential smoothing, variance analyses (ANOVA), and other applied statistics techniques.

For data visualization (along with the basic charts/graphs), the "Insert" tab provides options for pivot tables and data slicers. These items allow users to filter the data set, creating customized visual representations.

Additional resources and how-to guides can be found on these Microsoft websites:

Excel Help & Learning: https://support.microsoft.com/en-us/excel

Adding the Excel Toolpak: https://support.microsoft.com/en-us/office/load-the-analysis -toolpak-in-excel-6a63e598-cd6d-42e3-9317-6b40ba1a66b4

Pivot Tables Overview: https://support.microsoft.com/en-us/office/overview-of-pivot tables-and-pivotcharts-527c8fa3-02c0-445a-a2db-7794676bce96

Data Slicers (for data filtering): https://support.microsoft.com/en-us/office/use-slicers-to -filter-data-249f966b-a9d5-4b0f-b31a-12651785d29d

List of Acronyms

AAA	American Accounting Association
ABC	activity-based costing
ACA	Affordable Care Act
ACHE	American College of Healthcare Executives
ACO	accountable care organization
ACRC	American Cancer Research Center
ADA	Americans With Disabilities Act
AHIMA	American Health Information Management Association
AHRQ	Agency for Healthcare Research and Quality
AICPA	American Institute of Certified Public Accountants
AMA	American Medical Association
AONE	American Organization of Nurse Executives
APMs	advanced alternative payment models
AR	accounts receivable
ARRA	American Recovery and Reinvestment Act
AUPHA	Association of University Programs in Health Administration
BCBS	Blue Cross Blue Shield
BSC	balanced scorecard
CCC	corporate cost of capital
CCO	chief compliance officer
CDBG	Community Development Block Grant
CDC	Centers for Disease Control and Prevention
CEO	chief executive officer
CEP	community education program
CFO	chief financial officer
CHIP	Children's Health Insurance Program
CHRO	chief human resources officer
CIO	chief information officer
CMO	chief medical officer
CMS	Centers for Medicare & Medicaid Services
CNO	chief nursing officer
COO	chief operating officer
CPAP	continuous positive airway pressure
CPT	Current Procedural Terminology
CTO	chief technology officer
CUHS	Central University Health System
DCOH	days cash on hand

DHA	Defense Health Agency
DHS	Directorate of Health Services
DME	durable medical equipment
DRGs	diagnosis-related groups
DSRIP	Delivery System Reform Incentive Payment Program
EBIT	earnings before interest and taxes
EHR	electronic health record
EMR	electronic medical record
EOB	explanation of benefits
EPOs	exclusive provider organizations
ER	emergency room
ERP	Enterprise Resource Planning
ESRD	end-stage renal disease
ESRD QIP	End-Stage Renal Disease Quality Incentive Program
FAF	Financial Accounting Foundation
FASB	Financial Accounting Standards Board
FF&Es	furniture, fixtures, and equipment
FFS	fee for service
FMLA	Family and Medical Leave Act
FP&A	financial planning and analysis
FPL	federal poverty level
FSAs	flexible spending accounts
FTC	Federal Trade Commission
FTE	full-time equivalent
FV	future value
FY	fiscal year
GAAP	generally accepted accounting principles
GASB	Governmental Accounting Standards Board
GL	general ledger
GPCI	Geographic Practice Cost Indices
HAC	Hospital-Acquired Conditions Reduction Program
HCPCS	Healthcare Common Procedure Coding System
HEP	health education and promotion
HFMA	Healthcare Financial Management Association
HHS	U.S. Department of Health and Human Services
HHVBP	home health value-based purchasing
HIMSS	Health Information and Management Systems Society
HIPAA	Health Insurance Portability and Accountability Act
HITECH	Health Information Technology for Economic and Clinical Health
HLA	Healthcare Leadership Alliance
HMOs	health maintenance organizations
HR	human resources
HRRP	Hospital Readmissions Reduction Program
HSAs	health savings accounts
HVAC	heating, ventilation, and cooling
IASB	International Accounting Standards Board
ICD	*International Classification of Diseases* code
IHI	Institute for Healthcare Improvement

IRR	internal rate of return
IRS	Internal Revenue Service
IT	information technology
KFF	Kaiser Family Foundation
KPIs	key performance indicators
KSAs	knowledge, skills, and abilities
LLC	limited liability company
LLP	limited liability partnership
LTC	long-term care
MACRA	Medicare Access and Chip Reauthorization Act
MCOs	managed care organizations
MGMA	Medical Group Management Association
MIPS	merit-based incentive payment system
MMC	Mountain Medical Center
MSSP	Medicare shared savings program
NGOs	nongovernmental organizations
NPV	net present value
OPM	Office of Personnel Management
P4P	pay for performance
PAR	patient accounts receivable
PCP	primary care physician
PHHS	Preventive Health and Health Services Block Grant
PI	profitability index
PMPM	per member per month
POSs	point-of-service plans
PPACA	Patient Protection and Affordable Care Act
PPOs	preferred provider organizations
PV	present value
RBRVS	resource-based relative value scale
RHS	regional health system
ROA	return on assets
ROE	return on equity
ROI	return on investment
RVUs	relative value units
SCM	supply chain management
SDOH	social determinants of health
SEC	Securities and Exchange Commission
SHRM	strategic human resources management
SMART	specific, measurable, attainable, relevant, and time-bound
SNF	skilled nursing facilities
SNFVBP	Skilled Nursing Facility Value-Based Purchasing
SSBC	Social Services Block Grant
TQM	total quality management
TVM	time value of money
VBP	hospital value-based purchasing program
VHA	Veterans Health Administration
VM	value modifier program
WHO	World Health Organization

Glossary

access to care: The availability of health services to individuals, considering such issues as illness, location, and clinician availability.

accountable care organization: Groups of providers and facilities that work together to coordinate the healthcare for an assigned population of patients.

accounting breakeven: A breakeven calculation that is made with no profit included.

accounting cycle: A designed process for collecting and organizing accounting data with built-in checks and balances, as well as a meticulous time schedule.

accounting equation: A calculation that summarizes all facets of a company's financial activity and states them in terms of assets, liabilities, and equity.

accounting period: A block of time during which accounting data is reviewed, such as monthly, quarterly, or annually.

accrual accounting: A method of financial accounting in which financial transactions are recorded at the time they occur, regardless of when the actual payment arrives.

activity-based budgeting: A very detailed budgeting approach that includes the analysis and costing of individual activities; most prevalent in departments that have multiple methods of performing a specific task or process.

activity-based costing: A costing approach that analyzes the individual units of work performed that contribute to the total cost of a process.

acuity: The severity of an illness.

adjudication: To judge or decide a final ruling based on the evidence provided.

adjusting journal entries: Changes made to accounts to correct financial records by inserting any revenues or expenses previously unrecognized such as accruals, deferred items, and prepaid items.

adverse selection: A philosophy that states those who need healthcare insurance will secure it.

American Recovery and Reinvestment Act: U.S. legislation created following the 2009 Great Recession that was intended to both create new jobs and preserve existing ones, as well as provide financial relief in areas such as education, healthcare, and various other programs.

Americans With Disabilities Act: U.S. legislation created to ensure reasonable accommodations are made in the workplace as well as public spaces to assist those with disabilities to perform at their ideal level.

analysis worksheet: A spreadsheet created to reconcile the account debits and credits.

annualization: A process of reporting financial figures used for volume, supplies, salaries, or any other expense.

asset management: Process of assessing the healthcare organization's utilization and growth of items with value, such as cash, owned inventory, research patents, machines and equipment, buildings, and so on.

assets: Items of economic value that are owned by the organization, such as cash, equipment, property, supplies, trademarks, or patents.

asynchronous training: Educational sessions that rely on internet-based modules and presentations to deliver the information; there is no immediate instructor communication or collaboration with colleagues in this training delivery method, since employees take the training at a time convenient to them.

balanced scorecard: A tool commonly used to measure performance in a multifaceted organization, known for its flexibility.

balance sheet: A financial summary of an organization's assets and liabilities, showing stakeholders what is owned and what is owed.

base stock: Routine supplies used for every patient or consumer transaction.

benchmarking: The process used by organizations as they compare themselves to competitors to strive for optimal performance; it assists with the decision-making process throughout the entire organization, not just the financial performance.

benefits: Nonsalary items offered to company employees in addition to their base pay, such as insurance coverage, vacation and personal time, bonuses, and so on.

billing and coding process: The method organizations use to not just bring in money, but to secure resources for current and future routine operations and strategic initiatives.

block grants: Large sums of funding provided by the federal government to each state to fund a variety of state and local initiatives.

bottom-up budgeting: A budgeting approach in which the flow of budgeting information is communicated from front-line leadership to the executive team, which captures the nuances, special circumstances, and operational challenges that those without direct responsibility would not be aware of.

breakeven: The baseline of most pricing strategies that answers the question: Have we established an adequate price that meets our financial goals?

budget: An organization's estimation of future revenues, expenses, and profits as realized through projected patient visit volume or patient encounters.

budgeting: The process through which an organization estimates its revenues and expenses for the upcoming fiscal year or other specified time period.

budgeting approach: A method of developing an organization's budget, determined by governance structure, type of product or service produced, and age of the organization.

budgeting process: The method for creating estimations of an organization's expected revenues and expenses.

bundled payments: A payment method that reimburses a provider with a predetermined lump-sum payment covering one specific episode of care; also called episode-based payments.

business analytics and financial reporting: Investigation of an organization's past performance to identify strengths, challenges, and opportunities for improvement.

business process: The organization's mission, vision, and values—the drivers of the organization's purpose and scope of responsibilities.

capital budget: The planned funding of new, nonoperating expenditures and investments that are not included in the operating budget and are supported by separate sources of funding.

capital investments and management: Determination of the likelihood of success for new investments and large projects; "capital" refers to the value of a project or initiative and is typically defined by the dollar value of the investment.

capital project analysis: The evaluation process that examines the feasibility and profitability of long-term projects.

capital rationing: The concept of having more capital projects than available capital funding, which results in an evaluation and selection process.

capital structure: The organization's mix of equity and debt financing; a determination of the ideal financing by comparing the return on equity results for the anticipated equity financing percentage and the anticipated debt financing percentage.

capitation: A payment method that pays a provider a predetermined amount for each patient seen, no matter how many services are provided.

carrying costs: Costs incurred by an organization for storing and maintaining an inventory.

cash accounting: A method of financial accounting in which financial transactions are recorded when the item is paid or reflected on the banking/account statements.

cashflow: The movement of cash as specifically related to the implementation and ongoing activities of a project.

cash management process: A method of controlling both cash inflows and cash outflows to ultimately improve an organization's overall financial position.

Centers for Medicare & Medicaid Services: A government agency that serves as the administrator for Medicare benefits and provides guidelines and updates to the plan.

central tendency: A quantitative analysis method that describes individual data points in relation to an entire data set.

change in net assets: The percentage change of net assets from the previous fiscal year to the current fiscal year; this document details the increase or decrease in the value of assets over a specified period.

change management: The process of transitioning the organization to meet its strategic goals or into its future state by guiding everyone involved through the various stages of the change.

charge-based reimbursement: A payment approach that pays the medical provider for services rendered according to the provider's established rates or fee schedule; a provider is only paid up to the published rate, leaving any costs incurred above it out of the total reimbursed amount.

chargemaster: An organization's list of established services and procedures used to bill payers.

chart of accounts: A numbering system that organizes the accounts and types of transactions specific to the organization.

chief financial officer: Individual who provides oversight to financial functions; this ultimately includes the operation and performance of every unit and subunit within the organization.

Children's Health Insurance Program: U.S. legislation implemented in 1997 to provide health insurance coverage to children in families above the federal poverty line, as well as families that would otherwise be uninsured.

Civil Rights Act of 1964:   U.S. legislation implemented to prohibit discrimination on the basis of race, color, sex, religion, or national origin, for public accommodations and federally funded programs.

claims adjudication process: The initial claims review in which the submitted claim is checked for spelling errors in the patient's or provider's data, designed to ensure that the most important data that filters through and impacts other decisions is correct.

claims denial: A refusal to pay for services provided by a health insurance company, which may be due to missing preauthorization or primary care physician referral, incorrect or misaligned coding, or duplicative billing.

claims rejection: A transitory billing step when a claim is denied on initial review, with the intention of receiving corrections and moving forward with the remaining steps in the claims adjudication process.

claims scrubbing: A claims review process designed to identify any errors or missing information that may result in the rejection of denial of a claim.

clean claims: Medical claims that, following review, are deemed to be free of errors.

clearinghouse: A company outside the organization that specializes in quick electronic review, correction, and submission of medical claims.

collections aging schedule: An indicator that reflects accounts receivable balances in intervals according to the timing of payments.

compensation: The monetary value of a job or position paid to an employee for job performance.

consignment: An inventory method that leaves ownership of the supply item with the supplier while the consumer borrows it for use; this is seen in situations where the borrowed item is expensive and only needed for a limited time.

controller: Individuals whose purpose is to capture the financial position of an organization at a given point in time; sometimes called a comptroller.

copay: The portion of a medical payment that the insured is responsible for providing.

copayment: An amount of money paid by the insured at the start of each medical service visit.

corporate cost of capital: Calculation used to determine the cost to maintain an organization's capital structure, using debt and equity percentages and the required interest rate or rate of return for each; the weighted combination of the cost of equity and the cost of debt.

corporation: A business entity that has been established to be legally separate from its owners.

cost accounting: An analysis of inputs used in managerial accounting.

cost allocation: The distribution of indirect costs to revenue-generating areas.

cost-based reimbursement: A form of retrospective payment to the medical provider for costs incurred during the provision of healthcare goods and services.

cost center: An area of an organization that incurs expenses and adds to the organization's total liability but does not generate revenue; although unrelated to patient care, they are necessary for the operation of the healthcare organization.

cost driver: The basis for a cost allocation, the allocating department's unit of measure.

cost of debt: The interest rate applied by external lenders to borrowed funds.

cost of equity: The rate of return required by owners or shareholders to finance capital investments.

cost pool: The costs to be allocated within an organization, typically indirect costs or overhead costs.

costs: The expenses incurred by an organization to produce a healthcare good or service.

credit: An accounting entry that either decreases an asset or expense account, or increases a liability or equity account (revenue/payment received).

Current Procedural Terminology (CPT) code: Billing system code created by the American Medical Association that supports the *International Classification of Diseases* (*ICD*) code by identifying treatments and procedures for an identified diagnosis.

current ratio: A liquidity measure calculated by dividing current assets by current liabilities.

days cash on hand: An estimation of how long an organization can continue to operate by using only its cash.

debit: An accounting entry that either increases an asset or expense account, or decreases a liability or equity account (expense/payment made).

debt management: A ratio that analyzes the healthcare organization's use of debt in financing its operations and initiatives.

debt ratio: Calculation that analyzes the amount of debt an organization owes and if it has enough assets to cover its liabilities.

debt service coverage ratio: A measure of an organization's cashflow in relation to its debt; the greater the cashflow, the more liabilities covered.

decision-making process: A step-by-step method in making choices designed to accomplish different tasks toward problem mitigation and resolution.

deductible: An amount of money that must be paid by an insured before health insurance coverage is applied for healthcare services.

Delivery System Reform Incentive Payment Program: An initiative that offers flexibility and modification in payment for the Medicaid program based on medical judgments and evidence-based clinical management.

Delphi method: A method of forecasting demand that uses industry experts to predict the parameters and outcomes for the organization's supply chain.

demand: The desire of a consumer to purchase a particular good or service.

depreciation: A decrease in an asset's value over time, allowing the organization to incur the lost value gradually rather than all at once.

descriptive analytics: A statistical summation of historical data, highlighting the main characteristics or categories of the collected information.

diagnosis-related groups: Billing codes applied at the end of a patient's hospital stay that assign a value to the provider's resources used during the inpatient stay; each code represents a fixed reimbursement amount, no matter the costs incurred by the provider.

direct costs: Costs that are immediately identified as key to the production of healthcare services, or to the task at hand.

DuPont analysis: A profitability measure that combines multiple ratios to assess profitability and return on equity.

economic breakeven: A breakeven calculation that accounts for a marginal profit amount.

effectiveness: A qualitative target used as an indicator of achieving an intended outcome.

efficiency: A quantitative target answering the question of whether or not the organization is providing the best possible product or service at the least possible cost.

e-learning training: *See* asynchronous training

electronic health record: A comprehensive transcription and documentation tool that electronically captures medical information for a patient from all providers, specialists, and services.

electronic medical record: A transcription and documentation tool that electronically captures medical information for a patient at a specific provider's location.

employee retention: An organization's ability and efforts to keep its employees, minimizing turnover.

Equal Pay Act: U.S. legislation designed to eliminate pay disparities based on an employee's sex.

equity: The net worth of the organization, or the remaining assets after all liabilities are paid.

exclusive provider organization: A managed care organization similar to an HMO, but with the added requirement of preauthorization for services.

expense: Cost that an organization incurs for the production of goods and services provided.

expense budget: An estimation of an organization's expenses as they will be incurred during the budgeted time frame.

explanation of benefits: A summary of a healthcare service visit including the diagnosis and treatment, as well as the charges for the service and amounts covered by the insurance plan.

Fair Labor Standards Act: U.S. legislation passed in 1938 that introduced the minimum wage and overtime pay criteria.

Family and Medical Leave Act: U.S. legislation passed in 1993 that requires employers to guarantee employment and unpaid leave (up to 12 weeks) to employees in the event of family medical concerns.

federal poverty level: A measure of income used as an eligibility guide for various funding programs.

fee-for-service reimbursement: A payment structure that reimburses the healthcare organization or provider for services performed without regard to quality or service value.

financial accounting: The reporting of an organization's financial position at a given point in time.

financial analysis: Stage of the project analysis that shows the project details in operating and financial terms.

financial management: The combination of accounting and finance information for decision-making purposes in achieving the organization's goals and objectives.

financial planning and analysis: The process of using an organization's budgeted information to assess its financial health and develop strategies for sustained growth and viability.

financial reporting package: A series of routine monthly financial statements for the purposes of external reporting and compliance; these include the statement of financial position or balance sheet, statement of operations or income statement, statement of cash flows, and statement of shareholder's equity.

financial statements: Documents created to summarize all the accounting activity for an organization's reporting period, often shown in comparison to previous periods.

financing activities: Statement of cash flows section focused on payments of existing debt as well as newly financed purchases or projects.

fixed budgeting: A static budgeting method in which the previous values are transferred into the current projections with no change or adjustment.

fixed costs: Costs that remain static with changes in volume.

flexible budgeting: A budgeting approach that considers changes to patient volume, pricing, and expense updates, as well as seasonality; allows the organization to adjust operations based on expected conditions, increased patient volume, or updated reimbursement legislation.

flexible spending account: A mechanism by which insureds can save money over time, which is typically offered by an employer, with employees given the opportunity to save a specific dollar amount or percentage from each paycheck in preparation for out-of-pocket expenses.

for-profit: Investor-owned entities that focus on maximizing profits for shareholders through dividends.

forensic accounting: Process that examines accounting and financial records for erroneous, missing, or fraudulent data.

formative evaluation: A systematic analysis that includes review of all goals, objectives, and activities that contribute to the anticipated outcomes; a measure of the effectiveness and efficiency of a department, program, or initiative.

frequency: The number of patient visits, or the number of procedures performed in a particular medical category annually.

fringe benefits: Items offered to employees in addition to salary and wages, such as health insurance coverage, memberships and subscriptions, free parking, or other items of value to the employee.

full-cost pricing: Establishing a price that covers direct fixed costs, direct variable costs, and overhead, which includes indirect expenses incurred that have been applied using the allocation process.

full-time equivalents: Expenses associated with full-time employees, which may also include bonuses or fringe benefits.

fund accounting: A specialization that focuses on the financial operations of nonprofit organizations.

future value: A determination of the worth of a current asset at some specific moment in the future based on an assumed growth rate.

general journal: A listing of all accounting transactions as evidenced by the source documents.

general ledger: A summary of all account activity, which includes all journal entries as well as the account balances.

grants: Gifts given to an organization that may take the form of money or other valuable items that support the overall mission or possibly a specific purpose.

healthcare: The professional provision of medical services to address the emotional, mental, and physical well-being of a population.

Healthcare Common Procedure Coding System (HCPCS) code: Billing system code created by the Centers for Medicare & Medicaid Services that supports CPT code by providing the next level of documentation and coding for a medical diagnosis, denoting items such as personal medical supplies, services, and equipment not typically captured in other codes.

healthcare delivery system: An organized stand-alone network of healthcare organizations providing all-inclusive care to a specific patient population.

healthcare financial management: The application of financial management practices in the healthcare sector.

healthcare providers: Entities that come from a variety of disciplines and typically cover specific types of healthcare need, either working independently to care for the patient or operating as a team to provide a wider range of treatment.

healthcare sector: The people, organizations, and activities that contribute to promoting, restoring, or maintaining health.

healthcare suppliers: Entities that provide a wide range of materials utilized in the delivery of healthcare, including both inpatient and outpatient services.

Health Information Technology for Economic and Clinical Health (HITECH) Act: U.S. legislation enacted to promote the use of electronic health records, as well as comply with Health Insurance Portability and Accountability Act (HIPAA) Privacy and Security Rules.

health insurance: Mechanism designed to cover a myriad of health-related expenses, including preventive care and treatment for existing illness, as well as maintenance for longer-term illnesses.

Health Insurance Portability and Accountability Act (HIPAA): U.S. legislation designed to preserve patient privacy that created national standards to protect sensitive patient health information from being disclosed without the patient's consent or knowledge.

health maintenance organization: An economical but restrictive managed care plan which attempts to keep services within a specific network of providers.

health savings account: A mechanism by which insureds can save money over time through savings plans designed to accompany high-deductible health insurance plans.

horizontal integration: Ownership of healthcare organizations that perform the same services within the healthcare system.

income ratio: Calculation that analyzes the money coming into an organization, generated by assets and investments.

income statement: A report of an organization's activities as related to revenues, expenses, and profit.

incremental budgeting: A method of budgeting in which the previous year's budget is used as a foundation or baseline and then increased by a specific dollar amount or percentage; although not as restrictive as fixed budgeting, it tends to limit the amount of financial flexibility of the healthcare organization.

indirect costs: Costs that an organization incurs that are not tied to the final good or service purchased or consumed.

inflows: Money coming into an organization.

in-person training: A traditional approach to instruction in which an instructor and employees are present in the same workspace.

insurance premium: The total amount an insured pays for health insurance policy coverage annually.

insured: The person covered by a health insurance policy.

insurer: The company responsible for underwriting a health insurance policy and financial coverage for services.

integrated healthcare delivery system: A consolidated system comprised of multiple healthcare providers and/or suppliers arranged to either meet a series of healthcare needs or to resolve access and resource issues.

internal audit: A process that provides checks and balances within an organization, ensuring effectiveness and efficiency as well as compliance to regulatory guidelines and reporting requirements.

internal auditing: Process of examining an organization's internal processes, procedures, and systems to identify areas of improvement through uncovering evidence of misuse of resources and missed opportunities caused by inefficiencies.

internal rate of return: A financial assessment that measures the capital project's annual growth and profitability.

International Classification of Diseases (ICD)-10 **code:**   Billing system code maintained by the World Health Organization that identifies a patient's diagnosis or reason for a medical consultation, as required for all healthcare payers.

inventory management: The ordering, procurement, utilization, and recordkeeping of an organization's purchased goods.

inventory turnover ratio: A measure of the time between inventory purchase and inventory sales; the turnover determines how many times the organization has sold and repurchased its supplies.

investing activities: Statement of cash flows section focused on large equipment purchases, partnership ventures, and stock market and securities investments.

job analysis: A review of an available position and the related requirements; the first step in the recruitment and selection process

job description: The written narrative shared both inside and outside an organization that explains the details of the position.

job evaluation: A determination of a job's value by gathering relevant data from internal and external sources; may involve job classifications, quartile systems, point systems, and/or industry pricing.

journal entries: Records of financial transactions in ledgers, one as a debit and one as a credit, which balance the accounting equation.

just-in-time: An inventory system that delivers the needed supplies as close to the time of utilization as possible.

key performance indicators: Various performance measures that reflect the actual performance of the patient care and financial and operational functions in comparison to internally established targets, as well as in comparison to competitor and industry standards.

liabilities: Debts owed by the organization to creditors, such as loans, notes payable, or any other accounts payable item.

limited liability company: *See* limited liability partnership

limited liability partnership: A business structure that combines the benefits of partnership and collaboration with the limited liability of a corporation.

liquidity: An organization's ability to quickly convert assets to cash.

liquidity ratio: Calculation that gauges an organization's ability to use short-term assets to cover its short-term liabilities.

logic model: Visual representations of inputs, activities, and outcomes that operationalize an organization's goals and objectives.

long-term debt to capitalization: A measure that assesses an organization's capital structure and its long-term financing.

managed care organization: An administrative service that maintains a contracted provider network to manage healthcare costs, associated risks, and beneficiary volumes.

managerial accounting: The analysis and utilization of accounting data for decision-making purposes.

marginal-cost pricing: Establishing a price that covers additional units of service, but not all costs incurred; in this pricing strategy, just the variable costs are covered, making this a short-term approach.

market research: An approach to demand forecasting that analyzes the organization's demand and inventory practices in the context of current industry competition.

mean: Mathematical average of a set of data.

median: The number or value that sits in the middle of a data set.

Medicaid: A program implemented in 1965 to provide healthcare insurance coverage to those with limited income.

medical claim: A request for reimbursement from a health insurance provider for services performed.

medical claims process: The steps involved in securing funding from an insurance provider for services rendered.

Medicare: A program implemented in 1965 to cover healthcare expenses for persons 65 years of age or older.

Medicare Access and Children's Health Insurance Program (CHIP) Reauthorization Act: U.S. legislation that implemented financial incentives for providers with the creation of the quality payment program, which was designed to improve quality of patient care for Medicare and CHIP beneficiaries.

Medicare shared savings program: A program created by accountable care organizations under the Patient Protection and Affordable Care Act as a mechanism to foster improved medical outcomes for Medicare beneficiaries and reduce the overall cost of care.

mode: The number in a data set that appears most frequently.

moral hazard: An overreliance on healthcare services due to the existence or possession of health insurance; in other words, insureds may seek healthcare services just because they have health insurance and would not have to pay for care.

moving average: A data analysis method that involves creating subsets of smaller time frames and identifying trends in the data.

needs assessment: Stage in project analysis that examines the need or demand for a specific product or service.

net present value: The summation of the present value of a series of cashflows, providing the overall value for the financial portion of the capital project.

nonoperating revenue and expense categories: Balance sheet section that captures activities that may not routinely occur, such as contributions, fundraising activities, marketing materials, and investment income.

not-for-profit/nonprofit: Entities that are not investor owned but are instead owned by the community stakeholders they serve; these companies have a tax-exempt status and do not have federal tax obligations.

Occupational Safety and Health Act: U.S. legislation enacted in 1970 to reinforce safe working conditions and workplace health standards.

open enrollment period: The annual time frame during which employees can change health plans or other benefits coverage for the next calendar year.

operating activities: Statement of cash flows section focused on revenue and expense items that occur during routine business practices such as asset management and contributions.

operating budget: *See* budget

operating income: *See* profit margin

operating margin: A measure of an organization's operational efficiency; generally, 10% to 15% is considered efficient.

organizational training: Development process that provides information on company policies and industry regulations to all employees.

outflows: Money leaving an organization.

partnership: A business entity that has two or more owners and is relatively easy to form.

patient accounts receivable: The average time for collection of outstanding reimbursement for services already rendered, using the organization's aging schedule as an element in its calculation.

patient encounter: A personal, face-to-face interaction between a care provider and a patient.

patient mix: The demographic breakdown or categorization of the patient population or community served.

Patient Protection and Affordable Care Act (PPACA):   An act of comprehensive healthcare legislation implemented in 2010 that mandated coverage and benefits for those that would have otherwise not had healthcare insurance coverage at all.

payback period: The length of time it will take to recover the amount of an organization's initial investment.

pay for performance: A reimbursement plan that uses established metrics as the benchmarks to incentivize and penalize providers' trended performances.

payroll services and tax management: Financial processes that include compensation of employees and contractors, as well as annual filing of the organization's income taxes.

per diem: A type of all-inclusive, daily payment usually applied to inpatient hospital stays or residential/long-term care overnight settings; the facility is paid one predetermined, contracted amount for all services provided.

performance appraisal: A routine assessment of an employee's performance and progress compared to established goals and targets.

performance management: The process of controlling the activities that support an organization's mission, goals, and objectives.

performance measurement: Indicators and standards by which performance is measured.

per member per month: A capitated payment made monthly; for example, if an insurer has set a per member per month rate of $25, and a provider has 100 patients, each month the provider will receive $2,500.

point-of-service plan: A managed care organization similar to a PPO, with increased out-of-pocket costs to the patient; all services under this plan require a copayment, and services must be preauthorized by the insurance provider to be considered for reimbursement.

pooling: A grouping of insureds in an organization who are all charged the same premium for coverage regardless of their individual level of health.

preferred provider organization: A managed care organization that provides both in-network and out-of-network options, all of which require preauthorization from the insurance provider.

present value: The current worth of a sum of money as compared to what its value would be in the future assuming a certain rate of growth; for example, $125 in 10 years may have a present value of $100 assuming a 25% interest rate.

price: The amount an organization will charge consumers or patients to utilize the services provided.

price shifting: The process of charging higher pricing to one group of consumers to cover the financial shortfall of another group of consumers.

primary care: Initial, nonemergent medical care that allows a provider to assess a patient and determine if additional services are needed.

primary care physicians: Medical professionals who are the first point of contact for a patient and often provide referrals to specialists.

product: An item created for sale or consumption.

product life cycle: The time frame from initial purchase through a product's expiration date or required replacement.

profit: The income remaining after all expense obligations have been satisfied.

profitability index: A calculation used to gauge the value of a project, determined by dividing the net present value by the investment costs.

profitability ratio: Calculation that measures not only the revenues retained after debts are paid (net income), but also the underlying policies that support revenue generation.

profit estimations: Projections derived from the remaining revenue after all expenses have been covered in addition to any adjustments required to reach leadership-identified profit targets.

profit margin: A measure of the amount of money remaining after all operating expenses are covered.

program budgeting: A method of budgeting that considers all service lines to ensure the capture of all related inputs and outcomes; it addresses revenue and expense estimates of an entire program and its associated initiatives.

program theory: The modeling process of how a project, initiative, or department workflow begins and ends.

project: An initiative to expand service lines, improve horizontal efficiency, or restructure current operations.

project analysis: Process that examines all of the factors impacting a project's implementation and expected outcomes.

projected outcomes: Stage of project analysis that uses the information gathered in previous stages to determine the project's viability.

projections: The data analysis and decision-making processes that will guide the organization forward.

prospective reimbursement: A payment method that pays the provider before healthcare services are actually rendered, based on expected costs.

purchasing and supply chain: Functions that secure the products and goods needed to provide services within an organization.

quality of care: The level of health services that lead to an increase in positive health outcomes.

quick ratio: A liquidity measure calculated by dividing liquid current assets only by current liabilities.

ratio analysis: An evaluation designed to assess an organization's overall financial position; it also provides insight to operating efficiency and competitiveness.

receivables balance: The outstanding patient revenue.

Rehabilitation Act: U.S. legislation implemented in 1973 to prohibit discrimination in the workplace against persons with disabilities.

reimbursement mechanism: The payment methodology that guides the reimbursement process for a given payer and provider.

relative value units: Physician reimbursement method that involves three categories of costs: the physician's direct labor costs, the physician's overhead costs, and the physician's malpractice costs.

reorder point: The designated level of supplies in inventory that prompts an automatic order or restock.

resource-based relative value scale: A type of quality-based reimbursement utilized by healthcare providers and payers that assigns relative value units to each CPT code and the healthcare provider's related expenses.

restricted assets: Donations used for a specific purpose within the organization's operations, such as funds specifically donated for cancer research; in such an instance, the restricted funding cannot be used for any other purpose, no matter where a shortfall or need may be occurring.

restricted funding: Grants or other monies that can only be used for a specifically defined project or initiative.

return on assets: A measure of how efficiently an organization uses its assets to generate revenue.

return on investment: A financial assessment that measures the capital project's total life span growth and profitability.

revenue: The income generated by the provision of goods and services.

revenue budget: A projection of an organization's revenues based on the projected patient volume or healthcare product sales.

revenue center: An area of an organization that incurs expenses, but also generates revenue for the organization; this may be patient care-related revenue or other operating revenue, such as from the hospital gift shop, cafeteria, or parking garage.

revenue cycle and cash management: Accounting functions such as billing and collections activities as well as short-term transactions.

risk: The exposure to a negative financial outcome as influenced by financing decisions, particularly with borrowing or debt financing.

risk management: A finance department function that involves identifying and mitigating threats to the organization's operations, such as fraud, waste, abuse of funds, system breaches, and noncompliance; often done in conjunction with accounting.

role-specific training: Development process that prepares employees for the daily tasks and duties they are required to perform.

rolling budgeting: A method of budgeting that begins with the basic flexible budgeting approach, but is routinely updated as changes are considered.

safety stock: Additional inventory items beyond the expected amount maintained on hand to avoid running out if a greater need arises.

salvage value: The sales price of the items purchased for the capital project after the useful life with the organization.

secondary care: Medical care provided for more serious health conditions requiring hospitalization or minor surgery.

selection: The process of choosing the ideal candidate for a job opening.

sensitivity analysis: An assessment that examines the changes in project value and net present value as the inputs for the project, such as interest rates and initial investments, change.

service-line budgeting: A unique type of financial analysis that captures data based on the actual service line and workflow of the care provided; it captures revenues and expenses generated for a healthcare service across all departments that contribute to the delivery of that care.

shareholders: The owners and/or financial investors of a company.

SMART goals: Performance benchmarks that are **s**pecific, **m**easurable, **a**ttainable, **r**elevant, and **t**ime-bound, and designed to highlight employee strengths as well as opportunities for improvement.

social determinants of health (SDOH):   The nonmedical factors that impact a person's health and wellness outcomes, such as economic stability, education, healthcare, physical environment, and community.

sole proprietorship: A business entity wholly owned by one individual.

source documents: The actual evidence of financial transactions—receipts, invoices, purchase orders, checks received, cash payments, and so forth.

stakeholders: Those individuals impacted by the success of the organization.

statement of cash flows: Financial document that contains consolidated information on an organization's incoming and outgoing cash transactions.

statement of owner's equity: Financial document that presents an organization's value or net worth in the context of the shareholder's or owner's investments.

statistics budget: A projection of an organization's volume of activities and output based on an organization's actual performance, with adjustments made to include anticipated increases or decreases to standard operations.

stockless: An inventory system that skips on-site storage completely and delivers requested items directly to the unit or department; this is common in departments with extremely high volume and supply turnover.

stop-loss provision: A contract inclusion designed to control the amount of increased expense a payer would have to cover; they can be implemented as limits to excess charges or as limits to rate increases.

strategic human resources management: The application of the organization's strategic plan to the human resources functions to ensure that the healthcare workforce meets the needs of the organization by receiving proper training, development, and compensation.

strategic planning: The process of setting goals for an organization, then planning the steps and details required to achieve those goals.

superbill: A detailed list of a patient's diagnosis, treatments, supplies, provider charges, and any other costs directly related to a patient visit used for billing.

supply chain: The manufacturing and distribution process from raw materials to the final sale of goods and services.

supply chain length: A key performance measure used to analyze the efficiency of a supply chain; shorter chains are considered more efficient than longer ones.

supply chain management: The process of successfully overseeing the manufacturing and distribution process from raw materials to the final sale of goods and services.

T-account: A basic T-shaped accounting graphic with debits listed on the left side and credits on the right side.

tax accounting: An accounting specialization that may be used in healthcare organizations to manage complex tax scenarios that arise.

tertiary care: Medical care provided by specialists whose focus is one specific area or type of care.

time-series analysis: An analysis method that uses data from a previous time frame to estimate future demand.

time value of money: A concept that states money today is more valuable than the same amount of money in the future.

top-down budgeting: A budgeting process in which the executive team informs the functional areas of exactly what their budget will be, based on leadership's assessment of historical data, goals, and objectives.

total asset turnover: A ratio used to determine how well the organization uses its assets to generate revenue or income; calculated as total revenues divided by total assets.

total cost: The combination of an item's fixed cost (those that do not change with changes in volume) and variable cost (those that do change with changes in volume).

total population: The total number of patient visits, or the number of procedures performed across all categories of care.

total quality management: A tool commonly used to measure performance in a multifaceted organization that focuses on internal organizational changes as a catalyst for improved outcomes.

transaction: The interaction between providers and consumers—the sale and/or purchase of a good or service.

treasurer: Individual responsible for financial decision-making and the projection of anticipated financial performance.

trial balance: A process run to review account balances to assess the debit and credit totals; if entered correctly, all accounts will have a zero balance.

TRICARE: A health insurance program that covers active-duty service members, military retirees, and their families.

Triple Aim: Three key healthcare sector goals: (a) improving the quality of (changing) patient care, (b) maintaining sound financial operations and viability, and (c) addressing issues with access to healthcare services.

underlying cost structure: The relationship between costs and volume, represented by the equation: Total Costs = Fixed Costs + Total Variable Costs.

unrestricted assets: Donations that can be distributed or utilized in any way the organization deems necessary.

unrestricted funds: Grants or other monies that can be applied to any program at the discretion of the organization's leadership.

utility rate: A calculation of service utilization deduced from the frequency and total population.

value creation: The process of creating or developing a good or service that meets the needs of the consumer.

variable compensation: The awarding of pay (or other items of value) for increased performance or to promote fairness.

variable cost rate: An established set cost assigned per unit for each unit of volume.

variable costs: Costs that are dependent and change with variations in volume.

variance analysis: The comparison of actual figures to planned or budgeted estimates; large variances could signal an emerging event, or possibly missed information during the budgeting process.

vertical integration: The ownership of organizations that perform various functions at various levels within the healthcare delivery system.

Veterans Health Administration: Organization that provides medical coverage for all U.S. veterans who served at least two consecutive or continuous years without a dishonorable discharge.

videoconferencing: A meeting between two or more individuals that takes place at a designated time online; may be used for instructional purposes or information transfer.

virtual synchronous training: Instructor-led learning sessions that take place at a designated time online.

workload calculation: An estimate capturing anticipated labor expense for a project or process, which requires knowledge of the tasks that comprise the project, completion time for each task, frequency and duration of tasks, and the pay rate of the employee completing the tasks.

write-off: The process of eliminating a recorded debt or amount owed due to noncollection, often done when no other viable collection options are available.

zero-based budgeting: A budgeting approach that requires current justification for all budgeted items; rather than relying on prior performance, it instead requires "ground-up" calculations for all expenses and revenues starting from zero.

Index